AF344421

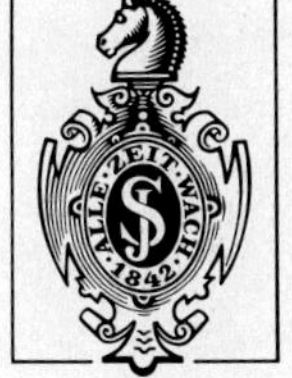

J. Fleischer (Ed.)

Leukemias

With 76 Figures

Springer-Verlag
Berlin Heidelberg New York London Paris
Tokyo Hong Kong Barcelona Budapest

Prof. Dr. J. FLEISCHER
Med. Akademie "Carl Gustav Carus"
Klinik für Innere Medizin
Abt. Hämatologie und Onkologie
Fetscherstrasse 74
0-8019 Dresden, FRG

ISBN 3-540-54782-7 Springer-Verlag Berlin Heidelberg New York
ISBN 0-387-54782-7 Springer-Verlag New York Berlin Heidelberg

Library of Congress Cataloging-in-Publication Data Leukemias / J. Fleischer (ed.). Includes bibliographical references and index. ISBN 3-540-54782-7 (alk. paper): DM98.00. — ISBN 0-387-54782-7 (alk. paper) 1. Leukemia—Cytopathology—Congresses. 2. Leukemia—Treatment—Congresses. I. Fleischer, J. [DNLM: 1. Cytokines—physiology—congresses. 2. Interferons—therapeutic use. 3. Leukemia—pathology—congresses. 4. Leukemia—therapy—congresses. 5. Macrophages—physiology—congresses. QZ 350 L6515] RC643.L448 1993 616.99'419—dc20 DNLM/DLC

Typesetting: Best-set Typesetter Ltd., Hong Kong
25/3130-5 4 3 2 1 0 – Printed on acid-free paper

Preface

Current problems in research and treatment of leukemias as discussed at the symposium of the International Society of Haematology on leukemias in Dresden (Germany) are dealt with in detail in this volume.

The characterization of leukemic cells and the evaluation of their function are themes, with the first hints emerging of the possibility of relating them to the intensity of treatment required. The cytokines, responsible for cooperation between cells, are also of great importance, and the beginnings of therapeutic applications can be discerned here.

Not only are the cytokines themselves very interesting, but also the application of cells producing cytokines according to the range of macrophages found. The emphasis on cell-to-cell relationship is thus a main topic of the book. Of course, other treatment such as bone marrow transplantation and interferon therapy play an important part, too, and the latest results of chemotherapy are reported.

A further essential area covered is the diagnosis and therapy of chronic leukemic diseases, the inclusion of which suitably rounds off the book. I am very grateful to the outstanding specialists from both the West and the East who contributed to the symposium and this book: an important sign of collaboration and integration for the future.

J. FLEISCHER

Contents

Cytokines and Macrophages

Bone Marrow Transplantation

Chemotherapy of Acute Leukemias

Contents XIII

**Chronic Myeloproliferative Diseases
and Chronic Lymphatic Leukemia**

List of Contributors

The Blast Cell of Acute Leukemias

Prognosis of Myelodysplastic Syndromes

O. Krieger[1] and D. Lutz

In a retrospective study 133 patients (64 men, 69 women) with myelodysplastic syndromes (MDS) were analyzed. The patients were middle-aged to elderly (median 70 years; range 38–88 years), and according to the French-American-British Group (FAB) criteria they were diagnosed as having: refractory anemia (RA), 36; refractory sideroblastic anemia (RAS), 16; RA with excess of blasts (RAEB), 23; chronic myelomonocytic leukemia (CMML), 46; and RAEB in transformation (RAEBT), 12.

The clinical picture, hematological findings, FAB subgroup, scoring systems (Bournemouth score), immunological findings, and cytogenetic abnormalities were correlated with leukemic transformation and survival. Three different groups could be defined: (1) RA including RAS with a long survival (58 months); (2) RAEB including RAEBT with a high risk of mortality (surviving 13 months); and (3) CMML with a variable clinical course of two subtypes, (a) CMML-dysplastic type (WBC < 10.0 G/liter) and (b) CMML-proliferative type (WBC > 10.0 G/liter), related to myeloproliferative disorders.

Overall survival time of CMML patients was 17 months. The risk of leukemic transformation was different in the three groups (overall 48%). Chromosome anomalies were seen in 23 of 58 patients (40%) and were found in patients with poor outcome.

[1] 3rd Medical Department and Ludwig Boltzmann Institute for Leukemia Research and Hematology, Hanusch Hospital, Heinrich Collin Straße 30, A-1140 Vienna, Austria

Fleischer (Ed.) Leukemias
© Springer-Verlag Berlin Heidelberg 1993

Megakaryocytopoiesis in Patients
with Myelodysplastic Syndromes

M. PODOLAK-DAWIDZIAK,[1] D. GEDDES, and D. BOWEN

Introduction

Myelodysplastic syndrome (MDS) is a progressive preleukaemic condition caused by an abnormality of haemopoietic stem cells [1,10] and characterized by both genetic and functional changes [3,4]. Dysmegakaryocytopoiesis is a common feature in MDS and results in thrombocytopenia in about 50% of cases [4]. Megakaryocyte colony formation was found to be defective in many MDS patients [5,6]. Futhermore, MDS plasma displayed a low ability to support the clonal growth of normal megakaryocytopoietic progenitors [13]. Although the number of marrow megakaryocytes may be decreased, normal or increased, they are often morphologically abnormal with reduced size (micromegakaryocytes) [2,14,19] and small hypo- or nonlobulated nuclei [13,16]. The degree of dysmegakaryocytopoiesis along with the degree of dysgranulocytopoiesis has been introduced as an additional criterion aiming at better prediction of patients' survival than that based on the French-American-British Group (FAB) classification alone [1,18].

In our study we have examined megakaryocytic progenitors and plasma megakaryocytopoietic activity in MDS patients in relation to chromosomal abnormalities.

Material and Methods

Megakaryocyte colony-forming units (CFU-Mk) were assayed in the bone marrow of ten normal subjects, five women and five men aged from 30 to 67 years (mean 54.8 years) and ten consecutively admitted patients with MDS, four women and six men aged from 57 to 85 years (mean 69.5 years), four with refractory anaemia (RA), three with refractory anaemia with excess of blasts (RAEB) and three with sideroblastic anaemia (SA). The assay was based on the method of Messner et al. [11]. The project of the study was

---

[1] Department of Haematology, Medical Academy, Pasteura 4, 50-367 Wrocław, Poland

Fleischer (Ed.) Leukemias
© Springer-Verlag Berlin Heidelberg 1993

Table 1. Megakaryocyte progenitors and karyotype data in MDS patients

No.	Patient	Diagnosis	Sex	Age (years)	Megakaryocyte (% marrow cells)	Platelet count ($\times 10^9$/l)	CFU-Mk (marrow)		Karyotype data
							MDS plasma	N plasma	
1	E.W.	RA	F	57	0.10	41.0	6	8	ND
2	A.B.	SA	M	85	0.34	41.0	1	5	46,XY/45,XY,−7
3	I.W.	RAEB	M	62	0.06	158.0	0	7	46,XY
4[a]	R.I.	RA	M	62	0.16	175.0	0	2	46,XY/46,XY,del(5)(q13q33)
5[a]	C.W.	RAEB	M	57	0.18	40.0	0	4	46,XY/46,XY,del(5)(q12q13)
6[a]	D.J.	RA	F	79	0.60	391.0	0	5	46,XX/46,XX,del(5)(q13q33)
7	E.P.	SA	F	84	0.20	425.0	2	8	46,XX
8	J.F.	RAEB	F	59	0.15	58.0	1	6	ND
9	T.T.	SA	M	76	0.20	157.0	1	1	46,XY
10[a]	R.K.	RA	M	74	0.20	186.0	0	4	46,XY/45,X,del(5)(q13q33)
			$\bar{x}$	69.5	0.22	167.2	1.1	5.0	
			SEM	11.9	0.15	140.3	1.6	2.3	

MDS, myelodysplastic syndrome; RA, refractory anaemia; SA, sideroblastic anaemia; RAEB, refractory anaemia with excess of blasts; CFU-Mk, colony-forming units – megakaryocyte; ND, not done
[a] del(5q)

Table 2. CFU-Mk from normal bone marrow

No.	Patient	Sex	Age (years)	Megakaryocyte (% marrow cells)	Platelet count ($\times 10^9$/l)	CFU-Mk (normal bone marrow)	
						MDS plasma	N plasma
1	S.F.	F	30	0.30	368.0	5	20
2	L.R.	M	61	0.20	277.0	0	17
3	G.F.	F	52	0.15	205.0	1	16
4	E.L.	F	66	0.18	173.0	3	25
5	R.L.	M	67	0.20	310.0	0	19
6	H.C.	F	53	0.25	357.0	2	17
7	R.S.	M	40	0.20	312.0	4	15.5
8	G.M.	M	59	0.15	239.0	2	23
9	G.A.	F	64	0.30	349.0	2	19
10	B.V-G.	M	49	0.15	209.0	0	16
		$\bar{x}$	54.1	0.21	279.1	1.9	18.7
		SEM	11.9	0.05	70.0	1.6	3.0

CFU-Mk, colony-forming units – megakaryocyte; MDS, myelodysplastic syndrome

approved by the South Glamorgan Ethics Committee. The growth of CFU-Mk was supported by normal plasma (N plasma), MDS plasma and phyto-haemagglutinin-stimulated lymphocyte-conditioned medium (PHA-LCM). Megakaryocyte maturation was studied morphologically accordingly to Levine et al. [9]. Cytogenetic studies were performed on the bone marrow and peripheral blood by standard procedures. Chromosome identification and karyotypic nomenclature were in accordance with the recommendations of the Paris Conference [12]. Comparisons were made by the nonparametric Mann-Whitney test and association has been estimated by Spearman's rank-order correlation test.

Results

As shown in Tables 1 and 2, although bone marrow megakaryocyte counts in MDS and in normal marrow were similar, thrombocytopenia was present in four MDS cases and the mean platelet count was significantly lower in MDS patients than in controls ($p < 0.005$). There was a positive correlation between megakaryocyte and platelet counts in normal subjects ($r = 0.85$, $p < 0.005$), but not in MDS. The proportion of immature megakaryocytes was much higher in MDS (50%) than in normal marrow (16.8%). In all MDS patients megakaryocyte colony formation was decreased, and in five patients there was no megakaryocyte colony formation at all when MDS plasma was used in the cultures (Table 1). Four of the five MDS patients who did not grow CFU-Mk had a clonal deletion, del (5q), in bone marrow preparations. Three patients (nos. 4, 6 and 10) showed the classic deletion of q13–33, the fourth case (no. 5) had a minor deletion affecting q12–13. In MDS patients with del(5q) (q13–33) bone marrow megakaryocytes varied between 0.16% and 0.60%, with a high proportion of immature hypo-lobulated cells; but in all these patients the platelet count remained normal.

Discussion

The present results confirm our previous observation that the number of CFU-Mk from normal marrow was significantly lower when stimulated by MDS plasma than by N plasma [13]. It was found that MDS plasma stimulated patients' own progenitors to form megakaryocyte colonies less than N plasma. Although the mean number of megakaryocytes in MDS marrow was normal, the proportion of immature megakaryocytes was much higher than in normal marrow. Thrombocytopenia was present in four of ten MDS patients. All ten patients had defective megakaryocytic colony formation and five of them did not show any CFU-Mk growth. These findings are much the same as published by Juvonen et al. [5,6]. It is of interest that four of the five MDS patients who did not grow CFU-Mk had a clonal del(5q) in bone marrow preparations. In Juvonen's set of data [6], two of the five MDS patients with del(5q) as the only chromosomal abnor-mality showed normal megakaryocyte growth, two had a decreased number of colonies and one exhibited no colony growth. Four of five of our MDS patients with del(5q) had a normal platelet count.

Within this overall picture, those patients with del(5q) have a signi-ficantly greater failure of CFU-Mk growth, suggesting a specific relevance of this chromosomal region to megakaryocytopoiesis. Although the 5q-syndrome was initially described in morphological terms [15,17], it is now known that the affected segment of chromosome 5q contains the genes for interleukin-3 (IL-3) [7] and granulocyte-macrophage colony-stimulating factor and the human c-*fms* protooncogene (FMS) [8].

The present findings suggest a role for a protein coded in this region in megakaryocytopoiesis. Impairement of megakaryocytopoiesis in MDS may be due to a defect at the level of an early progenitor, but the contribution of the low plasma stimulatory activity should be also considered.

References

1. Bennett JM, Catovsky D, Daniel MT, Flandrin G, Galton DAG, Gralnick HR, Sultan C, The French-American-British (FAB) Co-operative group (1982) Proposals for the classification of the myelodysplastic syndromes. Br J Haematol 51:189–199
2. Bracher C (1974) Atypical megakaryocytes. A reflection of a stem cell disorder. In: Baldini M, Ebbe S (eds) Platelets: production, function, transfusion and storage. Grune and Stratton, New York, pp 94–103

3. Greenberg PL (1983) The smouldering myeloid leukemic status: clinical and biologic feature. Blood 61:1035–1044
4. Jacobs A (1985) Myelodysplastic syndrome: pathogenesis, functional abnormalities, and clinical implications. J Clin Pathol 38:1201–1217
5. Juvonen E, Partanen E, Knuutila S, Ruutu T (1986) Megakaryocyte colony formation by bone marrow progenitors in myelodysplastic syndromes. Br J Haematol 63:331–334
6. Juvonen E, Partanen E, Knuutila S, Ruutu T (1989) Colony formation by megakaryocyte progenitors in myelodysplastic syndromes. Eur J Haematol 42:389–395
7. LeBeau MM, Epstein MD, O'Brien SJ, Nienhuis AW, Yang Y, Clark SC, Rowley JD (1987) The interleukin 3 gene is located on human chromosome 5 and is deleted in myeloid leukemias with a deletion of 5q. Proc Natl Acad Sci USA 84:5913–5917
8. LeBeau MM, Westbrook CA, Diaz MO, Larson RA, Rowley JD, Gasson JC, Golde DW, Sherr CJ (1986) Evidence for the involvement of GM-CSF and FMS in the deletion (5q) in myeloid disorders. Science 251:984–987
9. Levine RF (1980) Isolation and characterization of normal human megakaryocytes. Br J Haematol 45:487–497
10. Linman JW, Saarni MJ (1974) The preleukemic syndrome. Semin Hematol 11:93–100
11. Messner HA, Jamal N, Izaguirre C (1982) The growth of large megakaryocyte colonies from human bone marrow. J Cell Physiol 1:45–51
12. Paris Conference (1971) Standarization in human cytogenetics. Birth Defects 8:1972
13. Podolak-Dawidziak M (1989) Stimulation of CFU-Mk colony growth by normal plasma and plasma from myelodysplastic patients. Leuk Res 13:213–215
14. Smith WB, Ablin A, Goodman JR, Brecher G (1973) Atypical megakaryocytes in preleukemic phase of acute myeloid leukemia. Blood 42:535–540
15. Sokal G, Michaux JL, van den Berghe H, Cordier A, Rodhain J, Ferrant A, Mariau M, De Bruyere M, Sonnet J (1975) A new hematologic syndrome with a distinct karyotype: the 5q-chromosome. Blood 46:519–533
16. Tricot G, Vlietinck R, Boogaerts MA, Hendriks B, De Wolf-Peters C, van den Berghe H, Verwilgen RL (1985) Prognostic factors in the myelodysplastic syndromes: importance of initial data on peripheral blood counts, bone marrow cytology, trophine biopsy and chromosomal analysis. Br J Haematol 60:19–32
17. van den Berghe H, Cassiman JJ, David G, Fryns JP, Michaux JL, Sokal G (1974) Distinct haematological disorder with deletion of long arm of no 5 chromosome. Nature 251:437–438
18. Varela BL, Chuang C, Woll JE, Bennett JM (1985) Modification in the classification of primary myelodysplastic syndromes: the addition of a scoring system. Hematol Oncol 3:55–63
19. Wiesneth M, Pflieger H, Kubanek B, Heimpel H (1980) Micromegakaryocytes in human bone marrow. Acta Haematol 64:65–71

Diversity of Bone Marrow Findings
in Chronic Myelomonocytic Leukemia

L.L. Yavorkovsky,[1] L.Y. Ryauzova, D.Y. Solovey,
and L.I. Yavorkovsky

Since the early 1970s, when chronic myelomonocytic leukemia (CMML) was described as a novel type of leukemia, this entity has drawn our particular interest. At the beginning the disorder was separated from chronic myelogenous leukemia and, for about 10 years, was indisputably classified with myeloproliferative diseases. In 1982 a French-American-British (FAB) cooperative group decided to include CMML in the larger group of myelodysplastic syndromes (MDS) and to define diagnostic criteria. According to the authors' conceptions, the disease is now included either among myeloproliferative syndromes, particularly Philadelphia chromosome- (Ph^1)-negative chronic myelocytic leukemia (CML), or among MDS. To our mind, the reason for such different approaches lies in the extreme biological and clinical diversity of features observed in these patients. As to blood, some opposite (diminished or increased) values in all three cell lines may occur. When examining the bone marrow smears, a significant diversity is usually observed both in the extent of myeloid hyperplasia and, especially, dysplasia. Finally, CMML as defined by the FAB group is associated with a variable survival rate, ranging from a few weeks to several years. Taking into account all the above data, we tried to find a reasonable explanation of these divers observations and, moreover, to identify subgroups within our patients.

We studied 30 patients seen in our department from 1982 to 1989. The diagnosis of CMML was established according to the FAB criteria. There were 23 males and 7 females (3.3:1); the median age at presentation was 73 years, range, 58–84 years. Percentage of blast cells in the bone marrow ranged from 1% to 21%. Persons presenting with similar but different conditions, such as acute myelomonocytic leukemia "with differentiation", chronic monocytic leukemia, or idiopathic myelofibrosis, undergoing leukemic (monoblastic) transformation and prolonged myelomonocytic reactions to unnoticed infections (tuberculosis) or tumor were eliminated from the study.

Bone marrow biopsy was integrated into this study as an essential diagnostic procedure owing to which we could both exclude patients with

[1] Latvian Academy of Medicine, 1007 Riga, Latvia

Fleischer (Ed.) Leukemias
© Springer-Verlag Berlin Heidelberg 1993

Table 1. Blood and bone marrow findings in hematological disorders recognized within FAB's CMML

	RA, RAEB, RAEB(t) with monocytosis	Myelomonocytic dysplasia	True CMML	
			Monocytic type	Granulocytic type
	MDS		Leukemia	
WBC count (10^9/l)	3.45 ± 0.6		12.8 ± 4.1	32.5 ± 9.6
Monocyte count (10^9/l)	1.30 ± 0.35		4.0 ± 1.6	1.3 ± 0.3
BMS dyserythropoiesis	Pronounced	Weak	Weak	Weak
BMB cellularity	Increased	Normal	Normal or increased	Increased
Megakaryocytosis	Often	Absent	Absent	Often
Lymphoid nodules and perivascular plasmocytosis	Pronounced	Rare	Rare	Rare
Sinuses with myeloid precursors	Absent	Absent	Present	Present

BMS, bone marrow smears; BMB, bone marrow biopsy. Cell counts are shown as mean ± SEM.

unrelated disorders and, particularly, confirm the significant diversity of patients, meeting the FAB criteria for CMML.

Having reviewed our cases, we were able to show that CMML as defined by FAB appear to represent not a single entity, but comprise at least three separate groups of hematological disorders. The first represents the well known types of FAB-classified MDS – refractory anemia (RA), RA with ring sideroblasts (RARS), and RA with excess of blasts (RAEB) with concomitant monocytosis. The second one is a novel, so far indistinguishable, syndrome, which we named as myelomonocytic dysplasia. Some cases, in spite of their dysplastic features, were regarded as myeloproliferative disorders rather than MDS, and we designated them as "true" CMML. It is of interest that we could further distinguish two subtypes of true CMML – with either granulocytic or monocytic predominance. Table 1 summarizes hematological findings in each of the aforesaid disorders. First, it should be noted that elevated WBC count was the parameter separating true CMML patients from patients with MDS characterized by low WBC count. In addition, WBC count and absolute monocyte count emerged as factors allowing us to distinguish CMML with monocytic predominance from granulocytic predominance, respectively.

The most significant diversity was observed in the bone marrow samples. Pronounced erythroid dysplasia was noted exclusively in the first category – RAs with monocytosis. Other categories were characterized by lack of, or only weak, dysplastic features in the erythroid series. The next distin-

Table 2. Proposals for reclassification of FAB's CMML

FAB classification	Proposed classification
1. Refractory anemia	1.1. RA
	1.2. RA with monocytosis
2. Refractory anemia with ring sideroblasts	2.1. RARS
	2.2. RARS with monocytosis
3. Refractory anemia with excess of blasts	3.1. RAEB
	3.2. RAEB with monocytosis
4. RAEB in transformation	4.1. RAEB(t)
	4.2. RAEB(t) with monocytosis
5. Chronic myelomonocytic leukemia (CMML)[a]	5. Myelomonocytic dysplasia

[a] Myeloproliferative disorder.

guishing feature was the bone marrow cellularity. It was either normal or only slightly increased in monocytic type of true CMML and particularly in myelomonocytic dysplasia, regardless of the stage of the disease. On the contrary, RAs and granulocytic type of CMML had, usually, significantly increased cellularity. Megakaryocytosis was shown to have an additional diagnostic value since it was prominent in granulocytic type of CMML as well as in the RAs group. Finally, two additional important findings were noted. On the one hand, lymphoid nodules and particularly perivascular plasmocytosis were pronounced only in patients with RAs, and on the other, sinuses with immature myeloid precursors were noticed exclusively in patients with true CMML both of monocytic and granulocytic types.

In conclusion, several points should be noted. Although the dysplastic features are essential for the diagnosis of MDS, their diagnostic importance should not be overemphasized. In fact, many hematological disorders, except MDS, are accompanied by dysplastic myelopoiesis. Therefore, the FAB group criteria for CMML, based only on morphologic data are, in our opinion, insufficient for an accurate diagnosis. Our study allows for the identification, within the FAB-defined CMML, of three separate hematological disorders. Table 2 provides our proposals for the reclassification of FAB's CMML. Instead of the known types of MDS – RA, RARS, RAEB, and RAEB in transformation [RAEB(t)] – we propose to subdivide them into those without or with monocytosis. Our data suggest that cases with elevated WBC count together with other myeloproliferative features should be appraised as apparent leukemia and, regardless of dysplastic features, should be excluded from the MDS category. Instead, the novel dysplastic syndrome – myelomonocytic dysplasia – should be incorporated into MDS.

Nucleolar Organizer Regions in Acute Leukemia

M. Trněný[1,2] and K. Smetana[1]

Introduction

Nucleolar organizer regions (NORs) are loops of DNA which occur in the cell nucleolus and contain ribosomal RNA genes [1]. These regions can be demonstrated by reaction of NOR protein components with silver [6,9]. In light microscopy they appear as intensely stained brown or black granules called either silver-NORs (Ag-NORs) or silver-stained granules (SSGs). Their number is apparently related to nucleolar biosynthetic activity with respect to ribosomal RNA transcription [9]. The number of SSGs has been studied in metaphases of normal and leukemic bone marrow, and the silver stainability in interphasic leukemic cells has been also investigated in several studies (e.g., 2, 7). There are, however, some differences in the results of these studies. The aim of our study was to provide more information on the number of nucleolar SSGs in interphasic leukemic myeloblasts in the peripheral blood.

Materials and Methods

We have used the standardized two-step silver staining method described previously [6]. We examined 9 previously untreated patients with acute myeloid leukemia (AML) (Table 1). At least 50 blasts in each peripheral blood smear were investigated for the determination of the number of SSGs per cell. We used bone marrow samples of five untreated patients with various non-neoplastic hematological diseases and normal blood cell counts as controls. In each sample 25 myeloblasts were investigated. The t-test was used to compare differences between these groups.

Results

The number of nucleolar SSGs per myeloid blast in peripheral blood of patients with AML varies between 4.5 and 10.1 (Table 1). Their mean

[1] Institute of Hematology and Blood Transfusion, U nemocnice 1, CS-12820 Prague, Czechoslovakia
[2] Present address: 1st Dept. Med. 1st Med. Fac., Charles University, U nemocnice 2, CS-12808 Prague, Czechoslovakia

Fleischer (Ed.) Leukemias
© Springer-Verlag Berlin Heidelberg 1993

Table 1. Characteristics of patients with AML

	Diagnosis	Patients		Leukocytes (10^9/l)	Leukemic blasts (%)	SSGs per blast
		Age (years)	Sex			
1	AML M1	23	M	7.1	88	6.2
2	AML M1	45	M	148.0	65	6.8
3	AML M2	32	F	196.0	88	4.5
4	AML M2	22	M	74.0	91	7.2
5	AML M2	22	M	118.0	84	10.1
6	AML M2	17	M	196.0	88	6.6
7	AML M4	62	F	80.5	85	5.4
8	AML M4	36	M	66.0	66	7.7
9	AML M4	52	F	71.0	43	4.6

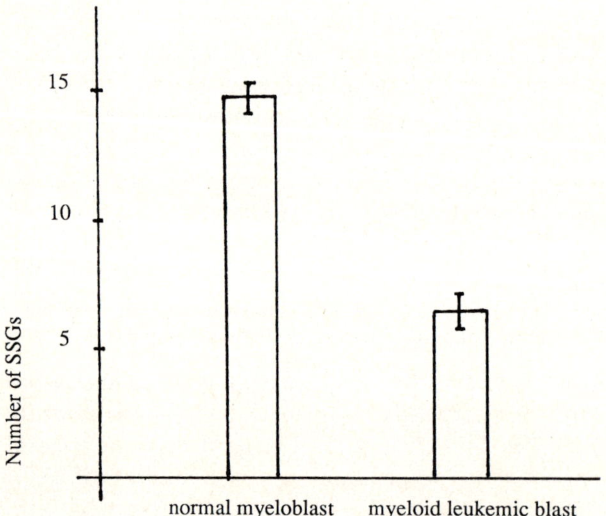

Fig. 1. Number of silver-stained granules per normal myeloblast and myeloid leukemic blast

number is 6.3, with standard deviation, 0.6. The mean number of nucleolar SSGs per normal myeloblast in bone marrow of patients from the control group is 14.9, with standard deviation, 0.6. The difference between number of nucleolar SSGs in normal myeloblast and leukemic myeloblast is significant at level 0.01 (Fig. 1). The differences between subtypes of AML are without significance.

Discussion

The present data indicate that the number of nucleolar SSGs (NORs) in interphasic leukemic myeloblasts in the peripheral blood is significantly smaller than in normal bone marrow myeloblasts. Since the number of nucleolar SSGs is related to the nucleolar biosynthetic activity and to the cell proliferation [3,5,6,9,10], myeloblasts of AML apparently seem to be less active with respect to these processes. This interpretation is in agreement with previous data published in the literature, according to which, the proliferation activity of myeloblasts of AML is reduced in comparison with normal myeloblasts [4,8]. In addition, as generally known, myeloblasts of acute leukemias have a diminished activity for further differentiation which might be reflected by a decreased number of SSGs (NORs) in these cells as compared with normal myeloblasts (present observations – Fig. 1).

References

1. Alberts B, Bray D, Lewis J, Raff M, Roberts K, Watson JD (1983) Molecular biology of the cell. New York, Garland Publishing, Inc. pp 422–428
2. Arden KC, Bucana CD, Johnston DA, Pathak S (1989) Computer-assisted image analysis of silver staining in normal and leukemic bone marrow. Int J Cancer 43:395–398
3. Crocker J, Macartney JC, Smith PJ (1988) Correlation between DNA flow cytometric and nucleolar organizer region data in non-Hodgkin's lymphomas. J Pathol 154:151–156
4. Gavosto F, Pileri A, Bachi C, Pegoraro L (1964) Proliferation and maturation defect in acute leukemia cells. Nature 203:92–94
5. Hall PA, Crocker J, Watts A, Stansfeld AG (1988) A comparison nucleolar organizer region staining and Ki-67 immunostaining in non-Hodgkin's lymphoma. Histopathology 12:373–381
6. Likovský Z, Smetana K (1981) Further studies on the cytochemistry of standardized silver staining of interphase nucleoli in smear preparations of Yoshida ascitic sarcoma cells in rats. Histochemistry 72:301–313
7. Mamaev NN, Mamaeva SE, Grabovskaya IL, et al (1987) The activity of nucleolar organizer regions of human bone marrow cells studied with silver staining. II. Acute leukemia. Cancer Genet Cytogenet 25:65–72
8. Smetana K, Gyorkey F, Gyorkey P, Busch H (1969) On the ultrastructure of nucleoli in human leukemic myeloblasts. Exp Cell Res 58:303–311
9. Smetana K, Busch H (1979) Studies on silver staining components, in Busch H, Croohe ST, Daskal Y (eds): Effects of drugs on the cell nucleus. New York, Academic Press pp 89–105
10. Smetana K, Likovský Z (1984) Nucleolar silver-stained granules in maturing erythroid and granulocytic cells. Cell Tissue Res 237:367–370

A Further Note on the Ultrastructure
of Human Leukemic Cells

K. Smetana[1] and I. Jirásková

At present, electron microscopy for classification of blastic cells has been replaced by immunological typing, which is faster and apparently more exact. On the other hand, conventional transmission electron microscopy remains the only procedure for investigation of various cell components within single cells, including abnormalities due to pathological processes or drug effects. In this area, electron microscopy cannot be replaced by any other procedure.

The most frequent abnormality of a leukemic cell is represented by maturation or differentiation anarchy – asynchrony or maturation arrest [1]. The nucleus may exhibit a fine, immature chromatic structure in a partially or fully differentiated mature cytoplasm. The chromatin structure may be already mature, condensed in a highly immature undifferentiated cytoplasm with an abundant number of ribosomes [4]. The asynchrony may be noted even within the cell nucleus. Nucleoli may be inactive or less active – represented by the presence of ring-shaped nucleoli or micronucleoli in a nucleus with a fine, highly immature chromatin structure. In contrast, active nucleoli such as compact nucleoli without segregation of nucleolar components or nucleoli with nucleolonemata are present in a nucleus with a condensed mature chromatin structure. In leukemic lymphoblasts, monoblasts with both active and inactive nucleoli were noted in the same nucleus [2]. Recent cytochemical electron-microscopic examination of the nucleolar structural organization resulted in the visualization of active and inactive nucleolus organizer regions in the same nucleolus of a leukemic lymphoblast (Smetana and Jirásková, in preparation). Similar asynchrony or maturation arrest was detected for perichromatin and interchromatin granules in relation to the chromatin structure or nucleolar type. In this case, the correct interpretation is very difficult since the function of interchromatin or perichromatin granules has not been completely clarified.

The evaluation of the nuclear shape is more efficient using the light microscope. However, cytoplasmic invaginations, nuclear clefts, pockets, and abnormalities of the nuclear envelope in leukemic cells, particularly malignant lymphocytes, can be easily seen in ultrathin section with the

[1] Institute of Hematology and Blood Transfusion, U nemocnice 1, CS-12820 Prague, Czechoslovakia

Fleischer (Ed.) Leukemias
© Springer-Verlag Berlin Heidelberg 1993

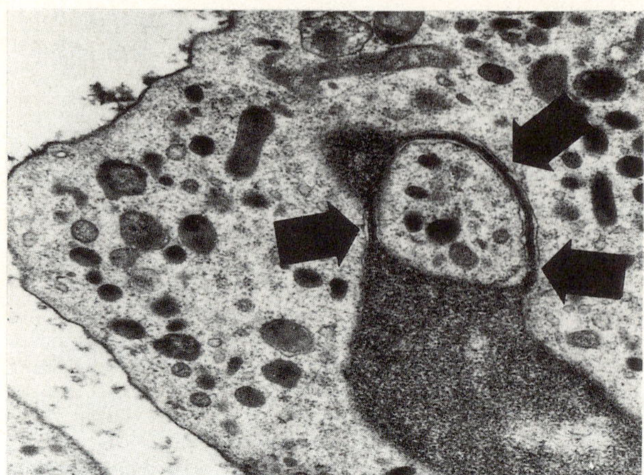

Fig. 1. Nuclear pocket (*arrows*) in a leukemic granulocyte. ×28 000

electron microscope (Fig. 1). In addition, a classification and quantitative data concerning such abnormalities are available in the literature. Some of these data might be important for monitoring chemotherapy [3].

Most frequent abnormalities of mitochondria are dilatations of the intercristal space which contain a variable amount of DNA filaments and mitochondrial ribosomes. Very interesting rodlet-like inclusions were noted in mitochondria of leukemic lymphocytes. By a high-magnification analysis and cytochemistry it has been shown that such inclusion bodies represent supertwisted DNA. In this connection it should be mentioned that mitochondrial rodlet-like inclusions were found in lymphocytes of a married couple suffering from chronic lymphocytic leukemia [7]. A very unusual abnormality of mitochondria and the cell nucleus has been observed in Sézary cells in mycosis fungoides or Sézary syndrome [6]. In some of these cells mitochondria fused with the cell nucleus; moreover, a mitochondrion has been found within the cell nucleus of a Sézary cell. Other mitochondrial abnormalites such as abnormal mitochondrial shape and structure in leukemic cells are not unusual.

Distinct abnormalities of the Golgi apparatus or centrioles are rare. Dilatations of Golgi tubules were found in leukemic lymphocytes [5]. Annulate lamellae were observed more frequently in lymphoma than leukemic lymphocytes. Abnormalities of the formation of granules are relatively frequent in immature leukemic and less differentiated cells. Generally known abnormalities are represented by Auer rodlets or bodies. The positivity for peroxidase of the endoplasmic reticulum – particularly at the cell nucleus – may be detected earlier by electron microscopy than by light-microscopic cytochemistry. Endoplasmic reticula also participate in the formation of focal cytoplasmic degradation bodies by encapsulating various cell components (e.g., ribosomes) and virus-like particles.

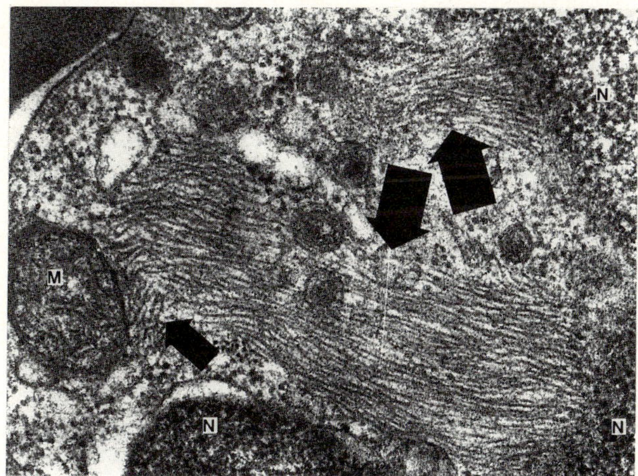

Fig. 2. Bundles of microfibrils (*arrows*) in a blastic cell of acute myelomonocytic leukemia. Some fibrils of the large bundle seem to be associated with the nucleus (*N*) and mitochondrion (*M*). ×90 000

Cytoplasmic microfilaments are either dispersed or form bundles and highly organized structures known as fibrillar bodies or fibrillar formations. The latter are present particularly in blastic cells of acute leukemias. Bundles of microfilaments are frequently connected with and external membrane of the cell nucleus or mitochondria; bundles of microfilaments interconnecting the cell nucleus and mitochodria were also observed [8]. Such phenomena were noted in blastic cells of acute leukemias with a relatively large incidence in acute myelomonocytic leukemia (Fig. 2).

Various inclusion bodies represent a further abnormality of leukemic cells [1,4,9]. However, their interpretation is usually difficult or impossible at present. Some of them may be classified as lysosomes. The presence of various virus-like particles in our collection of electron mirographss of human leukemic cells is rare rather than frequent.

Concerning abnormalities of the cell surface and structures related to the cell membrane, they are unusual except for characteristic cells of hairy-cell leukemia.

Conclusions

The presented data, based on the evaluation of electron micrographs of leukemic cells from the authors' archive, as well as of those published in the literature, demonstrate that leukemic cells are characterized by a broad variety of abnormalities. However, excepting a few abnormalities, most of them are not specific for a leukemic cell.

References

1. Bessis M (1973) Living blood cells and their ultrastructure. Springer, Berlin Heidelberg New York
2. Busch H, Smetana K (1970) The nucleolus. Academic, New York
3. Schuurmans Steehoven J, Holland R (1986) Nuclear pockets and clefts in the lymphoid cell population of bone marrow and blood of children with acute lymphoblastic leukemia. Am J Pathol 123:39–45
4. Smetana K (1970) Electron microscopy of lymphocytes. Methods Cancer Res 5:455–477
5. Smetana K, Heřmanský F, Janele J, Busch H (1968) A further note on the ultrastructure of leukemic lymphocytes. Folia Haematol (Leipzig) 89:1–14
6. Smetana K, Daskal Y, Gyorkey F, Gyorkey P, Lehane D, Rudolph AH, Busch H (1977) Cancer Res 37:2036–2042
7. Smetana K, Heřmanský F, Koblížková M (1978) Intramitochondrial rodlet-like inclusions in human leukemic lymphocytes. Folia Haematol (Leipzig) 105:161–168
8. Smetana K, Jirásková I, Roath S (1987) Studies on microfilaments (fibrillary structures) in blast cells of human acute leukemias. Hematol Rev 1:367–373
9. Zucker-Franklin D, Greaves MF, Grossi CE, Marmont AM (1981) Atlas of blood cells. Ermes, Milan

Cell Kinetics of Human Acute Leukemia: In Vivo Study with Bromodeoxyuridine and Flow Cytometry*

M. Danova,[1] M. Giordano, G. Mazzini, and A. Riccardi

Clinical investigators have been attracted by the possibility that cell kinetics could be a parameter for cancer prognosis and chemotherapy planning. Gross differences in proliferative activity are known to exist among various human tumors. Unfortunately, substantial overlap occurs, and the kinetic characteristic are largely unpredictable in the individual patient. The direct measurement of cell kinetics, however, is not easy in clinical settings. For example, the necessity of using radioactive tracers restricted the in vivo measurement of the labeling index (LI) of human tumors to only a few cases and led to the development of in vitro techniques for labeling biopsy material.

With the development of flow cytometry (FCM), rapid analysis of the DNA distribution of cell populations has become feasible. With this technique it has been possible to evaluate the S phase size of a tumor population by determining the percentage of cells with DNA content intermediate between the diploid ($2n$) and the tetraploid ($4n$) values. DNA FCM has not become entirely clinically feasible because of two major problems: first, the accuracy of the $2n:4n$ cell percentage in estimating the S phase has been hampered by the presence of S-phase-arrested cells which are considered as proliferating by DNA FCM, while they actually are not; second, the proliferative activity cannot be evaluated by DNA FCM when an aneuploid population is present because all the mathematical computer programs tend to overestimate the S phase size.

Bromodeoxyuridine (BUDR) is a thymidine analogue that is incorporated into the DNA of proliferating cells. Since the dose of BUDR needed to label cells is not toxic, cell labeling can be accomplished in vivo, by infusing the substance in patients. The in vivo administration of BUDR, coupled with bivariate FCM for measurements [7], allows a complete kinetic picture of human cancer to be obtained easily [1,2], and we report here the kinetic data, with some clinical correlations, obtained by this method in patients with acute non lymphoblastic leukemia (AnLL).

* Research supported by C.N.R. (Consiglio Nazionale delle Ricerche-Roma, Progetto Finalizzato Oncologia, grant no. 88.00841.44), by C.N.R. Target Project "Biotechnology and Bioinstrumentation," by A.I.R.C., and by I.R.C.C.S. Policlinico San Matteo, Pavia.
[1] Istituto di Clinica Medical, Dipartimento di Medicina Internae Terapia Medica, I-27100 Pavia, Italy

Table 1. Kinetic characteristics (determined by in vivo administration of BUDR) of patients with AnLL according to clinical outcome

Patients	n	LI	p	TS	p	Tpot	p	FTR	p
Responsive AnLL	20	6.4	<0.06	10.2	<0.05	5.7	0.07	17.1	0.08
Nonresponsive AnLL	14	7.8		12.5		7.5		15.9	
CR <8 months	8	5.4	<0.02	10.0	0.30	6.8	<0.05	14.6	0.07
CR >8 months	12	10.9		10.5		5.3		18.7	

Patients and Methods

Thirty-four consecutive patients with AnLL (median age, 51 years; range, 16–78 years; male to female ratio, 19:15) were classified according to French-American-British Group (FAB) subtypes: M1, 5 patients; M2, 6 patients; M3, 5 patients; M4, 11 patients; M5, 5 patients; M6, 1 patient; M7, 1 patient. DNA ploidy was as follows: diploid, 28 patients, aneuploid, 6 patients. The patients were uniformly treated with a standard protocol which included remission [CR] induction with two to three courses of sequential vincristine, arabinosylcytosine, and adriamycin, and maintenance treatment with monthly courses of different cytostatics. They received in vivo BUDR infusion for kinetic studies before cell specimens were obtained for diagnostic purposes, including cytologic and histologic examination. Administration of BUDR was authorized by the Ethical Committee at the Department of internal Medicine of the University of Pavia, and written informed consent was obtained from each patient.

Patients were given a 15- to 20-min infusion of BUDR, $250\,\text{mg/m}^2$ 100 ml sodium chloride (prepared by the Department of Phamacology, I.R.C.C.S. Policlinico San Matteo). All tumors were sampled 4–6 h after completion of the BUDR infusion. Two-ml bone marrow (BM) samples were obtained by sternal aspiration. The complete procedure for obtaining single-cell suspensions for FCM from tissue samples, as well as the methods used to detect BUDR and to obtain the BUDR LI the DNA, synthesis time (TS), the potential doubling time (Tpot), and the fractional turnover rate (FTR), have been detailed elsewhere [3,5,7].

Results

No immediate toxicity was seen following BUDR infusion. To obtain the LI and TS values, the complete in vivo BUDR procedure took 8–9 h from the start of BUDR infusion and 2–3 h from the BM sampling. Proliferative activity was greater in responsive than in nonresponsive patients. Responsive patients who experienced CR for more than 8 months had proliferative activity higher than those with shorter CR, mainly due to higher LI values (see Table 1).

Discussion

The evaluation of BUDR incorporation into DNA of proliferating cells by means of the anti-BUDR monoclonal antibody (MoAb) makes the study of cell kinetics in humans easier and more complete. Administering BUDR in vivo is ethically possible, in that immediate toxicity is not observed and DNA damage is unlikely. A quite complete kinetic pattern of tumors (including S phase size and duration, and Tpot and production rate) can be obtained within a few hours when in vivo BUDR administration is coupled with bivariate FCM to simultaneously measure BUDR incorporation and DNA content, using a single cell sample. Administering BUDR to patients and employing bivariate FCM to measure simultaneously BUDR incorporation and DNA content has allowed a complete panel of kinetic parameters to be obtained for several human tumors in a short time, while using only one tumor sample.

In a preceding paper [5] we thoroughly discussed the advantages of using the in vivo BUDR method for studying (in clinical settings) cell kinetics in a variety of human tumors. The first reason favoring this over the traditional cytokinetic methods is that it furnishes an S phase evaluation which is easier and more accurate than that obtained from both tritiated thymidine ($[^3H]$TdR) cytoautoradiography and DNA FCM. With respect to $[^3H]$TdR cytoautoradiography, the in vivo BUDR procedure is more rapidly accomplished and a much greater number of cells are evaluated. With respect to DNA FCM, an accurate estimation of the S phase can be obtained in both diploid and aneuploid tumors. A second advantage of the in vivo BUDR method is that it also furnishes the rate at which proliferating cells synthesize DNA, i.e., the TS, a parameter which is exceedingly difficult to obtain with the traditional techniques. With in vivo BUDR the TS is simply evaluated by measuring the degree of progression rate toward the G_2 phase of the cell cycle of the BUDR-labeled cells in the interval (4–6 h) between BUDR infusion and tumor sampling.

There are no reports of immediate adverse reactions following BUDR infusion; only one tumor sample is required for the study, and this is needed anyway for diagnostic or therapeutic purposes.

In the present study a preliminary attempt was made at correlating kinetic with clinical data in patients who had both LI and TS determinations. In 34 uniformly treated AnLL patients, proliferative activity, as measured from Tpot and FTR, was greater in responsive than in nonresponsive patients and in those who experienced CR for over 8 months than in those who had a shorter CR, suggesting that high proliferative activity is a favorable prognostic factor in this disease. We believe that these data on acute leukemia (AL) are of true clinical relevance. For many years investigators have tried to evaluate the clinical interest of proliferative activity in previously untreated AL by evaluating the S phase with [³H]TdR cytoautoradiography or DNA FCM. A number of them reported that CR was more frequent with high S phase values; others failed to confirm this finding, but none reported an advantage with low S phase values [6]. In this series, LI was not different in responsive and nonresponsive patients, but the responsive ones had a shorter Tpot and greater FTR due to a shorter TS. A response advantage for AL patients with shorter TS was also reported using in vivo BUDR coupled with immunohistochemistry [4]. From these data the concept that a high proliferative activity favors CR in AnLL, due to a high S phase value and/or a short TS can be accepted. Of course, the prognostic significance of proliferative activity must be better ascertained from the multivariate analysis of other clinical and laboratory features.

Acknowledgements. The authors appreciate the cooperation of Dr. L. Autelli from the Department of Pharmacology, I.R.C.C.S. Policlinico San Matteo, Pavia, for supplying the BUDR used in this study.

Dr. M. Danova was visiting fellow at the National Institute for Cancer Research (I.S.T.) Genova, Italy, supported by a Grant from I.R.C.C.S. San Matteo, and Dr. M. Giordano was a recipient of a fellowship of the "Ferrata-Storti" Foundation.

References

1. Begg AC, McNally NJ, Shrieve DC (1985) A method to measure the duration of the DNA synthesis and the potential doubling time from a single sample. Cytometry 6:620–625
2. Danova M, Wilson G, Riccardi A et al. (1987) In vivo administration of bromo-deoxyuridine and flow cytometry for cell kinetic studies in human malignancies. Haematologica 72:115–121
3. Danova M, Riccardi A, Gaetani P et al. (1988) Cell kinetics of human brain tumors: in vivo study with bromodeoxyuridine and flow cytometry. Eur J Cancer Clin Oncol 24:873–880
4. Raza A, Maheshwari Y, Preisler HD (1987) Differences in cell cycle characteristics among patients with acute nonlymphocytic leukemia. Blood 69:1647–1651
5. Riccardi A, Danova M, Wilson G et al. (1988) Cell kinetics in human malignancies studied with in vivo administration of bromodeoxyuridine and flow cytometry. Cancer Res 48:6238–6243
6. Riccardi A, Danova M, Montecucco CM et al. (1986) Acute nonlymphoblastic leukemia: reliability and prognostic significance of bone marrow S phase size determined with propidium iodide DNA flow cytofluorometry. Scand J Haematol 36:11–19
7. Wilson GD, McNally NJ, Dunphy E, Pfragner R, Karcher H (1985) The labelling index of human and mouse tumours assessed by bromodeoxyuridine staining in vivo and in vitro and flow cytometry. Cytometry 6:641–645

Clinical, Biochemical and Cytokinetic Parameters for Distinguishing Smouldering and Rapidly Proliferating Variants of Acute Leukemia

V. Nüssler,[1] H. Sauer, R. Pelka-Fleischer, D. Hölzel, and W. Wilmanns

Problems

The term "smouldering leukaemia" (SML) was first described in 1963 by Rheingold et al. [16]. They reported a variant of an acute myelogenous leukaemia (AML) for which a long survival time (8 months–3 years) without intensive therapy was found to be characteristic. Up to now there has been no clear distinction between myelodysplastic syndromes (MDS) and SML. In the literature the following expressions have been used to define SML: preleukaemia [5,7,14,15,17,23], oligoblastic leukaemia [1,18], subacute myelogenous leukaemia [9,24], chronic myelomonocytic leukaemia [24], chronic erythromonocytic leukaemia [4], hypocellular acute leukaemia [10] and MDS (dysmyelopoietic syndromes) [5, 7, 12].

In this work the leukaemic cell populations were also characterized by means of biochemical and cytokinetic studies. High thymidine kinase (TK) activity is a marker in about 80% of acute leukaemic cell populations [21].

This report was undertaken with the aim of defining the term smouldering leukaemia and to find a suitable tool for the recognition of the transition to the rapidly proliferating type of AML, in order to make a decision concerning aggressive treatment. In addition, the investigation of the efficacy of treatment of SML patients was an objective of this study.

Patients and Methods

Ten patients with a clinically defined smouldering form of AML ($>30\%$ myeloblasts in bone marrow, BM) were examined retrospectively. In most cases the patients survived for a long period (median, 16 months; five patients, more than 22 months; five patients, between 2.3 and 6.3 months) without any aggressive treatment. The reason for a decision to change to nonaggressive treatment was the reduced cytosolic TK, thymidine (dTR) and deoxyuridine (dUR). Three patients with SML were treated with low-dose cytosine arabinoside (Ara-C) because of an increasing thrombo-

[1] Medizinische Klinik III, Klinikum Grosshadern, Ludwig-Maximilians-Universität, W-8000 München 70, FRG

Fleischer (Ed.) Leukemias
© Springer-Verlag Berlin Heidelberg 1993

Table 1. TK, dTR, dUR, %S and blast count in BM (mean, m, and standard deviation, SD) of patients with SML compared with AML patients and healthy individuals

Parameters	Normal values (m ± SD) $n = 30$	Values for SML patients (m ± SD) $n = 10$	Values for AML patients (m ± SD) $n = 38$
TK nmol/min.10^{10} cells	12.02 ± 8.5	6.39 ± 2.43	74.91 ± 45.66
dTR nmol/min.10^{12} cells	66.95 ± 32.50	24.87 ± 13.68	74.19 ± 43.66
dUR nmol/min.10^{12} cells	60.0 ± 34.0	18.94 ± 12.59	61.93 ± 38.94
%S	9.34 ± 2.73	3.08 ± 2.04	8.86 ± 5.4
Blast Count in BM (%)	<5	54.0 ± 8.0	56.0 ± 11.0

cytopenia; the first after 3.03 months, the second after both 2.3 months and 6.8 months, the third after 2.1 months. A comparision was made with 38 patients having a typical, rapidly proliferating AML who were primarily treated by means of aggressive chemotherapy [AML-5-protocol or AML-6-protocol of the European Organisation for Research on Treatment of Cancer (EORTC)] and with 30 healthy individuals.

SML patients were registered between 1982 and 1987, and AML patients, between 1985 and 1987. The age, sex, symptoms and median survival, as well as the biochemical-cytokinetic parameters in human bone marrow cells, i.e., TK, dTR, dUR, percentage of cells in S phase (%S) and myeloblast count were determined. The values at the time of initial diagnosis were compared with the AML group and healthy individuals. The remission of patients with AML and SML was estimated using the criteria of the International Union Against Cancer (UICC). (For methods of TK, dTR, dUR and %S determination see Wilmanns et al., this volume, or Sauer and Wilmanns [6,19,20].

Results

The ten patients with SML were between 39 and 80 years old (mean, 58 years), with a predominance of females (70%). The 38 patients with AML were between 17 and 65 years old (mean, 46 years). In these cases the male sex was predominant (56%).

Comparison of biochemical-cytokinetic and morphological parameters of patients with SML, AML and healthy persons is shown in Table 1. The U test showed no significant differences in the blast count values between AML and SML patients. Moreover, there was no significant difference in the dTR, dUR and %S values between AML patients and healthy individuals; but there was a significant difference in the parameters TK, dTR, dUR and %S between the AML and SML patients ($p < 0.01$) and also between SML patients and healthy individuals ($p < 0.01$). The mean

Table 2. Type of treatment, treatment dosage and treatment duration and survival time after diagnosis of the ten patients with SML

Patients	Therapy	Dose. s.c. (mg/day)	Duration		Result		Survival time after SML diagnosis (months)
			Days	No. of courses	Type	Duration (months)	
P.A.	Supportive care	2.15	10	1	NC	3	4.6
	Ara-C after 91 days				NC	1.2	
W.A.	Supportive care				NC	2	22.4
	Ara-C after 68 days	2.15	10	3	PR	3.7	
	Ara-C after 205 days	2.10	8	2	PR	2	
S.F.	Supportive care				NC	2	6.3
	Ara-C after 64 days	2.15	10	3	NC	3.2	
W.H.	Supportive care				NC	23	23.9
S.P.[a]	Supportive care				NC	5.8	6.0
G.E.	Supportive care				NC	26	26.2
A.T.	Supportive care				NC	2.1	2.3
H.M.	Supportive care				NC	3.1	3.3
G.F.	Supportive care				NC	23	23.6
K.X.[a]	Supportive care				NC	23.1	24.4

NC, no change; PR, partial remission.
[a] After 6- and 24.4-months transition to AML.

TK level and blast count for AML patients were significantly increased in comparison to healthy individuals ($p < 0.01$).

At the time of diagnosis, none of the patients with SML showed clinical symptoms such as fever, night sweat, weight loss, hepato- and splenomegaly or lymphadenopathy. Only two patients with AML had no clinical symptoms. Comparison of the parameters TK, dTR, dUR, %S, myeloblasts, fever, night sweat, weight loss, hepato- and splenomegaly and lymphadenopathy by discriminant analysis in healthy individuals, AML patients and SML patients revealed a clear separation (100%) into these three groups under examination.

All SML patients had anaemia, 80% had thrombocytopenia, 40% leukocytopenia, 40% leukocytosis, and in 20% of the patients WBC counts were within the normal range. The AML patients exhibited no significant difference between these parameters.

Of the patients with SML 60% had a normocellular, 20% had a hypocellular and 20% a hypercellular bone marrow at the time of diagnosis. For

Table 3. TK, dTR, dUR, %S and blast count in BM of two SML patients at the time of diagnosis and at the time of transition to a rapidly proliferating acute leukaemia

Patients	TK (nmol/ min.10^{10} cells)	dTR (nmol/ min.10^{12} cells)	dUR (nmol/ min.10^{12} cells)	%S	Blast count in BM (%)
K.X. SML	7.0	10.0	18.4	4.5	58.0
AML	22.8	62.4	35.8	5.5	65.0
S.P. SML	7.4	27.3	21.5	3.5	62.0
AML	87.6	131.5	205.2	6.0	63.0

AML patients no significant difference was found. Results of the low-dose Ara-C treatment and supportive care of patients with SML are illustrated in Table 2.

The median survival time of the ten SML patients was determined by means of the Kaplan-Meier method and found to be 16 months. Four patients died from encephalorrhagia and four patients from sepsis. Two patients progressed to the rapidly proliferating form of AML. Biochemical-cytokinetic parameters and blast count in BM of two SML patients at the time of diagnosis and at the time of transition from SML to a rapidly proliferating AML are shown in Table 3. One of these patients died of encephalorrhagia in the aplastic phase after treatment, one was still living at the end of the period of investigation. This patient had been treated using the AML-6-protocol. (AML-6-protocol: day 1–3, daunorubicin 45 mg/m^2; day 2, vincristine 1 mg/m^2; day 1–7, Ara-C q 12 h 50 mg/m^2; and daily continuous infusion, 100 mg/m^2.)

Discussion

As described in the literature [8,12,13,16,22], the amount of myeloblasts in BM (10%–40%) together with a long survival time could be criteria for the definition of SML or for the characterization of progression to AML (>40% blasts in BM). Apart from the fact that this definition cannot be used as a clear differentiation between MDS and AML, in this analysis it could be shown that in SML the amount of myeloblasts in BM are meaningful only in so far as it is possible to use this value as an aid to diagnosis. The level of myoblasts in the bone marrow cannot, however, be used as a criterion for the assessment of progress to a rapidly proliferating form of AML. All SML patients exhibited the typical morphological criteria of AML (more than 30% blasts in BM) according to the French-American-British Group (FAB) classification [3]; thus SML is a particular variant of acute leukaemia.

The results of this investigation indicate that SML may be defined by low values of the biochemical-cytokinetic parameters TK, dTR, dUR and %S (Table 1) and by the absence of clinical symptoms such as fever, night sweat, weight loss, hepato- and splenomegaly or lymphadenopathy. Using this definition, it is possible to opt for supportive care only or to try low-dose Ara-C treatment.

An increase of TK activity above the normal range and a rise of dTR, dUR and %S from primarily low values during the course of the disease, however, are suitable criteria for diagnosis of a change from SML to AML. A consistent increase of TK above the normal range together with increasing dTR, dUR and %S values with time should be taken as indications for aggressive AML treatment, with due consideration for the clinical state of the patient.

In an AML study [11] a median survival time of 18.3 months was found for all 62 patients undergoing AML-specific treatment (AML-6) while the 47 patients with complete remission (CR) showed a median survival of 21.3 months. In our ten patients with SML the median survival time was 16 months, as determined by the Kaplan-Meier technique. Additionally, it should be emphasised that the median age of AML patients was 46 years, while that of SML patients was 58 years.

The MDS are defined according to Bennett et al. [2] and should be distinguished from SML as a variant of AML. The use of the above-mentioned terms for smouldering leukaemia is not recommended. In the literature this terminology always refers to a heterogenous group of patients (SML and MDS) or to a group of patients with MDS alone.

References

1. Barlogie B, Johnston DA, Keating M, Spitzer G, Hittelman WN, Nishioki K, Freireich EJ (1984) Evolution of oligoleukemia. Cancer 53:2115–2124
2. Bennett JM, Catovsky D, Flandrin G, Galton D, Gralnick H, Sultan C (1982) The French-American-British Co-operative Group. Proposals for the classification of the myelodysplastic syndromes. Br J Haematol 51:189–199
3. Bennett JM, Catovsky D, Daniel MT, Flandrin G, Galton DAG, Gralnick HR Sultan C (FAB Co-operative Group) (1976) Proposals for the classification of the acute leukaemias. Br J Haematol 33:451–458
4. Broun GO (1969) Chronic erythromonocytic leukemia. Am J Med 47:785–796
5. Dreyfus B (1976) Preleukemic states. Blood Cells 2:33–55
6. Fleischer W, Pelka R (1978) A practical analysis of DNA-histograms with a laboratory computer. Lutz D (ed) Pulse-Cytophotometry III. European Press, Ghent, p 137
7. Geary CG (1983) Clinical annotation. The diagnosis of preleukaemia. Br J Haematol 55:1–6
8. Greenberg PL (1983) The smouldering myeloid leukemic states: clinical and biologic features. Blood 61:1035–1044
9. Heimpel H, Drings P, Mitrou P, Queißer W (1979) Verlauf und prognostische Kriterien bei Patienten mit "Präleukämie". Klin Wochenschr 57:21–29
10. Howe RB, Bloomfield CD, McKenna RW (1982) Hypocellular acute leukemia. Am J Med 72:391–395
11. Jehn U, Knüppel W, Wilmanns W (1988) Intensive maintenance treatment in acute myelogenous leukemia (AML): single institution experience of a multicenter randomized trial. Onkologie 11:13–17

12. Joseph AS, Cinkotal KI, Hunt L, Geary CG (1982) Natural history of smouldering leukaemia. Br J Cancer 46:160–166
13. Knospe WH, Gregory SA (1971) Smouldering acute leukemia. Arch Intern Med 127:910–918
14. Koeffler HP, Golde DW (1980) Human preleukemia. Ann Intern Med 93:347–353
15. Linman JW, Bagby GC (1978) The preleukemic syndrome (Hemopoietic dysplasia). Cancer 42:854–864
16. Rheingold JJ, Kaufman R, Adelson E, Lear A (1963) Smouldering acute leukemia. N Engl J Med 268:812–815
17. Saarni MI, Linman JW (1973) Preleukemia; the hematologic syndrome preceding acute leukemia. Am J Med 55:38–48
18. Sanchez-Fayos J, Outeriño J, Calabuig T, Perez-saldaña R, Lite M, Figuera A, Perez-rus G (1984) Biological significance of nonlymphocytic oligoblastic leukemia. Acta Haematol 72:105–110
19. Sauer H, Wilmanns W (1977) Cobalmin dependent methionine synthesis and methyl-folate-trap in human vitamin B12 deficiency. Br J Haematol 36:189–198
20. Sauer H, Wilmanns W (1982) Thymidine kinase. ATP: thymidine 5'-phosphotrans-ferase, EC 2.7.1.21. Bergmeyer HU (ed) Methods of enzymatic analysis III. Verlag Chemie, Weinheim, p 468
21. Sauer H, Wilmanns W, Pelka-Fleischer R, Twardzik L, Vehling-Kaiser U, Jehn U (1987) DNA-metabolism in human bone marrow cells. Z antimikrob antineoplast Chemother 5:71–77
22. Slyck EJ Van, Rebuck JW, Waddell CC, Janakiraman N (1983) Smouldering acute granulocytic leukemia. Arch Intern Med 143:37–40
23. Weber RFA, Geraedts JPM, Kerkhofs H, Leeksma CHW (1980) The preleukemic syndrome; I. Clinical and hematological findings. Acta Med Scand 207:391–395
24. Zittoun R (1976) Annotation. Subacute and chronic myelomonocytic leukaemia: a distinct haematological entity. Br J Haematol 32:1–7

Dimethylsulfoxide and Retinoic Acid-Induced Differentiation and Commitment in HL-60 Cells*

P.A. Meyer,[1] C. Kleinschnitz, and F. Gieseler

Introduction

Leukemia can be viewed as a disorder of gene expression resulting in uncoupling of the control of cellular proliferation and differentiation. In this context, neoplastic cell lines which can be induced to terminal differentiation can be used to study the modification of this process, possibly providing new options for the treatment of leukemias.

Normal hematopoietic cell development is depicted as proceeding from a morphologically immature stem cell with unlimited self-renewal capacity to progenitor cells committed to a specific lineage with limited self-renewal capacity and terminally differentiated lineage-specific cells with restricted or no self-renewal capacity. The strategy of differentiation induction in tumors is based on the assumption that, by inducing differentiation, down-regulation and eventually loss of self-renewal capacity of the malignant clone is achievable.

The human myeloid leukemic cell line HL-60 [1] is a bipotential cell which can be differentiated by various agents either to the monocytic or granulocytic pathway [2]. Limited information is available on the question of how commitment to differentiation is achieved by induction of differentiation. Recent studies have addressed the question by separating early and late events of differentiation, which are not necessarily coupled [3–5], and by using clonal assays after exposing cells to dimethylsulfoxide (DMSO) and retinoic acid (RA) [6,7]. The present study takes a different experimental approach by using whole cell populations in liquid culture as differentiation targets. In addition to the nitroblue tetrazolium (NBT) assay, surface antigen expression of transferrin receptor (TfR) is used to monitor cellular differentiation.

Experimental Procedures

Cell Line and Culture Conditions. HL-60 cells were obtained from the American Tissue Culture Collection and routinely passaged at a density of

---

* Supported by the Deutsche Forschungsgemeinschaft (SFB 172, C3).
[1] Medizinische Poliklinik, Universität Würzburg, Klinikstraße 8, W-8700 Würzburg, FRG

Fleischer (Ed.) Leukemias
© Springer-Verlag Berlin Heidelberg 1993

2×10^5 cells/ml in RPMI 1640 (Seromed, FRG), 10% (v/v) preselected fetal calf serum (FCS; Gibco, FRG), 100 U/ml penicillin G (Seromed), and 100 mg/l streptomycin (Seromed) in a 5% CO_2 automatically controlled atmosphere. The doubling time of the cells in the present experiments was between 20 and 22 h.

Viability. The cell suspension was incubated with 0.1% trypan blue (Sigma, FRG) in 0.9% NaCl for 10 min. Trypan blue exclusion was determined by scoring 200 cells, using a light microscope.

NBT Assay. Using a commercially available NBT assay (Sigma), 0.1 ml cell suspension at a density of 10^6 cells/ml were mixed with 0.2 ml NBT solution and 0.1 ml stimulant and incubated for 25 min at 37°C. Subsequently, cytocentrifuge slides were prepared. NBT reduction to blue-black formazan (NBT-positive) after stimulation indicates oxidative bursts characteristic for mature granulocytic or monocytic cells. NBT-positive cells were determined by scoring 200 cells under a light microscope.

S phase Assignment. After 10^6 cells were washed in RPMI 1640, the pellet was resuspended in 0.6 ml staining solution (0.1% sodium citrate, 50 µg/ml propidium iodide, 0.1% Triton X-100, 0.05 mg/ml RNase) and incubated for 30 min at 37°C. Relative deoyribonucleic acid (DNA) content was determined by measuring propidium iodide fluorescence at 380 nm using a fluorescence-activated cell scanner (FACScan, Becton Dickinson, USA) and cells were assigned to S phase according to relative DNA content.

Experimental Design. HL-60 cells at a density of 2.5×10^5 cells/ml were incubated in liquid culture with $2 \times 10^{-6} M$ *cis*-RA for 12 h and 96 h or DMSO 1.1% v/v for 24 h and 96 h (incubation time). Controls were cultured without RA or DMSO. Cells were removed from the culture and assayed for viability, scored for NBT reduction, and assayed for TfR expression and DNA content. The remainder of the cells were washed 3 times in FCS-containing culture medium and reseeded in liquid culture at initial density without RA or DMSO. At 24, 48, 72, 96, and 120 h (reculture time), aliquots were removed from the cultures and cells assayed as described above. All experiments were done in triplicate; results are given as medians ($\pm$standard deviations).

Results

The present study, using HL-60 cells, addressed the question of commitment to differentiation after exposure to RA and DMSO. HL-60 cells in liquid culture were incubated with $2 \times 10^{-6} M$ RA or 1.1% v/v DMSO for 12, 24, and 96 h (incubation time) and subsequently recultured without RA or

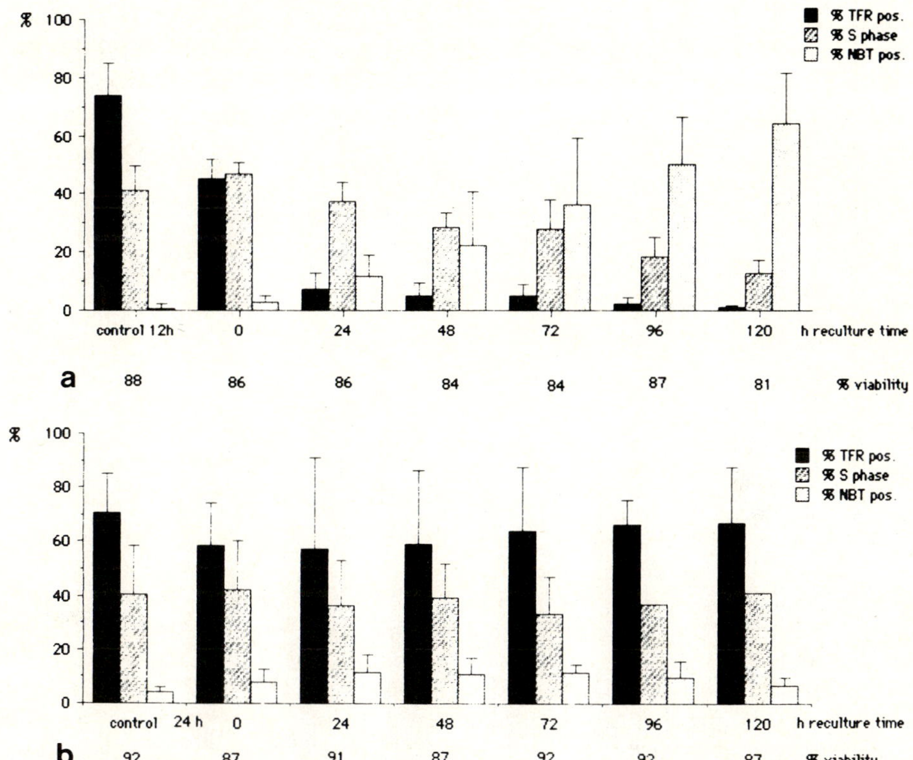

Fig. 1a, b. Kinetics of differentiation in HL-60 cells after **a** 12-h incubation with 2 × $10^{-6}M$ RA or **b** 24-h DMSO 1.1% v/v. Cells were assayed for NBT reduction, TfR expression, trypan blue exclusion, and number of S-phase cells after 24- to 120-h reculture time without RA or DMSO. Control 12 h denotes cells cultured for 12 h without RA or 24-h DMSO exposition. At 0 h cells were assayed directly after 12-h RA or 24-h DMSO incubation

DMSO then assayed for TfR expression, NBT reduction, and trypan blue exclusion at 24, 48, 96, and 120 h (reculture time).

Incubation of HL-60 Cells Without RA or DMSO (Controls). In control cultures 68%–74% of cells were TfR-positive, 41%–46% were in S phase, and 0%–0.8% were NBT-positive. Viability was 89%–91%. No difference in these parameters was apparent after different times (0–120 h) in liquid culture without RA or DMSO.

Reculture of HL-60 Cells After 12-h RA Incubation. Cells were incubated with RA for 12 h and recultured without RA for 24–120 h (Fig. 1a). Viability was 80%–88%. After 24-h reculture there was a slight increase in NBT-positive cells, and TfR-positive cells had decreased to 7% (6.0). With longer

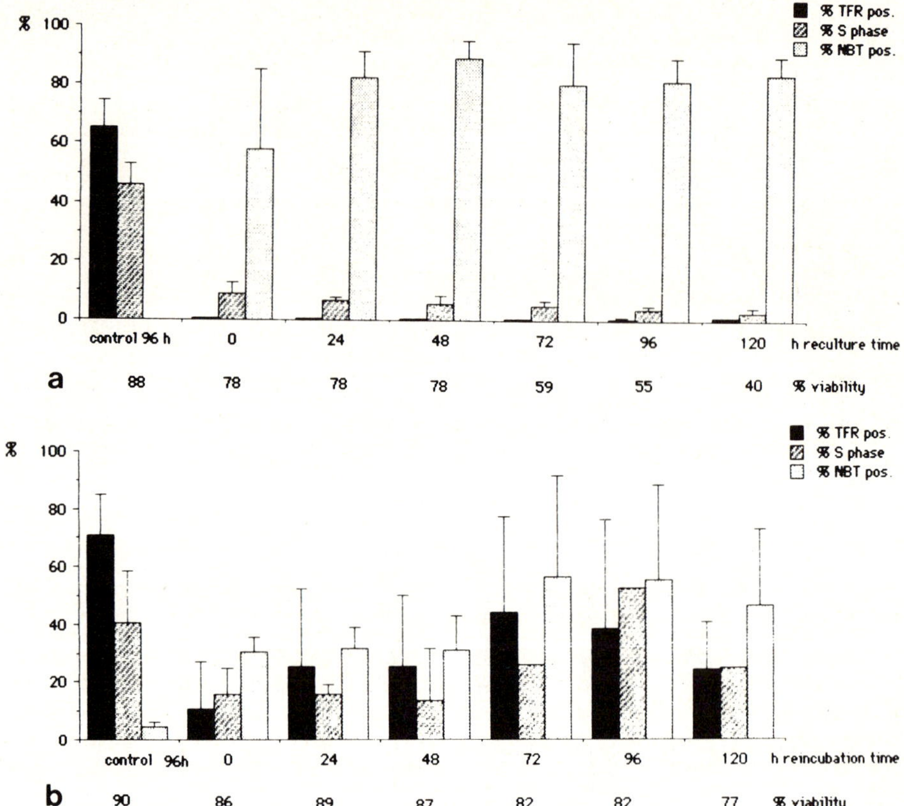

Fig. 2a, b. Kinetics of differentiation in HL-60 cells after **a** 96-h incubation with $2 \times 10^{-6} M$ RA or **b** 1.1% DMSO v/v. Cells were assayed for NBT reduction, TfR expression, trypan blue exclusion, and number of S-phase cells after 24- to 120-h reculture time without RA or DMSO. Control 96 h denotes cells cultured for 96 h without RA or DMSO exposition. At 0 h cells were assayed directly after 96-h RA or DMSO incubation

reculture time a progressive decrease of S phase cells to 12.75% (4.6) at 120 h and an increase of differentiated cells with 64.5% (12.2) NBT-positive cells was observed. Thus, after 12-h RA incubation and subsequent 96-h reculture, cells displayed a phenotype comparable to cells incubated for 96 h with RA. This suggests that after 12-h RA incubation HL-60 cells are committed to differentiation and continue to differentiate without RA in the culture medium, as did cells incubated for 96 h with RA.

Reculture of HL-60 Cells After 96-h RA Incubation. After 72-h reculture of HL-60 cells that had been incubated with RA for 96 h, viability had decreased significantly to 59.5% (21.9), and at 120 h viability had further decreased to 40.0% (17.0). The number of S phase cells remained low, between 6.5% (1.3) and 2.5% (1.7). NBT-positive cells remained virtually unchanged over the reculture time, between 81.3% and 88.7% (Fig. 2a).

Reculture of HL-60 Cells After 24-h DMSO Incubation. Cells were incubated with DMSO for 24 h and recultured without DMSO for 24–120 h (Fig. 1b). Viability was 87%–92%. TfR-positive cells were slightly decreased to 58%–59% at 0-h, 24-h, and 48-h reculture, but were not different from controls at 72-h, 96-h, and 120-h reculture time. NBT-positive cells and S-phase cells were not different from controls and baseline after 24-h DMSO incubation at 24-h, 48-h, 72-h, 96-h, and 120-h reculture without DMSO. There was no evidence for commitment to differentiation.

Reculture of HL-60 Cells After 96-h DMSO Incubation. After 96-h DMSO incubation NBT-positive cells increased to 31% (5) and had a further, although not significant, increase to 56% (35) at 72 h, 55% (33) at 96 h, and 46% (27) at 120-h reculture (Fig. 2b). S phase cells and TfR-positive cells were not different from baseline (0 h). Viability declined slightly from 90% (5) at 0 h to 77% (9) at 120-h reculture. There was no evidence for commitment to differentiation as the differentiated phenotype (NBT-positive cells) did not increase and proliferation markers (TfR-positive cells and S phase cells) did not decrease.

Discussion

The present study was done to address the question of commitment to differentiation of a whole population of cells after removing the inducer in a time-dependent manner. The experimental design also allowed for detection of regrowing of undifferentiated cells in a population for up to six generation times of the undifferentiated cells. The present study shows, as the first event of RA-induced differentiation, a decrease in TfR expression followed by a decrease in the number of S phase cells and later by phenotypic maturation to NBT reduction. Viability is not affected for up to 96-h RA incubation, suggesting that cell death does not occur to a significant degree during this time interval. With reculture after 12-h RA incubation the same series of events occurs. In addition, even after 120-h reculture, no regrowth of immature cells is detectable, as the number of S phase cells and TfR-positive cells remain very low suggesting "self-propelled" progression through the differentiation process. There is no evidence for regrowth of immature cells which could have escaped the effects of the inducer. Phenotypic differentiation seems to be determined after 12-h incubation with $2 \times 10^{-6} M$ RA: cells need an additional 96–120 h to proceed to terminal differentiation after termination of RA exposition. Incubation with DMSO for 24 h results in a decrease of TfR-positive cells, indicating downregulation of proliferation and no increase of the differentiated phenotype

(NBT-positive cells). At 96-h incubation NBT-positive cells increase as evidence for differentiation. Reculture after 24- and 96-h DMSO incubation does not result in further changes in the phenotype or proliferation markers, in contrast to results obtained with RA incubation. We were not able to show evidence for commitment to differentiation after DMSO incubation although DMSO-induced changes remained stable for up to 120-h reculture.

RA-mediated commitment to differentiation could be a result of altered gene transcription by RA. Alternatively, RA-mediated posttranscriptional effects or direct biochemical action of RA on cellular differentiation is possible. Commitment of HL-60 cells to terminal differentiation by DMSO and RA has been reported using the NBT assay and clonal growth in plasma clots after cells had been exposed to the respective inducer in liquid culture [7]. Evidence for commitment was that colonies became NBT-positive and contained fewer cells than control cultures. Data derived from sequential daughter cell transfer in semisolid medium, allowing determination of the fate of clones derived from one single cell [6], suggested that reversible losses of self-renewal capacity precede irreversible phenotypic differentiation. The limitation of the experimental approach in both cases is that it does not allow for detection of regrowth of relatively few cells in liquid culture after prolonged reculture without inducer. From both types of experiments it was concluded that commitment to differentiation occurred in HL-60 cells. Further analysis using semisolid cultures in the present experimental setting is necessary to determine the correlation of changes in clonal growth with the parameters reported here. If leukemic cells in vivo can be commited to differentiation with differentiation inducers, a novel therapeutic modality for the treatment of leukemias becomes available.

Acknowledgement. We gratefully acknowledge the excellent technical assistance of M. Haupt and B. Sommer.

References

1. Collins S, Gallo RC, Gallagher RE (1977) Continuous growth and differentiation of human myeloid leukemic cells in suspension culture. Nature 270:347–349
2. Collins SJ (1987) The HL-60 promyelocytic leukemia cell line: proliferation, differentiation, and cellular oncogene expression. Blood 70:1233–1244
3. Yen A, Forbes M, DeGala G, Fishbaugh J (1987) Control of HL-60 cell differentiation lineage specificity, a late event occurring after precommitment. Cancer Res 47:129–134
4. Yen A, Freeman L, Fishbaugh J (1987) Hydroyxyurea induces precommitment during retinoic acid induced HL-60 terminal myeloid differentiation: Possible involvement of gene amplification. Leuk Res 11:63–71
5. Yen A, Powers V, Fishbaugh J (1986) Retinoic acid induced HL-60 myeloid differentiations: dependence of early and late events on isomeric structure. Leuk Res 10:619–629

6. v Melchner H, Hoeffken K (1985) Commitment to differentiation of human promyelocytic leukemia cells (HL-60): an all-or-none event preceded by reversible losses of self-renewal potential. J Cell Physiol 125:3–12
7. Tsiftsoglou AS, Wong W, Hyman R, Minden M, Robinson SH (1985) Analysis of commitment of human leukemia HL-60 cells to terminal Cancer Res 45:2334–2339

Immunophenotyping of Adult Acute Leukemia by Immuno-Alkaline Phosphatase Labeling

J. OERTEL,[1] B. OERTEL, S. KLEINER, and D. HUHN

Introduction

The French-American-British (FAB) classification system has provided a popular classification for acute leukemias based on cell morphology and cytochemistry [1]. However, difficulties with some diagnostic criteria are evident. The major difficulties include distinguishing M1 from L2 in cases where peroxidase staining is negative [10]. Immunophenotyping using fluorescence microscopy or flow cytometry has emerged as an essential tool for the categorization of acute leukemias. A number of more recent papers have described the use of immunocytochemical labeling employing the alkaline phosphatase/anti-alkaline phosphatase (APAAP) method and light microscopy [4,6,9,16]. Immunocytochemistry has some advantages: simultaneous staining for immunoprofile and morphology, small sample quantity, enhanced sensitivity, long-term storage, and no expensive instrumentation. In this paper we describe the diagnostic value of the APAAP technique in 61 consecutive patients with acute leukemia.

Material and Methods

Blood and bone marrow samples were obtained from patients attending the Hematology Department of the Klinikum Rudolf-Virchow Charlottenburg Berlin or referred from other hospitals in Germany. 61 adult patients with acute leukemia diagnosed over the last 3 years were classified by the FAB classification using May–Grünwald–Giemsa-stained smears and cytochemical stains. Cases of chronic myeloid leukemia in blast crisis were not included in this study.

The cytochemical stains used included myeloperoxidase, α-naphthyl acetate esterase, and periodic acid–Schiff (PAS) according to standard methods. For immunocytochemical staining air-dried blood and bone marrow smears and cytocentrifuge preparations were fixed in acetone

[1] Hämatologische Abteilung im Klinikum Rudolf-Virchow-Charlottenburg der Freien Universität Berlin, W-1000 Berlin, FRG

Fleischer (Ed.) Leukemias
© Springer-Verlag Berlin Heidelberg 1993

Table 1. Antibodies used in this study

Antibody	CD number	Expression	Source
Leu 4	3	T cells	Becton Dickinson
Leu 9	7	T cells	Becton Dickinson
J5	10	C-ALL	Coulter
My 7	13	Granulocytes	Coulter
My 4	14	Monocytes	Coulter
B 4	19	B cells	Coulter
B 3	22	B cells	Coulter
My 9	33	Granulocytes	Coulter
HPCA 1	34	Blasts	Becton Dickinson
BMA 210	65	Granulocytes	Behringwerke Marburg
	61	Platelets	Immunotech
HTdT mix		ALL	Molecular Genetic Resources
Myeloperoxidase		Granulocytes	Dako
Anti-human light chain lambda		B cells	Immunotech
Anti-human light chain kappa		B cells	Immunotech
Anti-glycophorin A		Erythroblasts	Dako
Anti-human IgM		Pre-B cells	Dako

(10 min) and washed in Tris-buffered saline (TBS). It is possible to storage the preparations at −20°C for up to 24 months. Immunolabeling was performed according to the APAAP method [5]. We used a three-stage technique, as previously described [14]. The criterion for marker positivity was expression by at least 20% of blasts. The specific antibodies (obtained from commercial sources) used in this study are given in Table 1. Specificity controls included omission of primary antibody, and reactivity with normal blood cells was ascertained.

Results

61 patients with acute leukemia were analyzed. In 32 cases peroxidase activity was demonstrated cytochemically in more than 3% of blasts. Two patients with acute monocytic leukemia M5 were peroxidase negative and showed esterase positivity. These cases were classified as acute myeloid leukemias (AML). The diagnosis was accomplished using the standard FAB criteria of cell maturation. All patients expressed at least one of the myeloid markers CD13, CD33, and CD65. Table 2 illustrates the reactivity of the three antibodies with leukemic cells from these patients. The antibodies CD13 and CD33 were positive in 24/34 and 20/34 cases, respectively, while CD65 was positive in 14/34 cases. Six patients expressed only the marker CD65. We found coexpression of lymphoid markers CD19 in 6 AML cases CD7 in 7, CD3 in 3, CD10 in 2, and TdT in 11.

Table 2. Immunotyping of 61 acute leukemias using cytochemistry and immunocytological methods (APAAP technique)

I. *Cytochemical*: 32 peroxidase positive and 2 only esterase (diffuse) positive
    = 34 AML M1–M7
    Immunocytological (APAAP):
       10 CD13$^+$ CD33$^+$
        7 CD13$^+$
        6 CD65$^+$
        6 CD13$^+$ CD33$^+$ CD65$^+$
        3 CD33$^+$
        1 CD13$^+$ CD65$^+$
        1 CD33$^+$ CD65$^+$
II. *Cytochemical*: 27 peroxidase and esterase (diffuse) negative
    Immunocytological (APAAP):
        = 20 ALL
        8 TdT$^+$ CD19$^+$ CD10$^+$ (= c-ALL) including 3 pre-B-ALL with cytoplasmic
          μ chains
        4 TdT$^+$ CD19$^+$ CD10$^-$ (= O-ALL)
        4 TdT$^+$ CD3$^+$ CD7$^+$ (= T-ALL)
        4 TdT$^-$ CD19$^+$ Ig$^+$ (= B-ALL)
        = 7 AML-MO
        3 CD3$^+$
        2 CD65$^+$
        1 CD13$^+$ CD33$^+$
        1 CD33$^+$

---

27 patients had fewer than 3% peroxidase-positive blasts and were esterase (diffuse) negative. 16 of these cases were TdT positive, and 12 of these patients showed reactivity with CD19. Eight cases were diagnosed as common acute lymphatic leukemia (c-ALL) and four cases were of null-ALL phenotype (CD10$^-$). Four were of T-cell origin (CD3$^+$, CD7$^+$). We found four cases of B-ALL (TdT$^-$, CD19$^+$) showing immunoglobulins with restriction of kappa or lambda light chains. It is necessary to use cytocentrifuge preparates because it is not possible to investigate the immunoglobulins in blood or bone marrow smears. 14 of the 16 CD19-positive ALL cases showed cytoplasmic expression of CD22. Seven of the ALL cases expressed myeloid markers (3 CD13; 4 CD65; 1 CD14).

In seven cases, blasts did not show peroxidase or diffuse esterase activity and were negative with monoclonal antibodies used as lymphoid markers (TdT, CD19, CD22, CD3, CD7). These leukemias expressed myeloid antigens (CD13, CD33 or CD65) and were designated AML-MO [2].

Mixing of the antibodies CD13, CD33, and CD65 allowed detection of myeloid leukemias including AML-MO. All AML cases reacted with the mixture of these three antibodies. We did not find reactivity in ALL patients (excluding the cases with myeloid markers). Immunocytochemical analysis of myeloperoxidase using the APAAP technique demonstrated positivity with anti-myeloperoxidase in 38 of 41 AML patients (including AML-MO).

Four AML patients (= 10%) and one ALL patient (= 5%) had a biphenotypic leukemia according to the criteria of Catovsky et al. [3]. The score was between 2 and 3.

Discussion

Morphological classification of acute leukemia is based on criteria established by the FAB Cooperative Study Group [1]. Cytochemical studies include peroxidase and nonspecific esterase. Using immunoflourescence, 80% of the AML patients reacted with the myeloid antibodies CD13, CD33, or CD65 [7]. We used the APAAP method and found reactivity with one or more of these antibodies in all patients with peroxidase- or esterase-positive AML. Mixing of the three antibodies and staining of one blood or bone marrow preparation allowed detection of myeloid origin in all cases.

We found 21 AML cases with expression of myeloid antigens and TdT, CD19, and/or CD7. This is in agreement with results in the literature. Using several methods, a variable percentage of the AML cases showed TdT, CD19, and/or CD7 positivity [8,15]. However, a typical marker constellation of ALL was demonstrated only in biphenotypic cases.

AML-MO is a form af AML with minimal myeloid differentiation not included in the FAB classification. A diagnosis on morphological grounds alone is not possible [2]. The percentage of peroxidase-positive blasts using cytochemistry is less than 3%. The leukemic cells did not show reactivity with antibodies against specific lymphoid antigens (CD19, CD10, cytoplasmic CD3, or CD22). At least one of the myeloid markers CD13 or CD33 is positive. We found seven patients with AML-MO using the myeloid antibodies CD13, CD33, and CD65. The antibody CD65 is also able to demonstrate the myeloid origin of leukemic cells [12]. Two cases of AML-MO showed positivity only with this myeloid marker.

Cases of acute leukemia without morphological and cytochemical differentiation and without specific lymphatic markers were designated as acute undifferentiated leukemia. Most patients showed expression of CD34 and IA. However, these antigens are unspecific with expression on myeloid and lymphatic blasts. Our study of 61 patients with acute leukemia demonstrates that differentiation between myeloid and lymphatic leukemia was possible in all cases. This is in agreement with the study of Kaplan et al. [11]. These authors investigated 59 adult patients with acute leukemia and found 51 AML and 8 ALL. Neame et al. [13] analyzed 138 cases and were able to distinuish between AML, ALL, and mixed lineage in all cases. Further studies are necessary to confirm these results in a large number of patients with acute leukemia.

References

1. Bennett JM, Catovsky D, Daniel MT et al. (1976) Proposals for the classification of acute leukemias. Br J Haematol 33:451–458
2. Bennett JM, Catovsky D, Daniel MT et al. (1991) Proposals for the recognition of minimally differenciated acute myeloid leukemia (AML-MO). Br J Haematol 78:325–329
3. Catovsky D, Matutes E, Buccheri V et al. (1991) A classification of acute leukemia for the 1990s. Ann Hematol 62:16–21
4. Chen Z, Sigaux FS, Miglierina R et al. (1986) Immunological typing of acute lymphoblastic leukemia: concurrent analysis by cytofluorometry and immunocytology. Leukemia Res 10:1411–1417
5. Cordell JL, Falini B, Erber WN et al. (1984) Immunoenzymatic labeling of monoclonal antibodies using immuno complexes of alkaline phosphatase and monoclonal antialkaline phosphatase (APAAP) complexes. J Histochem Cytochem 32:219–229
6. Davey FR, Erber WN, Gatter KC et al. (1987) Immunophenotyping of acute myeloid leukemia by immuno-alkaline phophatase (APAAP) labeling with a panel of antibodies. Am J Hematol 26:157–166
7. Drexler HG (1987) Classification of acute myeloid leukemias – a comparison of FAB and immunophenotyping. Leukemia 1:697–705
8. Erber WM, Mason DY (1987) Immunoalkaline phosphatase labeling of terminal transferase in hematologic samples. Am J Clin Pathol 88:43–50
9. Hanson CA, Gajl-Peczalska KJ, Parkin JL et al. (1987) Immunophenotyping of acute myeloid leukemia using monoclonal antibodies and the alkaline phosphatase-antialkaline phosphatase technique. Blood 70:83–89
10. Head DR, Savage RA, Cereza I et al. (1988) Reproducibility of the French-American-British classification of acute leukemia. Am J Hematol 18:47–52
11. Kaplan SS, Penchansky L, Stolc V et al. (1989) Immunophenotyping in the classification of acute leukemia in adults. Cancer 63:1520–1527
12. Majdic O, Bettelheim P, Stockinger H et al. (1984) M2, a novel myelomonocytic cell surface antigen and its distribution on leukemia cells. Int J Cancer 33:617–623
13. Neame PB, Soamboonsrup P, Browman GP et al. (1986) Classifying acute leukemia by immunophenotyping: a combined FAB-immunologic classification of AML. Blood 68:1355–1362
14. Oertel J, Oertel B, Lobeck H et al. (1988) The value of immunocytochemical staining of lymph node aspirates in diagnostic cytology. Br J Haematol 70:307–316
15. Parreira A, Pompo de Oliveira S, Matutes E et al. (1988) Terminal deoxynucleotidyl transferase positive acute myeloid leukemia: an association with immature myeloblastic leukemia. Br J Haematol 69:219–224
16. Vago JF, Hurtubise PE, Martelo OJ et al. (1987) Immunohistochemical classification of acute leukemias using peripheral blood smears. Leukemia Res 11:475–480

Diagnostic and Prognostic Value of Immunological Leukemia Phenotyping

J. Hołowiecki,[1] B. Stella-Hołowiecka, D. Lutz, S. Krzemień,
V. Callea, M. Brugiatelli, V. Schranz, R. Ihle, G. Kelenyi, K. Jagoda,
G. Barceanu, and T. Ławniczek

Unique, monoclonal antibody (MoAb) defined cell differentiation antigens are increasingly accepted as markers for certain cell lines and for particular differentiation stages [1,2]. However, while we clearly do not know many answers, we do have some new questions dealing with clinical application of monoclonal antibodies. In this report we shall try to gather information on the following of these problems: (1) How MoAbs should be used; (2) the diagnostic utility of MoAb; and (3) evidence that some phenotypes may serve as novel prognostic indices, useful for the so-called risk-adopted strategy of therapy of acute leukemia (AL).

Previously, the most frequently used method of immunophenotyping was indirect fluorescence. During the last few years immunoenzymatic staining of hematological samples with MoAb has been introduced as an alternative. The most interesting one appears to be the alkaline phosphatase anti-alkaline-phosphatase (APAAP) immunoenzyme method. In our institution we compared, therefore, the results obtained with these two methods in 60 patients with de novo AL.

In brief, the most important advantages of the APAAP technique were the following: (1) the possibility of correlating the cytoimmunological reactions to morphology; (2) its use with normally prepared smears, even if only very few cells are available; and (3) the possibility of storage and reevaluation.

Nevertheless, we learned that the interpretation of the findings obtained using APAAP should be particular while this method not only detects the antigens existing in the membrane, as in immunofluorescence (IF) staining of cell suspensions, but also stains the antigens within the cytoplasm. This was demonstrated in our studies of the correlation between these two methods. We found that the results obtained with IF and APAAP displayed a good correlation only with antigens present in the cell membrane, whereas those antigens which are expressed for the most part or, also, within the cytoplasm, show a distinctly higher positivity with the APAAP technique

---

[1] International Society for Chemo-Immunotherapy Cooperative Group (IGCI) – Vienna, Austria; Katowice, Poland; Reggio Calabria, Italy; Budapest, Hungary; Berlin, FRG; Pecs, Hungary; Bucharest, Romania

Fleischer (Ed.) Leukemias
© Springer-Verlag Berlin Heidelberg 1993

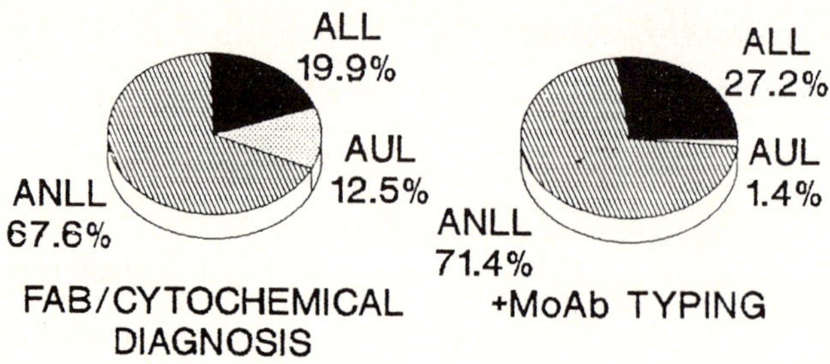

Fig. 1. Morphocytochemical (FAB) classification versus monoclonal antibody immuno-phenotyping – results based on analysis of 830 untreated adult acute leukemia patients. (*AUL*, acute undifferentiated leukemia)

(such as Ia, CD3, CD22). The correlation for some of the most important antigens will be presented later.

In order to define the value of MoAb phenotyping of leukemia we organized a cooperative study, which was entered by 1054 untreated patients with AL. All patients were subclassified according to French-American-British Group (FAB) criteria and immunophenotyped by means of 6–21 MoAb (mainly delivered by W. Knapp, Vienna, Austria) [2]. Then the laboratory data and the clinicial follow-up were analyzed using specially prepared computer programs and the BMDP statistics package.

To prove the usefulness of MoAb for making exact diagnosis of leukemia, we compared, in 830 cases, morphocytochemical diagnosis with immunophenotype. We found that the immunophenotyping reduced the proportion of unclassifiable cases from 12.5% after morphocytochemical evaluation up to 1.4%. It means that 98.6% of acute leukemia cases can be properly subclassified if the FAB diagnosis is combined with immuno-phenotyping with a panel of 8–10 MoAb (Fig. 1).

A question arises regarding the composition of a minimal panel of MoAb which could be accepted for clinical use. A series of comparative analyses helped us to select reagents necessary for differentiation between acute lymphoblastic leukemia (ALL) and acute myeloid leukemia (AML) as well as those important for further subclassification (Table 1).

In our experience the best screening marker for granulomonocytic line-derived acute leukemia is the VIM-2 MoAb which detects the CDw65 antigen. In turn, for identification of M5 and M4, the CD14 and, to a lesser extent, CD11b antigen were revealed to play a decisive part.

Seeing that most of the groups use, for screening of AML, a combina-tion of two antibodies detecting CD13 and CD33 antigens [3], we per-formed, in 125 patients treated in Vienna and Katowice, a comparative study of CDw65 versus CD13 and/or CD33.

Confronting the results obtained with each of these reagents separately, we found the CDw65 antigen to give the highest rate of positive results in

Table 1. Proposal for a diagnostic panel for acute leukemia (IGCI Study Group 1982–90)

Subtype	First set			Second set
	Screening		Classification	
AUL	Ia, CD34			
AML	Peroxidose, Sudan B	FAB M4, M5	– CD14, ANAE	CD15 prognosis
	CDw65 or	FAB M6	– Clyc. A, Gero.	CD38 prognosis?
	CD13 + CD33	FAB M7	– CD41	CD11b
ALL		B line	– cCD22/CD19/CD24	CD20
	Tdt		CD10, cytμ, SmIg,	CD21
	PAS	T line	– cCD3/CD7, CD2/Erec.	CD5, CD1
			CD4, CD8	

the group, equaling 90.4%. Using two or all three reagents the positivity rate could be only slightly improved: CD65 plus CD33 gave 94.4% and the triple combination CD65+33+13 gave up to 96% of positive results. These trials proved, therefore, CDw65 to be the most reliable marker of the granulomonocytic line, as effective as the combination of two markers, CD33 and CD13, which were most frequently used up to now [5]. In a separate study we confirmed that VIM-2, detecting the CDw65 antigen, can be used both with the IF and APAAP methods because the results obtained using these two methods displayed a significant correlation.

Regarding markers for the lymphoid lines, there are differences depending upon the method of staining. Some determinants such as Ia, CD3, and CD22 could be more strongly demonstrated using the APAAP technique rather than IF, because these determinants are expressed at first in cytoplasm. Thus, if the APAAP method is being used, a screening marker for T cells can be cCD3 and for B cells cCD22. If, however, the IF techniques are employed, the relevant markers are CD7 for T cell line- and CD19 for B cell line-derived malignancies. It should, however, be kept in mind that these two determinants have been recently found, also, in some patients on AML blasts.

Finally, we propose the following composition of markers for screening and, further, also for accurate subclassification of acute leukemias: (1) CDw65 or CD13 plus CD33 as a screening marker for granulomonocytic line; (2) CD14 as an indicator of the monocytic line; (3) glycophorin A for erythroid line; (4) CD41 for megakaryocytic line; (5) cCD3 or CD7 for T cell line; (6) cCD22, CD19, and, possibly, CD24 for B cell line. Additionally, second line reagents are occasionally helpful for more accurate diagnosis.

Prognostic significance of immunophenotypization became increasingly interesting since the so-called risk-adopted strategies were introduced into the therapy of AL.

Table 2. Expression of antigens and patient outcome in 424 de novo adult ANLL patients (age 16–82 years)

Antigen CD (+/−)		CR (%)	(n)	Survival Median Days	(n)	1-year	2-year	Disease-free survival Median Days	(n)	1-year	2-year
Ia	+	47	221	203	60	0.26	0.08	296	97	0.4	0.23
								$p < 0.01$			
	−	47	152	216	237	0.29	0.16	415	63	0.56	0.33
CD38	+	51	92	229	101	0.29	0.16	252	45	0.31	0.18
								$p < 0.01$			
	−	41	179	206	181	0.28	0.14	415	70	0.55	0.32
Trf rec.	+	41	52	203	60	0.26	0.08	184	21	0.28	0.08
								$p < 0.01$			
	−	48	227	216	237	0.29	0.16	365	100	0.49	0.32
CD15	+	50	282	200	302	0.37	0.14	365	136	0.49	0.28
		$p < 0.01$		$p < 0.01$							
	−	36	242	103	157	0.26	0.14	352	41	0.46	0.33
CDW65	+	46	309	241	334	0.4	0.23	344	132	0.45	0.29
	−	38	40	253	47	0.4	0.23	485	14	0.79	0.34
11	+	43	155	237	153	0.35	0.23	323	61	0.46	0.3
	−	47	179	255	201	0.37	0.23	415	78	0.54	0.3
CD14	+	52	61	242	66	0.3	0.23	344	29	0.41	0.32
	−	45	121	246	204	0.3	0.23	415	75	0.56	0.34
Glyc. A	+	31	10	161	12	0.18	0.05	443	3	0.1	0
	−	45	282	217	303	0.32	0.24	385	116	0.51	0.33

+, >15% positive blasts
Tests statistics: X^2, Wilcoxon-Breslow, Mantel-Cox
Trf rec., transferrin receptor; Glyc. A, glycophorin A

Some 3 years age we published a first paper [4] indicating that CD15 expression on ANLL blasts has positive prognostic significance for achieving complete remission (CR) and our results have been confirmed recently by L. Campos et al. [1].

At present we are able to confirm these observation in 456 newly diagnosed acute nonlymphoblastic leukemia (ANLL), using the mutli-variate logistic regression method (Table 2). The first analysis demonstrated that CD15 expression has a significance independent from other MoAbs and the following one proved that it is also independent of other important factors such as age, WBC, and the proportion of blasts.

A longer follow-up of 456 patients indicates that not only the CR rate but also the product limit survival is better in patients with CD15 positivity than in CD15-negative cases. The median survival of the CD15-positive group is about twice as high as in the CD15-negative cohort, and the differences between curves are highly significant, as shown by Wilcoxon and Mantel Cox tests. Using the multivariate analysis according to Cox, we confirmed that the CD15 expression has an independent predictive value for survival but not for the disease-free survival (DFS). These findings seem to confirm our preliminary hypotheses, i.e., that CD15 expression reflects at least to some degree the maturity of leukemic cells, and its impact on CR and survival could be dependent upon worse functional capacity of the granulocytic cells.

Apart from CD15 we found also some interrelationships between the CD11, CD14, and CD65 expression and survival, but the results were either insignificant or age dependent.

Recently we demonstrated that the expression of CD38, Ia, and of transferrin receptor displays a negative correlation to DFS. A further multivariate analysis employing the Cox model proved, however, that out of these three antigens only CD38 is independent as a prognostic index predicative for a shorter DFS in patients with a higher expression of these markers.

In ALL the common acute lymphoblastic leukemia antigen expression was found to be a positive prognostic index for DFS, but this topic will be presented separately [6].

Our trial allows us to draw the following conclusions: (1) The proposed panel of first line MoAb allows a classification of over 98% of cases; (2) the expression of CD15 on ANLL blasts offers a new independent factor displaying a positive correlation to CR rate and sruvival; (3) in contrast, the expression of CD38 appears to be an independent index predicting a shorter DFS.

References

1. Campos L, Guyotat D, Archimbaud E, Devaux Y, Treille D, Larese A, Maupes I, Gentilhomme O, Ehrsam A, Fiere D (1989) Surface marker expression in adult AML: correlations with initial characteristics, morphology and response to therapy. Br J Haematol 72:161–166
2. Knapp W, Majdic O, Stockinger H, Bettelheim P, Liszka K, Köller V, Peschel C (1984) Monoclonal antibodies to human myelomonocyte differentiation antigens in the diagnosis of AML. Med Oncol Tumor Pharmacother 1:257–262
3. Pombo de Oliveira MS, Matutes E, Rani S, Morille R, Catovsky D (1988) Early expression of MCS2 (CD13) in the cytoplasm of blast cells from AML. Acta Haematol 80:61–64
4. Hołowiecki J, Lutz D, Krzemień S, Stella-Hołowiecka B, Graf F, Kelenyi G, Schranz V, Callea V, Brugiatelli M, Neri A, Magyarlaki T, Ihle R, Jagoda K, Rudzka E (1986) CD15 Antigen detected by the VIM-D5 monoclonal antibody for prediction of ability to achieve complete remission in ANLL. Acta Haematol 76:16–19
5. Hołowiecki J, Lutz D, Callea V, Brugiatelli M, Kelenyi F, Stella-Hołowiecka B, Krzemień S, and Jagoda K (1992) Myelomonocyte differentiation antigens in the diagnosis of acute nonlymphocyte leukemia. Jn: Hiddemann W. et al. Acute leukemias. Springer, Berlin Heidelberg New York (Haematology and Blood Transfusion) 34: 222–227

6. Hołowiecki J, Koehler M, Zintl Z, Kardos G, Lutz D, Krzemień S, Rewesz T, Brugiatelli M, Callea V, Kachel Ł, Jagoda K, Stella-Hołowiecka B, Zgagacz A (1992) Childhood acute lymphoblastic Leukemia immunophenotypes and their prognostic significance: Experience of the IGCI-Study in 389 children. Leukemia and Lymphoma 7:225–234

Immunoelectron Microscopy of Megakaryoblasts in Megakaryoblastic Transformation of Chronic Granulocytic Leukemia

A. Matolcsy,[1] V. Kalász, and O. Majdic

Problems

The cells undergoing blastic transformation of chronic granulocytic leukaemia (CGL) are considered to be of pluripotent stem cell origin [1,4]. As in acute haemoblastosis, several types of blasts may be identified by cytochemical methods [10]. In the blastic transformation of CGL, myeloblasts are predominant in about 60% and lymphoblasts in 20% of cases. The lymphoblastic and other uncommon types of transformation cannot be identified by cytochemical methods alone [12]. In the diagnosis of megakaryoblastic transformation the electron-microscopic platelet-peroxidase reaction (PPO) and antibodies against platelet glycoproteins and against factor VIII antigens may be of help. Owing to these methods the number of cases with megakaryoblastic proliferation has increased substantially in the past few years [2,6,11]. According to San Miguel et al. (1985), the frequency of megakaryoblastic transformation within the poorly differentiated types of blastic transformation of CGL exceeds 30% [9]. Electron-microscopic study of the binding of monoclonal antibodies against platelet glycoproteins makes it possible to analyse simultaneously the ultrastructural features and the immunophenotype of megakaryoblasts.

Using monoclonal antibodies to platelet glycoproteins, megakaryoblasts in the blastic transformation of CGL in five patients have been examined by electron microscopy.

Materials and Methods

Patients. Five patients with megakaryoblastic transformation of CGL were studied.

Antibodies. The VI-PL2 monoclonal antibody against platelet glycoprotein IIIa (GpIIIa) employed in this study was provided by Prof. Dr. W. Knapp of the Institute of Immunology, University of Vienna, Austria.

---

[1] Department of Pathology, University Medical School of Pécs, Pécs, Hungary

Fleischer (Ed.) Leukemias
© Springer-Verlag Berlin Heidelberg 1993

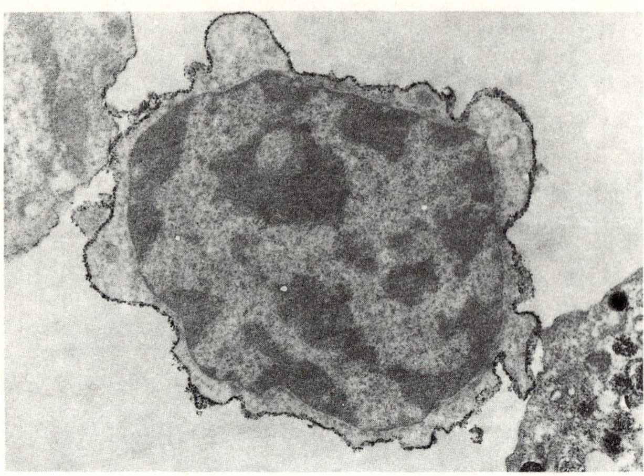

Fig. 1. Immature "lymphocyte-like" megakaryoblast (cell type 1) illustrating the presence of GpIIIa (VI-PL2) on the cell surface. This lymphocyte-like cell lacks the morphological features of megakaryoblastic differentiation. Without uranyl acetate and lead citrate, ×20 000

Electron-Microscopic Immunocytochemistry. Washed mononuclear cells (5×10^6 cells) were fixed for 5 min in $1.0 M$ phosphate buffer (PBS), pH 7.2, containing 1.0% glutaraldehyde (Manara et al. [7]). The fixed cells were washed three times in PBS, pH 7.2, and treated for 1 h at 4°C with 100 µl of monoclonal antibodies diluted 1:10 with PBS. After three washes in PBS the cells were incubated for 1 h with 100 µl peroxidase-conjugated goat antimouse Ig (DAKO) diluted 1:50 with PBS. After three washes with the same buffer, the cells were fixed in PBS containing 1.0% glutaraldehyde. After a further washing in PBS, peroxidase activity was revealed in 2 mg/ml DAB medium (Graham and Karnovsky [5]). The cells were then postfixed in osmium tetroxide, dehydrated and embedded in Epon. Ultrathin sections were examined in a Jeol 100 electron microscope.

Results

Light Microscopy. In the blood smears of all five patients the cytological findings were indicative of blastic transformation. The percentage of blasts ranged between 20% and 44%. The blast cells showed different morphological features: some showed a relatively wide basophilic cytoplasm with several ear-shaped protrusions, and some blasts were like small lymphocytes, i.e., small round cells with narrow basophilic cytoplasm.

Electron Microscopy. Megakaryoblasts incubated with antiplatelet glycoprotein antibodies exhibited a distinct linear electron-dense reaction at the cell surface membranes (Figs. 1–3).

On the basis of their ultrastructural features and immunophenotype, three types of megakaryoblasts were distinguished. Cell type 1 is 10–12 µm in diameter and reminiscent of small lymphocytes with a narrow cytoplasm poor in organelles. Only few mitochondria are present. The nuclear to cytoplasmic ratio is high in these cells, and the small amount of heterochromatin lies near to the nuclear membrane. The nucleolus is prominent. This type of cell was identified by cell surface GpIIIa positivity (Fig. 1).

Cell type 2 has the size of a myelocyte, its cytoplasm is wider and the cell surface uneven (Fig. 2). Cytoplasmic organelles are scattered along the nuclear membrane and separated by the membrane structures from other compartments of the cytoplasm which is poor in organelles (Fig. 2 inset). VI-PL2 antibody is bound on the cell surface and is also present in a cytoplasmic membrane system which resembles the demarcation membrane system (Fig. 2 inset). These are paired membranes localized outside the perinuclear cisternae around the nucleus.

On the surface of cell type 3, round cytoplasmic fragments "butt off" (Fig. 3). They are demarcated from the cytoplasm by the membranes. The alpha-granules and vacuoles characteristic of megakaryocytes are situated around the nuclear membrane. Polysomes are scattered in deep indentations of the nuclear membrane. The heterochromatin is adjacent to the nuclear membrane and the nucleolus is prominent.

Discussion

The increase in the incidence of megakaryoblastic leukaemia or megakaryoblastic transformation of chronic myeloproliferative diseases can be attributed to the advent of new histochemical and immunological methods [3,8,11]. Based on their light-microscopic features, these cells may be suspected to be of megakaryoblastic origin (wide basophilic agranular cytoplasm, peculiar protrusion of the cytoplasm, vacuolisation [12]). The megakaryoblastic origin can be proved by immunocytological demonstration of platelet glycoproteins on the surface of the blasts and by the PPO reaction [11]. The cells stained by the two procedures are not identical [9]. The differences between them may be attributed to the various degrees of maturation of the megakaryoblasts even in blastic transformation [12].

Based on their differing ultrastructural features, reflecting maturation stages, we recognized three types of megakaryoblasts. At the earliest stage of maturation (narrow cytoplasmic rim, few cellular organelles), the origin of the cell can be determined on the basis of positivity of GpIIIa antigen at the cell surface membrane. These "lymphoid-like" cells have been shown to express only GpIIIa (VI-PL2). These findings support the ideas that GpIIIa is the most sensitive marker for the identification of these precursors [13].

In the course of further maturation, specific organelles (alpha-granules, demarcation membranes) appear in the cytoplasm and eventually cells more or less resembling mature megakaryocytes can also be seen. In a few cells

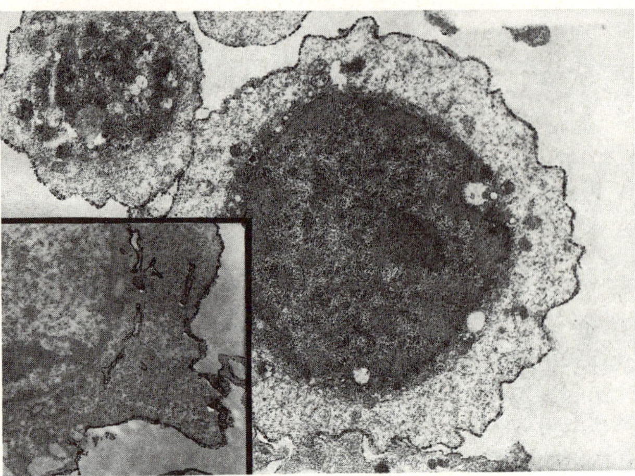

Fig. 2. Megakaryoblast, cell type 2, stained with VI-PL2, showing organelle-free peripheral cytoplasm, central clustering of the organelles. Reaction product is present on the cell surface membrane as well as in the demarcation membrane system (*inset*). Without uranyl acetate and lead citrate, ×19 200

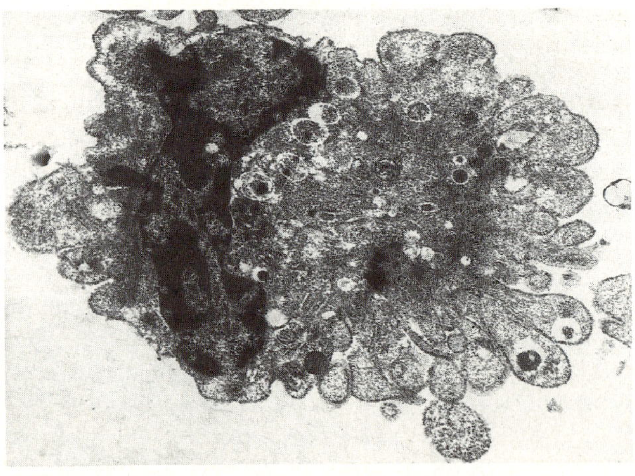

Fig. 3. Megakaryoblast of type 3 has irregular cell surface with pseudopodia, composed of organelle-free cytoplasm. The alpha-granules and vacuoles are situated around the nuclear membrane. Monoclonal antibody to the GpIIIa complex (VI-PL2) is bound on the cell surface. Uranyl acetate and lead citrate, ×10 000

localization of the antigen in the demarcation membrane system was seen in the whole course of megakaryoblastic maturation.

On the basis of the ultrastructure and immunophenotype of mega-karyoblasts we observed that in the five patients the degree of differentiation of the leukemic cells varied from patients to patient. Thus, the three cell types of megakaryoblastic maturation were present in all of the five patients, but in variable numbers. In two patients, the immature cell types, in one the intermediate forms (cell type 2) and in one the relatively mature megakaryoblasts, predominated. Investigation of larger groups of patients would enable the different types of megakaryoblastic leukemias to be distinguished.

References

1. Barton JC, Conrad ME (1978) Current status of blastic transformation in chronic myelogenous leukemia. Am J Hematol 4:281–291
2. Breton-Gorius J, Reyes F, Vernant JP, Tulliez M, Dreyfus B (1978) The blastic crisis of chronic granulocytic leukaemia: megakaryoblastic nature of cell as revealed by the presence of platelet-peroxidase (A cytochemical ultrastructural study). Br J Haematol 39:295–303
3. Breton-Gorius J, Vainchenker W (1986) Immunological and cytochemical characterisation of megakaryocytic lineage leukaemia. In: Levine RF, Williams N, Levin J (eds) Megakaryocyte development and function. Liss, New York, pp 301–317
4. Fialkow PJ, Jacobson RJ, Papayannopoulou T (1977) Chronic myelocytic leukemia of clonal origin in a stem cell common to the granulocyte, erythrocyte, platelet and monocyte/macrophage. Am J Med 63:125–129
5. Graham RC, Karnovsky MJ (1966) The early stages of absorption of injected horseradish peroxidase in the proximal tubules of mouse kidney. Ultrastructural cytochemistry by a new technique. J Histochem Cytochem 14:291–302
6. Koike T (1984) Megakaryoblastic leukaemia: characterisation and identification of megakaryoblasts. Blood 64:683–692
7. Manara GC, Panfilis G, Ferrari G (1985) Ultrastructural characterisation of human large granular lymphocyte subsets defined by the expression of HNK-1 (Leu-1), Leu-11 or both HNK-1 and Leu-11 antigens. J Histochem Cytochem 33:1129–1133
8. Polli N, O'Brien M, Tavares de Castro J, Matutes E, San Miguel JF, Catowsky D (1985) Characterisation of blast cells in chronic granulocytic leukaemia in transformation, acute myelofibrosis and undifferentiated leukaemia. I. Ultrastructural morphology and cytochemistry. Br J Haematol 59:277–296
9. San Miguel JF, Tavares de Castro J, Matutes E, Rodrigues B, Polli N, Zola H, McMichael AJ, Bollum FJ, Thompson DS, Goldman JM, Catovsky D (1985) Characterisation of blast cells in chronic granulocytic leukaemia in transformation, acute myelofibrosis and undifferentiated leukaemia II. Studies with monoclonal antibodies and terminal transferase. Br J Haematol 59:297–309
10. Shaw MT (1982) Clinical and haematological manifestation of terminal phase. Chronic granulocytic leukemia. Praeger, East Sussex, pp 168–188
11. Tabilio A, Vainchenker W, Van Haeke D, Guichard J, Henry A, Reyes F, Breton-Gorius J (1984) Immunolgoical characterisation of the leukemic megakaryocytic line at light and electron microscopic levels. Leuk Res 8:769–781
12. Velez-Gracia E, Fradera J, Telmont ML, White JG (1985) Megakaryoblastic transformation of Ph positive chronic granulocytic leukaemia. Am J Clin Pathol 84:228–233
13. Vinci G, Tabilio A, Deschamps JF (1984) Immunological study of in vitro maturation of human megakaryocytes. Br J Haematol 56:589–605

Thymidine Kinase in Leukemic Cells: Significance for Characterization and Follow-Up of Acute Leukemia

W. Wilmanns,[1] H. Sauer, R. Pelka-Fleischer, and V. Nüßler

The enzyme thymidine kinase (TK) catalyzes the magnesium ions (Mg^{2+}) and adenosine triphosphate (ATP) dependent phosphorylation of thymidine (dTR) to thymidine monophosphate (dTMP) [10]:

$$dTR + ATP \xrightarrow[\text{TK}]{Mg^{2+}} dTMP + ADP \text{ (adenosine diphosphate).}$$

TK is a key enzyme of DNA synthesis. Its activity can be demonstrated in numerous rapidly proliferating cell populations and tissues [2–7,10–12]. Investigations we had carried out on cultured human cells from lymphoblastic leukemia (LS-2), which had been separated according to cell cycle phases, showed that TK is an S- and G_2 plus M-specific enzyme [8].

As early as 1967, we demonstrated TK activity in leukemic blood and bone marrow cells and we had characterized this enzyme according to its kinetic properties [15].

During the following years, these investigations were extended by the determinations of the incorporation of deoxyuridine (dUR), which is utilized in the thymidylate synthase reaction to synthesize dTMP de novo and of dTR, the substrate of TK in the salvage pathway [13,15]. By means of a simultaneous determining of the incorporation rates of these nucleosides and the activities of the involved enzymes it was possible to characterize leukemic cell populations according to their DNA metabolism and to test their sensitivity against distinct antileukemic drugs – primarily antimetabolites [14,16,17]. This was possible by carrying out the described investigations with leukemic cells from bone marrow and/or from peripheral blood in short time intervals after a single injection of the drug [11].

As a result of the development of new therapeutic strategies almost all intensive-treated patients reach an aplastic phase and the complete remissions rate has increased considerably. Under these conditions the importance of such investigations of the DNA metabolism for the follow-up of acute leukemias during and after intensive polychemotherapy – especially

[1] Medizinische Klinik III, Klinikum Grosshadern, Ludwig-Maximilians-Universität, W-8000 München 70, FRG

Fleischer (Ed.) Leukemias
© Springer-Verlag Berlin Heidelberg 1993

Table 1. Thymidine kinase activity in leukemic and nonleukemic bone marrow cells

Cell population	n	TK (nmol/min . 10^{10} cells)		Sensitivity (%) >$\bar{X}$+ 2s (>29.8)
		$\bar{X}\pm s$	Range	
AL	119	64.5 ± 47.4	5.2–259.6	78
First diagnosis	85	64.9 ± 50.4	5.3–259.6	80
Relapse	34	63.6 ± 38.9	5.2–145.2	74
diagnosis	91	64.7 ± 47.4	5.2–259.6	78
ANLL	28	63.8 ± 48.1	7.6–211.5	79
ALL/AUL				
AL in CR	164	21.2 ± 19.4	1.9–114.0	–
Controls	28	14.6 ± 7.6	2.8–34.4	–

in view of the aspect of diagnosing an early relapse – had to be examined again. The activity of TK in the cytosol of bone marrow cells and of leukemic cells of the peripheral blood was correlated with the incorporation rates of [^{3}H]dTR and [^{3}H]dUR into the DNA of intact cells and with the percentage of proliferating cells in the S phase of the cell cycle (%S).

Methods. The procedure was carried out in accordance with TK assay (see also in Sauer and Wilmanns [10]), [^{3}H]dTR, [^{3}H]dUR (in Sauer and Wilmanns [9]) and %S (in Fleischer and Pelka [1]).

Results and Discussion

TK in Leukemic and Nonleukemic Bone Marrow Cells

A total of 283 bone marrow specimens from patients with acute leukemia were assayed for their TK activity in the cytosol of isolated cells and the results were compared with 28 controls (14.6 ± 7.6 nmol/min . 10^{10} cells) (Table 1).

In about 80% of the leukemic bone marrow populations TK was increased by a factor of 4–5. These TK activities were similar at primary diagnosis (64.9 ± 50.4), at relapse (63.6 ± 38.9), in acute nonlymphoblastic leukemia (64.7 ± 47.4) and in acute lymphoblastic leukemia (63.8 ± 48.1). One hundred sixty-four specimens from patients in complete remission did not differ statistically from normal controls. Accordingly, an increased TK activity characterizes the respective leukemic cell population.

Few of the patients with acute leukemia were characterized by significantly reduced cytosolic TK activity, dTR incorporation and dUR incorporation into DNA as well as reduced amounts of DNA-synthesizing S phase cells (%S) in the bone marrow, compared with healthy individuals.

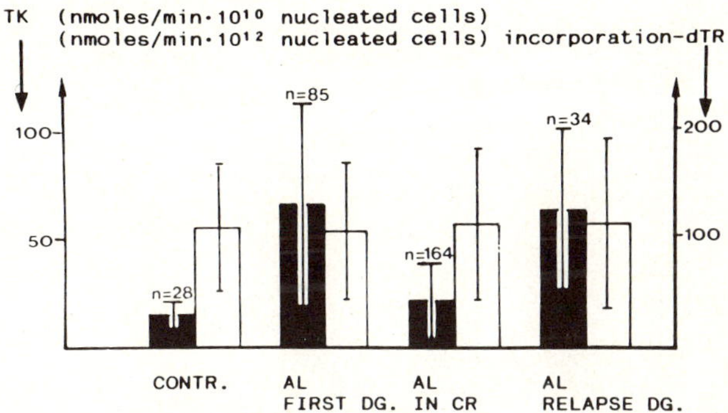

Fig. 1. Comparison of TK activity and incorporation of dTR into DNA of bone marrow cells of patients with acute leukemia: at first diagnosis (*AL first DG.*), in remission (*AL in CR*), and at relapse (*AL relapse DG.*). ■, TK activity; □, dTR incorporation; *CONTR.*, controls

This is so-called smoldering leukemia (SML). None of the patients showed clinical symptoms such as fever, night sweat, weight loss, hepato- and splenomegaly or lymphadenopathy at initial diagnosis. For characterization of SML we recommend the use of biochemical-cytokinetic parameters such as TK, dTR, dUR, and %S, together with the observed absence of the above-mentioned clinical symptoms. The definition and diagnosis of this form of *acute leukemia* is important, because these patients should not be treated by aggressive chemotherapy.

Comparison of TK With Other Proliferation Parameters

There is no correlation between TK and the number of blasts, the amount of proliferating cells, in the bone marrow. However, there is a significant correlation within the leukemic cell populations between TK, dTR, and dUR incorporation, the %S, and of S plus G_2M phase cells ($p > 0.01$).

These results raise the question of whether TK activity represents only a parameter for cell proliferation or it is an individual characteristic of acute leukemic cell populations comparable with a "tumor marker."

This question can be answered by comparing the different parameters in leukemic cell populations with normal controls and with bone marrow specimens during complete remission. In contrast to TK there was no significant difference between dTR and dUR incorporation rates and of %S in these cell populations. In Fig. 1 this is shown for the dTR incorporation.

Normal cell populations with equal high dTR incorporation rates (or dUR incorporation rates or %S cells) have a low specific TK activity. On the contrary, in leukemic cell populations this specific TK activity is significantly increased in comparison with these proliferation parameters. Thus, TK can be considered as a tumor marker for acute leukemias independent

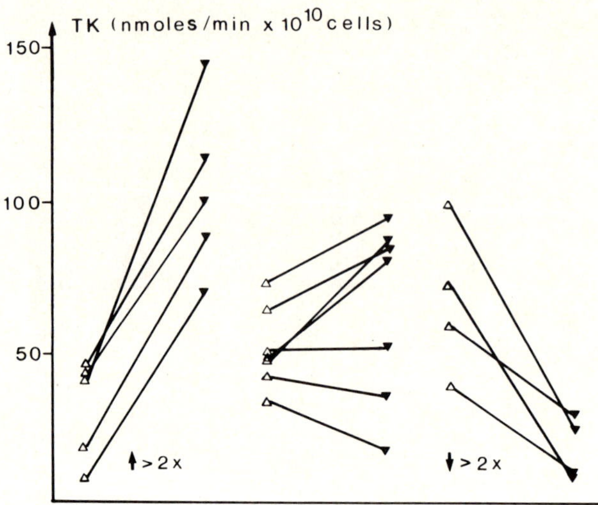

Fig. 2. Thymidine kinase (TK) activity in bone marrow cells of patients with acute leukemia at first diagnosis ($\triangle$) and at relapse ($\blacktriangledown$)

of the proliferation intensity, which does not mean that this marker is specific for acute leukemia only.

Prognostic Value

Out of 85 patients with acute leukemia (66 with acute nonlymphoblastic leukemia; 19 with lymphoblastic leukemia) who were treated after primary diagnosis with aggressive chemotherapy according to the European Organisation for Research on Treatment of Cancer (EORTC) and Bundesministerium für Forschung und Technologie (BMFT) protocol, 52 (61%) patients reached complete remission and 33 (39%) did not reach complete remission. Between both groups there was statistically no significant difference in TK activity or in the proliferation parameters before treatment. Thus, these parameters do not have any prognostic value. This is beyond our expectation, because as a result of the reduction of leukemic cells by cytocidal drugs, the aplastic phase is generally the first signal of a response of acute leukemia to specific treatment. Reaching a complete remission depends on the maturation of normal precursor cells in the bone marrow, thus on the regeneration of hematopoiesis from normal stem cells.

Implication of TK for the Follow-Up and for Early Detection of Relapse in Acute Leukemias

As mentioned above, the mean TK activities in leukemic bone marrow have the same degree at primary diagnosis and at relapse (Table 1). Three groups

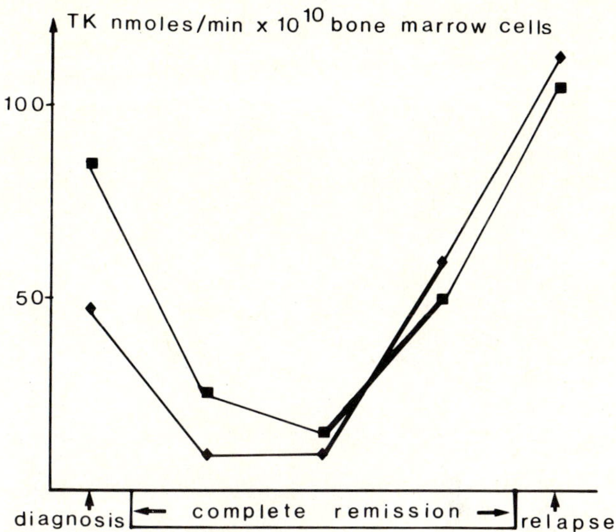

Fig. 3. Thymidine kinase (*TK*) activity in bone marrow cells of two patients with acute leukemia in the course of disease

can be characterized: (1) merely unimportant differences between first diagnosis and relapse (Fig. 2), (2) distinct increase of TK at time of relapse in comparison to first diagnosis (Fig. 2), (3) considerably lower TK at time of relapse in comparison to the beginning of the disease (Fig. 2).

This, in some cases considerably altered reaction of TK activity at relapse supports selection of a leukemic clone with different behavior of DNA metabolism in the course of disease.

Figure 3 shows that in a patient's individual course of acute leukemia an increase in TK activity can predict a relapse before bone marrow blasts increase again.

Now, the results of TK control investigations of 38 patients, who by 1987 reached a complete remission under specific treatment, are summarized. A relapse occurred in 15 patients. In 12 patients DNA metabolism was investigated in the course of disease. Six patients showed an increase of TK in the bone marrow 3 months prior to morphological manifestation of the relapse. The same number of patients did not show an increased TK activity in the cytosol of the isolated bone marrow cells. Out of 23 patients with persistent complete remission, 5 patients showed an increase of TK activity without a relapse within the following 3 months.

The described results are an indicator of the usefulness in controlling TK in the cytosol of bone marrow cells during remission in each bone marrow aspirate in order to judge the quality of the remission and to direct our attention to a possibly imminent relapse in patients where TK increases.

References

1. Fleischer W, Pelka R (1978) A practical analysis of DNA-histograms with a laboratory computer. In: Lutz D (ed) Pulse-cytophotometry III. European Press, Ghent, p 137
2. Gilette PC, Claycomb WC (1974) Thymidine-kinase activity in cardiac muscle during embryonic and postnatal development. Biochem J 142:685–690
3. Hartje J, Wilmanns W (1970) Autoradiographische und enzymatische Untersuchungen der DNS-Synthese in Leukämiezellen. I. Korrelation von Thymidin-Kinase und ^{3}H-Thymidin-Markierungsindex. Klin Wochenschr 48:780–788
4. Hopkins HA, Campbell HA, Barbiroli B, Potter VR (1973) Thymidine-kinase and deoxyribonucleic acid metabolism in growing and regenerating livers from rats on contolled feeding schedules. Biochem J 136:955–966
5. Kit S (1976) Thymidine-kinase, DNA-synthesis and cancer. Mol Cell Biochem 11:161–182
6. Nakai GS, Michael E, Peterson M, Craddack CG (1966) Thymidine and thymidylate kinase and thymidylate phosphatase in human leukemic leukocytes. Clin Chim Acta 14:422–425
7. Olsen I, Harris G (1975) Thymidine-kinase activity of mouse spleen cells in vivo and in vitro. Biochem J 146:489–496
8. Pelka-Fleischer R, Ruppelt W, Wilmanns W, Sauer H, Schalhorn A (1986) Relation between cell cycle stage and the activity of DNA-synthesizing enzymes in cultured human lymphoblasts: investigations on cell fractions enriched according to cell cycle stages by way of centrifugal elutriation. Leukemia 1:182–187
9. Sauer H, Wilmanns W (1977) Cobalamin dependent methionine synthesis and methyl-folate-trap in human vitamin B12 deficiency. Br J Haematol 36:189–198
10. Sauer H, Wilmanns W (1982) Thymidine kinase. ATP: thymidine 5'-phosphotransferase, EC 2.7.1.21. In: Burgmeyer HU (ed) Methods of enzymatic analysis III. Verlag Chemie, Weinheim, p 468
11. Sauer H, Wilmanns W, Pelka-Fleischer R, Twardzik L, Vehling-Kaiser U, Jehn U (1987) DNA-metabolism in human bone marrow cells. Z antimikrob antineoplast Chemother 5:71–77
12. Szikla K, Pokorny E, Hullà L, Holczinger L (1981) Variations of Thymidine-Kinase activity and DNA content in Ehrlich and L1210 Ascites tumor cells during tumor growth. Cancer Biochem Biophys 5:259–264
13. Wilmanns W, Neef V (1971) Die Thymidylat-Synthetase in weißen Blutzellen und im Knochenmark unter normalen und pathologischen Bedingungen. Klin Wochenschr 49:755–762
14. Wilmanns W, Wilms K (1972) DNA Synthesis in normal and leucemic cells as related to therapy with cytotoxic drugs. Enzyme 13:90–109
15. Wilmanns W (1967) Die Thymidin-Kinase in normalen und leukämischen Zellen. Klin Wochenschr 45:505–511
16. Wilmanns W (1971) Antimetabolite. Internist 12:127–135
17. Wilmanns W (1971) DNA-synthesis in leukemic cells under the action of cytotoxic agents in vitro and in vivo. In: Hall TC (ed). Prediction of response in cancer therapy. NCI Monogr 34:153

Bleeding Tendency in Acute Promyelocytic Leukemia: Reversal by Cell Differentiation?

P.W. Wijermans,[1] G.J. Ossenkoppele, P.C. Huijgens, and
M.M.A.C. Langenhuijsen

Introduction

Acute promyelocytic leukemia (APL) is a subvariety of acute myeloid leukemia (AML) and is associated with a high incidence of severe hemorrhage [7]. Tissue factor-like structures found on the leukemic blast cell, inducing disseminated intravascular coagulation (DIC), are often said to be responsible for this coagulopathy [2]. However, the observed bleeding disorder could not always be explained by DIC [5], and signs of fibrinolysis due to proteolytic lysosomal enzymes from the azurophilic granules were found [4]. Moreover, recently, specific fibrinolytic activity has also been described as a cause of the coagulopathy [6], and plasminogen activator has been found in the blast cells of patients with APL [3]. In a previous study [10] we investigated promyelocytic cell line cells (HL60) and blast cells from patients with APL and were able to show that in promyelocytes a combination of procoagulant activity (PCA) and proteolytic activity (lysosomal enzymes) exists that could be responsible for the observed bleeding tendency. Because HL60 cells are susceptible to differentiation in vitro to either more mature granulocytic or monocytic cells we are able to study whether combinations of PCA, proteolytic activity, and/or plasminogen activator activity exist in these cells, and whether these combinations are unique for the promyelocyte. We compared our findings with those obtained in blast cells of patients with different subtypes of AML.

Materials and Methods

HL60 cells were cultured as previously described [11]. The following differentiation-inducing agents were used: dimethylsulfoxide (DMSO) at a concentration of 1.25%; retinoic acid (RA) $10^{-7} M$; and 1,25-dihydroxy-vitamin D_3 (Vit D_3) $10^{-7} M$. A series of differentiation parameters were used as described previously [11]. Normal monocytes and polymorpho-

[1] Free University Hospital, Department of Haematology (BR 238), De Boelelaan 1117, NL-1081 HV Amsterdam, The Netherlands

Fleischer (Ed.) Leukemias
© Springer-Verlag Berlin Heidelberg 1993

nuclear leukocytes (PMN) were isolated as previously described. Leukemic blast cells were obtained from either peripheral blood or bone marrow and isolated by density gradient centrifugation on Ficoll Isopaque. Cells were lysed in medium with 1% Triton X-100 by freezing them three times in liquid nitrogen for the proteolysis experiments. For the determination of plasminogen activator activity, cells were lysed in the appropriate buffer by sonication; three bursts of 10 s at 0°C. Proteolytic activity of cell lysate was determined using fibrin plates as described previously [11]. Fibrinolysis as a parameter for proteolysis was measured as the area of lysis produced by 10 µl of cell lysate (πr^2) after 36 h of incubation at 37°C.

Specific fibrinolysis was also determined by the conversion of plasminogen into plasmin by cell lysate. Supernatant (150 µl) was added to 200 µl Tris buffer, pH 7.8, and 50 µl of S2251 chromogenic substrate was added and the increase in light absorption was measured at 405 nm with a spectrophotometer. The (PCA) was measured by the recalcification time. Pooled citrated normal human plasma (0.1 ml) was incubated with 0.1 ml of cell suspension (resuspended in Michaelis buffer, pH 7.4) for 6 min at 37°C. Then 0.1 ml of calcium chloride (30 mM) was added to the plasma and the clotting time was recorded. The PCA is expressed as minutes necessary for clot formation. We compared the activity with a standard curve of thromboplastin and expressed the observed mean clotting time in relative thromboplastin units (RTU).

Results

In Table 1 we show the influence of cell differentiation on the PCA. HL60 cells had a significantly higher PCA than human monocytes ($p < 0.01$) and PMN ($p < 0.001$). Granulocytic differentiation induced by both DMSO and RA led to a significant increase in recalcification time, thus indicating a decrease in PCA. No differences were found in the PCA after culturing the cells in the presence of Vit D$_3$. We stimulated the cells with phorbol ester (TPA) to show that a PCA increase was possible, as is known for human monocytes.

After incubation of the cells with concanavalin A (Con A) or with phospholipase C (Phos C) the PCA had almost completely disappeared in the HL60 cells (Table 1). Also, in the cells stimulated with TPA, these drugs induced a strong decrease in PCA activity.

With the fibrin plate technique we found a high proteolytic activity in the lysate of HL60 cells. Previously we were able to show that this activity was higher than that found in human monocytes but lower than in human PMN [11]. Table 2 shows the influence of cell differentiation on this proteolytic activity.

The observed proteolytic activity in HL60 cell lysate was not due to specific fibrinolysis because the fibrinogen used to make the fibrin plates

Table 1. Influence of cell differentiation on PCA

	Recalcification time (Seconds, mean ± SD)	PCA (RTU)
	$(1.2 \times 10^6$ cells)	
HL60 control	84 ± 9	320
HL60 Vit D$_3$	93 ± 16	225
HL60 RA	136 ± 10	82
HL60 DMSO	137 ± 18	80
HL60 TPA	53 ± 5	1450
Monocytes	132 ± 34	88
PMN	186 ± 13	32
	$(0.6 \times 10^6$ cells)	
HL60 control	105 ± 3	160
HL60 Con A	224 ± 20	10
HL60 Phos C	>300	<5
HL60 TPA	64 ± 1	720
HL60 TPA/Phos C	174 ± 3	39
HL60 TPA/Con A	90 ± 7	250

Table 2. Influence of cell differentiation on proteolytic activity and plasminogen activator activity.

	Proteolysis (mm^2)	Fibrinolysis (nkat/10^{-7} cells)
HL60 control	294 ± 79	0.136 ± 0.034
HL60 Vit D$_3$	0	0.098 ± 0.033
HL60 RA	284 ± 59	0.177 ± 0.020
HL60 DMSO	231 ± 140	0.325 ± 0.101

Values are mean ± SD.

was said to contain no plasminogen and the control experiments with streptokinase were negative. Moreover, when we added plasminogen to the fibrin plate no significant increase in proteolysis was observed (314 ± 74 mm^2) whereas the streptokinase control became positive (963 ± 129 mm^2). A small decrease in proteolytic activity was found after myeloid differentiation with DMSO ($p < 0.05$). A complete disappearance of the activity was seen after monocytic differentiation (Vit D$_3$). Table 2 also depicts the values found for the specific fibrinolysis. Low amounts of plasminogen activator activity were found in the cell lysate of HL60 cells. After monocytic differentiation we observed a significant decrease in the conversion of plasminogen to plasmin. After granulocytic differentiation, however, there was an increase in activity (RA $p < 0.03$, and DMSO $p < 0.01$). No increase

Table 3. Acute myeloid leukemia patients

FAB class.	Proteolytic activity (mm^2)	Procoagulant activity (s)	RTU
M1	0	236	12
M2	0	260	<10
M2	0	135	88
M2	113	230	10
M2[a]	314	181	35
M3	123	53	2400
M3	404	54	2350
M3	133	74	520
M3	77	85	290
M3	143	68	590
M3	346	40	5000
M4	0	206	22
M4	72	236	12
M5A	0	215	20
M5B	0	255	<10
M5B	50	171	45

[a] M2 subtype on morphological and cytogenetic findings but with a high percentage of promyelocytes.
FAB class., French-American-British Group classification.

in plasminogen activator activity was observed by adding soluble fibrin products.

We were able to study the PCA and the proteolytic activity in 15 AML patients of whom 6 showed the FAB M3 – promyelocytic – subtype. As can be seen in Table 3, only the patients with the M3 subtype showed both a high PCA and a high proteolytic activity.

Discussion

It seems possible from the available literature to assume that the bleeding disorder found in patients with APL is of multicausal origin [2,3,5,6,10]. In this study we show that promyelocytic cell line cells can induce coagulation (PCA) and exhibit also both a specific and an aspecific fibrinolytic activity. Because the PCA could be inhibited by Con A and Phos C it is likely that tissue factor-like structures are responsible for the coagulation induction. This is supported by the findings with TPA [8]. From the differentiation experiments it is clear that this combination of different activities is unique to the promyelocyte. Monocytic differentiation led to disappearance of the proteolytic activity, probably due to the decrease of lysosomal enzymes [9] and a decrease in plasminogen conversion. The PCA, however, remained stable, which is in agreement with the finding of PCA on human monocytes.

Granulocytic differentiation showed a diminishing of the PCA toward levels found in human PMN, the proteolytic activity remained stable but an increase was seen in the plasminogen activator activity. Our findings with soluble fibrin products and the observations in the literature [9] show that the plasminogen activator is of the urokinase type. The observed increase in fibrinolytic activity might than be explained by a decrease in plasminogen activator inhibitor type 2 [1].

We studied the blast cells of patients with AML. Only in patients with the APL subtype did we observe both a proteolytic activity and PCA, which supports our findings in the HL60 cells. It has become clear now that severe alpha-2-antiplasmin deficiency is associated with an increased risk of life-threatening bleeding [12]. In patients with APL, a combination of PCA, proteolysis due to lysosomal enzymes (such as elastase [10]), and fibrinolytic activity might easily lead to such a decrease in alpha-2-antiplasmin level.

References

1. Alving BM, Krishnamurti C, Lin YP, Lucas DL, Wright DG (1988) Stimulated production of urokinase and plasminogen activator inhibitor-2 by the human pro-myelocytic leukemia cell line HL60. Thromb Res 51:175
2. Andoh K, Kubota T, Takada M, Tanaka H, Kobayoshi N, Naekawa T (1987) Tissue Factor activity in leukemia cells. Cancer 59:748
3. Bennett B, Booth NA, Croll A, Dawson AA (1989) The bleeding disorder in acute promyelocytic leukemia: fibrinolysis due to u-PA rather than defibrination. Br J Haematol 71:511
4. Eckhardt T, Koch M (1986) Fibrinogen proteolysis in acute myeloid leukemia. Blut 53:39
5. Imaoka S, Ueda T, Shibata H, Masaoka T, Ogawa M, Sasaki Y, Iwanaga T, Terasawa T (1986) Fibrinolysis in patients with acute promyelocytic leukemia and disseminated intravascular coagulation during heparin therapy. Cancer 58:1736
6. Kahle LH, Avvisati G, Lamping RJ, Moretti T, Mandelli F, ten Cate JW (1985) Turnover of alpha-2-antiplasmin in patients with acute promyelocytic leukemia. Scand J Clin Lab Invest 45 [Suppl 178]:75
7. Kantorjian HM, Keating MJ, Walters RS, Estey EH, McCredie KB, Smith TL, Dalton WT, Cork A, Trjillo JM, Friereich EJ (1978) Acute promyelocytic leukemia: MD Anderson Hospital experience. Am J Med 80:789
8. Lyberg T, Pryds H (1981) Phorbol esters induce synthesis of thromboplastin activity in human monocytes. Biochem J 194:699
9. Takada A, Takada Y (1988) Physiology of plasminogen: with special reference to activation and degredation. Haemostasis 18 [Suppl 1]:25
10. Wijermans PW, Rebel VI, Ossenkoppele GJ, Huygens PC, Langenhuijsen MMAC (1989) Combined procoagulant activity and proteolytic activity of acute promyelocytic leukemic cells: reversal of the bleeding disorder by cell differentiation. Blood 73:800
11. Wijermans PW, Ossenkoppele GJ, Huijgens PC, Imandt LMFM, de Waal FC, Langenhuijsen MMAC (1987) Quantitative enzyme determination: a parameter for leukemic cell differentiation. Leuk Res 11:641
12. Williams EC (1989) Plasma alpha 2 antiplasmin activity: role in the evaluation and management of fibrinolytic states and other bleeding disorders. Arch Intern Med 149:1768

Risk Prediction of Therapy-Induced Leukemia After Cytostatic Treatment*

T. Raposa[1] and J. Várkonyi

Introduction

Due to the improved survival of cancer patients receiving chemo- and radiotherapy, the risk of developing a second primary tumor has become a problem in planning the management of patients with a first malignancy [3]. It has been established that up to 10% of all the acute leukemias are of therapy-induced type, i.e., arise as a consequence of the cytotoxic therapy for a tumor or immunopathological disorder [1]. It is therefore important to quantitate the degree of the carcinogenicity of such compounds, determine the range of patients most at risk of developing a secondary leukemia and outline the measures which should be made in order to minimize the carcinogenicity of various treatment modalities.

This study makes an attempt to estimate the genotoxicity and carcinogenicity of the potential human mutagenic and/or carcinogenic cytostatic agents. The genotoxicity studies on the cytostatic agents are performed in the in vivo-in vitro sister chromatid exchange (SCE) assay in the lymphocytes of cancer patients under cytostatic treatment [4]. As far as the validation of these genotoxicity data with regard to carcinogenicity of the same therapeutic protocols is concerned, the therapy-induced leukemias were used as a real human carcinogenesis model. The analysis of 999 therapy-induced leukemias from the pool of the published reports on therapy-related leukemias between 1930 and 1986 served as the basis of this comparison.

Material and Methods

SCE Analysis of Patients Under and Off Cytostatic Therapy

These data have been partly drawn from our earlier compilation of SCE studies on the SCE frequencies in phytohemagglutinin (PHA) stimulated

* This study was supported by grants: National Scientific and Research Foundation (OTUA) 1012 and Ministry of Welfare (ETT)
[1] III Department of Internal Medicine, Semmelweis University Medical School, 1121, Budapest, Eotvos u. 12, Hungary

Fleischer (Ed.) Leukemias
© Springer-Verlag Berlin Heidelberg 1993

Table 1. Influence of different cytostatics on the frequencies of SCEs in PHA-stimulated lymphocytes in vivo in man

Group 1: No SCE induction	Group 2: SCE induction
Aclacinomycin	Adriamycin
Actinomycin D[a]	Busulfan
Acyclovir	Chlorambucil
Azathioprine[a]	Cyclophosphamide
Bleomycin[a]	Melphalan
Cytosine arabinoside	Mitomycin-C
Dacarbazine	Nitrosoureas
5-Fluorouracil	Platinum complexes
Hydroxyurea	
Methotrexate[a]	
Tamoxifen	And combination with drugs from group 1
6-Thioguanine	(e.g. COPP, Cyclophosphamide +
Vincristine	Vincristine + Procarbazide +
Vinblastine	Prednisolone)
As well as drugs from group 2, 2–3 months after their administration	

[a] According to some data, slight increase in SCE.

lymphocytes of cancer patients [4–6], in addition to those studies performed in the past years, amounting to 524 SCE analyses in 154 patients. The diagnosis of the patients is as follows: Hodgkin's disease (HD), 20; non-Hodgkin's lymphoma (NHL), 36; multiple myeloma (MM), 12; solid tumors, 18; myelodysplastic syndromes (MDPS), 18; acute nonlymphocytic leukemias (ANLL), 17; acute lymphoblastic leukemia (ALL), 8; chronic myelogenous leukemia (CML), 8; immunopathological disorders, 17 cases. A total of 224 SCE studies were done in those cases when the patients were given monochemotherapy; the rest of the patients were treated with combination chemotherapy.

Data Identification of Secondary Acute Leukemias

Acute leukemias following cytotoxic therapy (tAL) reported between 1930 and 1986 were identified through computer searches using Medline and Cancerline and through extensive manual searches of bibliographies and identified books and articles. More than 180 studies that contained adequate information on clinical history, histological diagnosis, treatment details of the primary cancers (solid tumors, lymphomas, and immunopathological diseases), and the time interval to tAL, age, cytogenetics, and response to the therapy of the tAL were selected for this analysis.

The antineoplastic protocols used for the treatment of the primary malignancies were evaluated in the light of their SCE-inducing abilities and analyzed with regard to their leukemogenic potential as far as the total of 999 tAL, identified from the literature search, is concerned. The 324 tAL

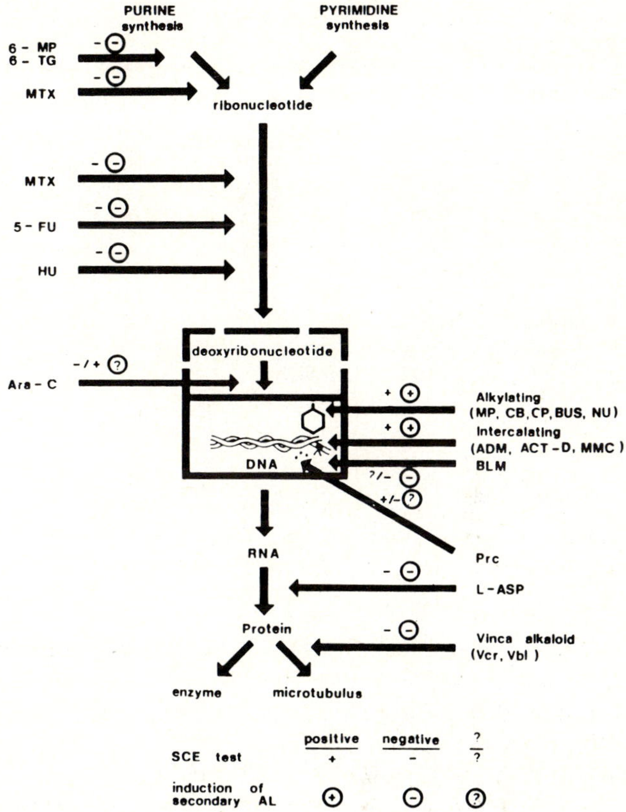

Fig. 1. Model of DNA synthesis showing the ability of the cytostatics to induce SCEs and secondary leukemias

following HD and MM contained sufficient information for an analysis between the age of the patients at the start of the therapy and the latency period to the tAL. The 182 tAL arising after monochemotherapy served as the basis of the analysis to assess whether the type of carcinogenic chemotherapy and the subtypes of the resulting tAL are causally related.

Results

SCE-Inducing Ability of Cytostatics with Regard to Their Mechanism of Action

Table 1 summarizes our experiences of the ability of many of the cytostatics currently used for the treatment of tumors as far as their SCE-inducing ability is concerned in the in vivo-in vitro SCE assay in PHA-stimulated

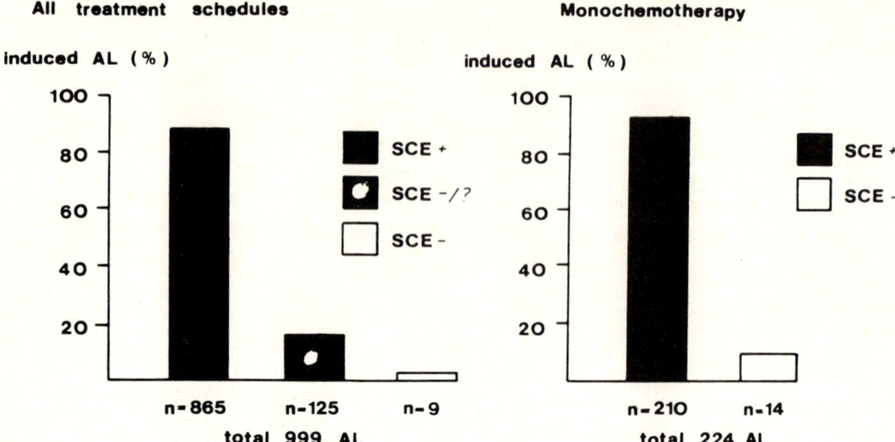

Fig. 2. The distribution of the therapy-induced acute leukemias with regard to the type of therapy for the first primary tumor and the SCE-inducing ability of this therapy. • includes also 115 induced AL after irradiation also

peripheral blood lymphocytes. The cytostatics fall into two categories, one with no ability to induce SCEs and the other with an obvious ability to elevate the baseline rate of SCEs. There seems to be a close relationship between the mechanism of action of a given cytostatic and its SCE-inducing ability. The cytostatic agents that have a strong SCE-inducing ability, such as alkylating agents, directly interact with the DNA, whereas those acting at the level of pyrimidine, purine, and protein or microtubule synthesis are only weak inducers of SCEs (Fig. 1).

Leukemia-Inducing Ability of Various Cytostatic Agents with Differing Ability to Induce SCEs

Out of the 999 tAL, 865 (86%) have been those which followed the administration of a drug or a combination of drugs which are positive in the SCE assay (Table 1). Less than 1% of all the tAL seem to be associated with the administration of an SCE-negative cytostatic protocol (Fig. 2).

Influence of Age of the Patients on the Latency Period to tAL

In the HD population (182), and among the multiple myeloma patients (142), tAL patients had sufficient information for an analysis between the age of the patients at the start of therapy for the first primary tumor and the time interval to the development of the tAL. There has been a strong tendency toward the older patients, above 40 years of age, having a shorter latency period to an induced acute leukemia, i.e., representing a subset

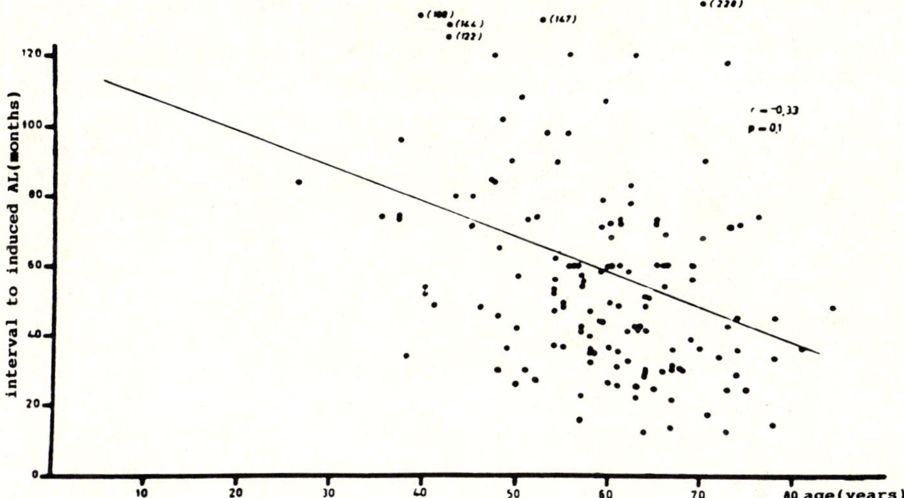

Fig. 3. The correlation between the age of the patients with multiple myeloma at the start of the therapy and the latency period to the tAL

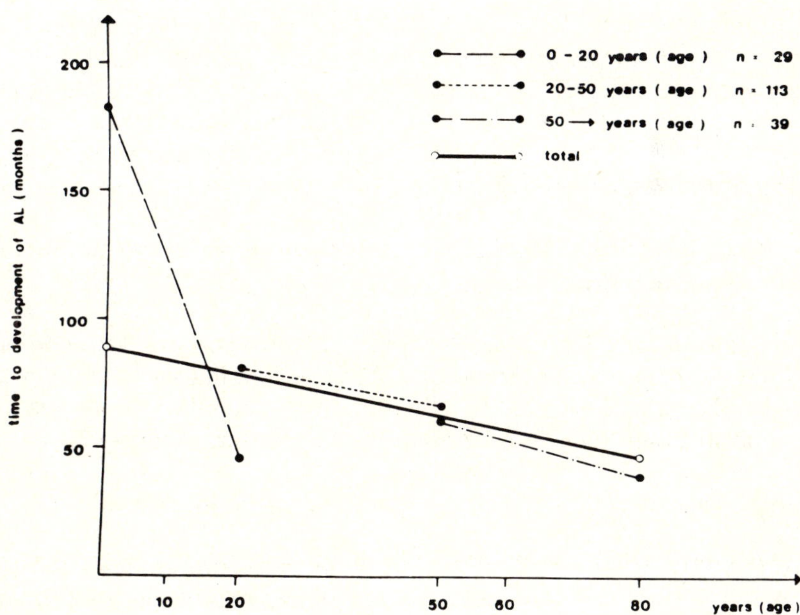

Fig. 4. Latency period to a tAL in the population of Hodgkin's disease patients. Patients older than 40 years of age have a shorter, whereas patients under the age of 20 have a longer latency period

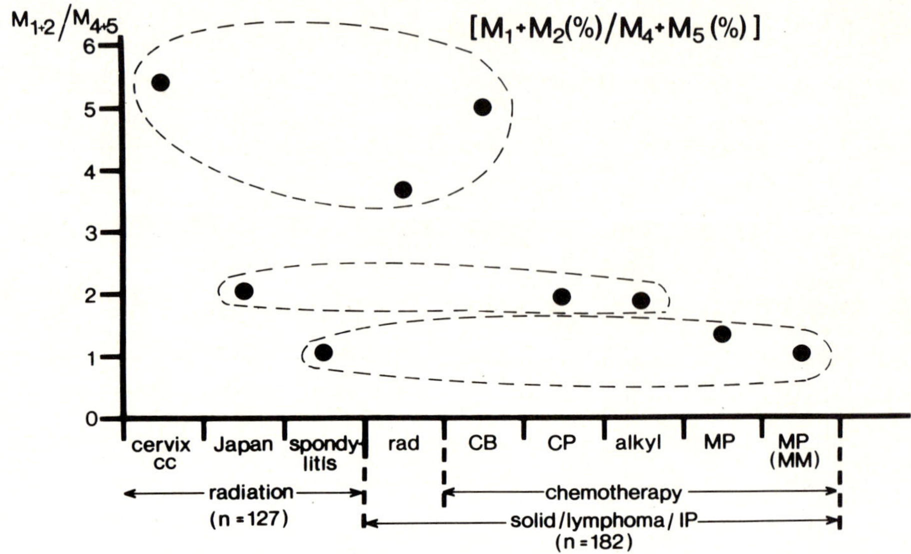

Fig. 5. Subtype distribution of tAL after various types of monotherapy, chemotherapy, and radiation (*rad*). (Some of the radiation data are adopted from Moloney [2])

of patients who are at higher risk for the development of the tAL (Figs. 3 and 4).

The Distribution of Subtypes of tAL with Regard to the Type of Therapy

Among the total of 999 tAL patients 182 were found who had received only one cytostatic drug. The therapy consisted of either cyclophosphamide, chlorambucil, or melphalan. The distribution of the monocytic and myeloid variants of tAL had a clear difference according to different protocols. Radiation alone and chlorambucil tended to induce myeloblastic rather than monoblastic subtypes. The administration of cyclophosphamide and melphalan, however, was followed by the preponderance of M4 + M5 acute leukemias. Leukemias following radiation seem to have a peculiar subtype distribution depending on the type of the radiation applied and the underlying disease [2]. The more frequent occurrence of M1 + M2 ANLL among the patients treated with radiation for cervical cancer and solid tumors as well as after chlorambucil in immunopathological disorders is in sharp contrast with the prevalence of M4 + M5 variants of ANLL among the patients with a previous multiple myeloma treated with melphalan or irradiated for spondylitis (Fig. 5). These data are very suggestive in the respect that a specific etiologic agent may induce specific subtypes of leukemias.

References

1. Kantarjian HM, Keating HJ, Walters RS, Beran M, McLaughin P et al. (1986) The association of specific "favorable" cytogenetic abnormalities with secondary leukemia Cancer 58:924–927
2. Moloney WC (1987) Radiogenic leukemia revisited. Blood 70:905–908
3. Penn I (1988) Tumors of the immunocompromised patient. Ann Rev Med 39:63–73
4. Raposa T (1978) Sister chromatid exchange studies for monitoring DNA damage and repair capacity after cytostatics in vitro and in lymphocytes of patients under cytostatic therapy. Mutat Res 57:241–251
5. Raposa T (1984) SCE induction by cytostatics and its relation to iatrogenic leukemogenesis. In-Hollander A, Tice RR (eds) Sister chromatid exchange. Twenty five years of experimental research. Plenum, New York, pp. 859–884
6. Raposa T, Várkonyi J (1987) The relationship between sister chromatid exchange induction and leukemogenicity of different cytostatics. Cancer Detect Rev 10:141–151

Cytokines and Macrophages

The Role of Cytokines in Experimental and Clinical Hematology

E.E. Polli[1] and P. Foa

Introduction

Cytokines are a family of molecules especially important in the physio-pathology of hematopoiesis. Besides that, the interest in these factors is further increased by the fact that this area of research is certainly one of the most rapidly evolving and therefore most appealing of modern hematology. While until a few years ago cytokines were poorly defined substances, the recent advent of sophisticated biochemical approaches and the progress of molecular biology led to a precise characterization of these molecules. Moreover, the use of recombinant DNA technology made available several of these factors on a scale large enough for both extensive biological research and clinical investigation. As a consequence, molecules such as interleukins, interferons, tumor necrosis factor (TNF), and colony-stimulating factors (CSFs) are presently being thoroughly studied in order to clarify their role in the physiopathology and eventually in the treatment of hematological diseases. This review will be focused on a single aspect of this broad field which seems to be especially promising, that is, the therapeutic use of CSFs. CSFs are glycoproteins essential for sustaining the proliferation and function of granulocyte-macrophage cells. So far, four distinct CSFs have been identified in man: granulocyte–CSF (G-CSF) and macrophage–CSF (M-CSF), which are released by monocytes, fibroblasts, and endothelial cells; granulocyte-macrophage–CSF (GM-CSF), which is produced also by T-lymphocytes; and finally, multi–CSF or interleukin-3 (IL-3), which is derived from activated T-lymphocytes [1–4].

The availability of CSFs as recombinant molecules made possible an extensive investigation into the biological activity of these factors both in vitro and in vivo in animals.

G-CSF was shown to stimulate both proliferation and function of normal granulocyte cells. As far as leukemic cells are concerned, interestingly and intriguingly enough, G-CSF can sometimes, but not always, induce terminal differentiation. Finally, when injected in animals, G-CSF induces neutrophilic leukocytosis. On the other hand, M-CSF does stimulate pro-

[1] Institute of Medical Sciences, University of Milan, Via F. Sforza, 35, I-20122 Milan, Italy

Fleischer (Ed.) Leukemias
© Springer-Verlag Berlin Heidelberg 1993

liferation and function of monocytes and synergizes with G-CSF, GM-CSF, and IL-3.

GM-CSF has quite a complex pattern of activities. It stimulates the proliferation of granulocytes, macrophages, and megakariocytes, and it supports blast cell proliferation.

Besides that, GM-CSF inhibits granulocyte motility but enhances all the other functional activities of these cells and it increases also eosinophil cytotoxicity. GM-CSF can also induce the production of cytokines such as TNF and IL-1, partly responsible for the toxicity of GM-CSF treatment. Finally, IL-3 can support the proliferation of almost any hematopoietic cell type. IL-3 synergizes with other CSFs, and when injected in animals followed by GM-CSF it increases neutrophil, monocyte, lymphocyte, and erythroid counts.

Based on the experimental data which have been previously summarized, it's not difficult to outline the potential therapeutic applications of the CSFs. CSFs can be used for stimulating the host defense against infections, especially in the immunocompromised patient; they can also be used with the aim of preventing or treating the hematopoietic toxicity induced by chemotherapy and/or radiotherapy. Further areas of therapeutic applications are acceleration of hematopoietic recovery after bone marrow transplantation and extinction of hematological malignancies by induction of terminal differentiation of the malignant cell clone.

Several studies have now been completed which explore the therapeutic role of CSFs, namely G-CSF and GM-CSF, in the clinical settings which have just been mentioned.

CSFs and AIDS

First to be taken into consideration will be the use of CSFs for improving the host defense of the immunocompromised patient [5]. GM-CSF at doses ranging from 1.0×10^3 to 2.0×10^4 U/kg body weight per day has been administered by continuous intravenous infusion to AIDS patients. A 14-day treatment with GM-CSF resulted in a dose-dependent increase of leukocyte counts; mature neutrophils, neutrophilic bands, and eosinophils accounted for most of the increase in the absolute number of circulating leukocytes. Interestingly enough, an enhancement of leukocyte function was also recorded. After discontinuation of GM-CSF administration, the white cell count returned to approximately the baseline values within about 1 week, clearly indicating that continuous treatment is required in order to sustain GM-CSF-induced hematological changes. Toxicity was mild; transient skin rash, facial flushing, and local phlebitis were usually observed. Based on these data, it can be therefore concluded that preliminary clinical trials in AIDS patients indicate that these patients are responsive and tolerate GM-CSF treatment well in spite of the underlying disease; more-

over, according to preliminary observations, a persistent increase of leukocyte number and function seems to be effective in reducing morbidity and
mortality due to infections.

CSFs in Cancer Patients

Another clinical setting where the use of CSFs seems to be as promising as
in AIDS is the treated cancer patient.

It is well known that hematological toxicity in cancer patients treated by
aggressive chemotherapy and/or radiotherapy, is a major factor contributing
not only to underdosing of patients but also to morbidity and mortality,
mostly due to infections. The efficacy of G-CSF in accelerating recovery
from therapy-induced myelosuppression or in preventing this untoward side
effect has therefore been explored by several groups [6–8].

G-CSF administration, either before or after anticancer treatment, has a
strong impact on hematological toxicity and related complications. G-CSF
treatment can effectively shorten the period of severe neutropenia which in
turn reduces the incidence and severity of infections. A significant decrease
of mucositis is also usually recorded. Even more important is that G-CSF
treatment greatly increases the percentage of patients able to receive their
full treatment on schedule. Since in cancer patients a positive correlation has
been shown between dose intensity and response, it is conceivable that
G-CSF supportive therapy might increase the response rate to cytostatic
treatment.

CSFs in Myelodysplastic Syndromes

One of the theoretically most appealing ways of exploiting CSFs' biological
activity is that one aimed at eradicating hematological malignancies by
inducing terminal differentiation of the neoplastic cell clone [9].

So far, this therapeutic approach has been evaluated in the myelodysplastic syndromes, stem cell disorders characterized by ineffective
hematopoiesis, refractory cytopenias with high risk of infections or bleeding,
and frequent evolution into overt acute myelogenous leukemia [10–12].

The myelodysplastic syndromes are therefore usually viewed as preleukemia states, often characterized by the presence of hematopoietic
malignant clone.

Supportive therapy with transfusions has been the mainstay of therapy,
while treatment with either cytotoxic drugs or differentiation-inducing
agents, such as vitamin D_3, retinoic acid, and interferons, has been only
partly successful.

Since GM-CSF not only stimulated growth and differentiation of
hematopoietic cells and enhanced functional activities of mature effector

cells, but also induced terminal differentiation of some myeloid leukemic cell lines, it became obvious that its therapeutic role in patients with myelodysplastic syndromes should be tested. GM-CSF treatment consisted of repeated cycles of 14 days' continuous intravenous infusion of the agent given every 4 weeks. As a result of this treatment schedule, a dose-dependent increase of leukocyte number was recorded, while no persistent improvement of reticulocytes and platelets was observed. Moreover, in the majority of patients, administration of recombinant GM-CSF resulted in a significant rise of both peripheral and bone marrow blasts. In general, the treatment was well tolerated. A minority of patients experienced slight fever, phlebitis at the injection site, and sometimes bone pain. Which are therefore the tentative conclusions which can be drawn from these preliminary clinical trials with GM-CSF in myelodysplastic patients?

Despite the initial promise, results were partly disappointing. Not only stimulation of normal hematopoiesis, especially erythropoiesis and megakaryocytopoiesis, turned out to be poor, but in addition GM-CSF treatment seemed to promote the proliferation of the leukemic cell clones.

Caution seems therefore warranted in treating myelodysplastic patients with CSFs, until more experience and longer follow-ups have been obtained.

CSFs and Bone Marrow Transplantation

As mentioned earlier on, GM-CSF has been shown to stimulate the proliferation of a variety of hematopoietic cell types. It is therefore quite obvious that a great deal of interest is being directed at evaluating the role of GM-CSF administration in accelerating hematopoietic recovery after bone marrow transplantation.

Preliminary experiments were performed in primate models [13,14]. Continuous subcutaneous infusion of GM-CSF at a dosage of 50 000 U/kg body weight per day into autologous bone marrow-transplanted monkeys, led to an accelerated recovery of peripheral blood neutrophils, monocytes, and platelets. No significant effect on erythropoiesis was detected, while the recovery of lymphocytes to normal level turned out to be prolonged in GM-CSF-infused animals. Treatment was usually well tolerated. Based on this data, clinical trials with GM-CSF in cancer patients treated with high-dose chemotherapy and autologous bone marrow support, were recently started at different institutions [15].

GM-CSF has been usually administered by continuous infusion over periods of 14 days at concentrations ranging from 2.0 to 32.0 µg/kg per day. Briefly, in most, but not all, treated patients GM-CSF administration caused a dose-dependent increase in granulocyte and, sometimes, platelet number. However, a 50% decrease in absolute cell counts was usually recorded within 48–72 h after discontinuing GM-CSF administration. As far as toxicity is concerned, pharmacological doses of GM-CSF were in general

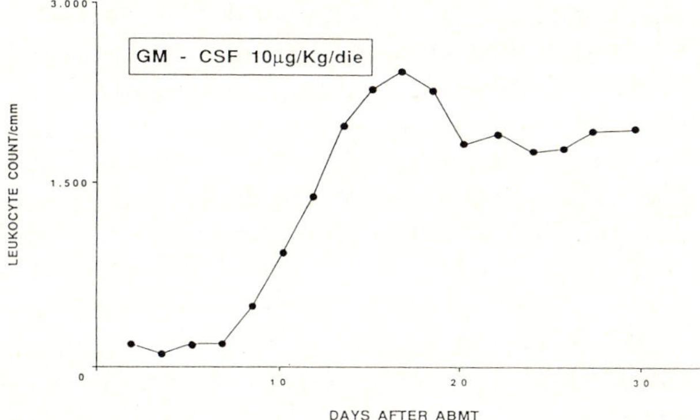

Fig. 1. Leukocyte count after autologous bone marrow transplant (*ABMT*) and GM-CSF treatment in a patient with acute lymphoblastic leukemia

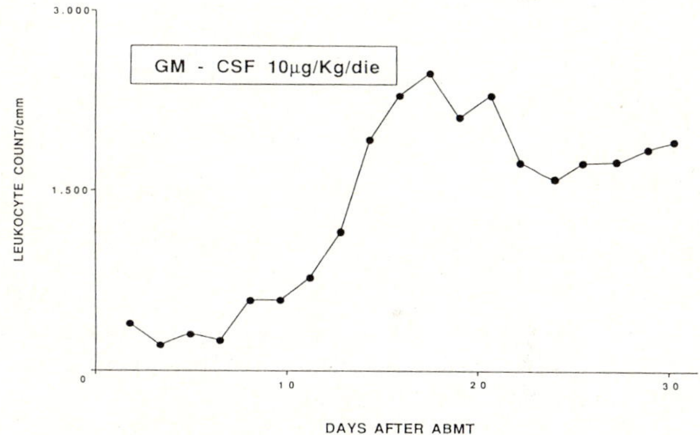

Fig. 2. Leukocyte count after autologous bone marrow transplant (*ABMT*) and GM-CSF treatment in a patient with Hodgkin's lymphoma

well tolerated. Transient rash, minor edema, fever, bone pain, and myalgia typically involving lower extremities were usually recorded. Severe drug-related toxic effects, consisting of erythroderma, pleural and pericardial effusions, generalized edema, and hypotension occurred only in patients receiving more than 30 µg GM-CSF/kg per day.

At our institute we used to treat, with GM-CSF, patients undergoing autologous bone marrow transplantation for acute leukemias, Hodgkin's (HG) and non-HG lymphomas, and having a previous history of aggressive chemotherapy followed by persistent bone marrow suppression.

Figure 1 shows the leukocyte counts of a patient submitted to bone marrow transplant owing to an acute lymphoblastic leukemia. GM-CSF treatment was started immediately after bone marrow transplant and resulted in a rapid recovery of leukocyte number.

Essentially the same type of result is shown in Fig. 2. This is an HG lymphoma patient submitted to autologous bone marrow transplant. Once again, early treatment with GM-CSF led to an accelerated recovery of leukocytes. In our experience, GM-CSF-induced toxicity is usually mild and transient and consists of bone pain, fever, skin rash, and localized edema.

Despite the fact that results of preliminary clinical trials with GM-CSF in bone marrow-transplanted patients sound promising, larger prospective trials are certainly needed in order to define more precisely both efficacy and safety of such a treatment. Moreover, a couple of concerns might be expressed: First of all, not all patients are responsive to GM-CSF and, therefore, further investigation is obviously required in order to clarify the reason for GM-CSF treatment-failure; second, receptors for GM-CSF have been shown not only on leukemic myeloid cells, but also on other cancer cells such as small-cell lung cancer and some lymphoid tumor cells. Caution seems therefore warranted in the use of GM-CSF at least in certain types of bone marrow-transplanted cancer patients.

References

1. Stanley ER, Jubinsky PT (1984) Factors affecting the growth and differentiation of hemopoietic cells in culture. Clin Haematol 13:329
2. Clark SC, Kamen R (1987) The human hematopoietic colony stimulating factors. Science 236:1229
3. Sieff CA (1987) Hematopoietic growth factors. J Clin Invest 79:1549
4. Pegoraro L, Avanzi G, Lista P (1988) Growth and differentiation factors in human hematopoiesis. Haematologica 73:525
5. Groopman JE, Mitsuyasu RT, De Leo MJ et al. (1987) Effect of recombinant human granulocyte-macrophage colony-stimulating factor on myelopoiesis in the acquired immunodeficiency syndrome. N Engl J Med 317:593
6. Bronchurd MH, Scarffe JH, Thatcher N, Crowther D, Dexter M (1987) Phase I/II study of recombinant human granulocyte colony stimulating factor in patients receiving intensive chemotherapy for small cell lung cancer. Br J Cancer 56:807
7. Gabrilove JL, Jakubowski A, Scher H, Sternberg C, Wong G, Grous J, Yagoda A, Fain K, Moore MAS, Clarkson B, Oettgen H, Alton K, Welte K, Souza L (1988) Effect of granulocyte colony stimulating factor on neutropenia and associated morbidity of chemotherapy for transitional cell carcinoma of the urethelium. N Engl J Med 318:1414
8. Morstyn G, Souza LM, Reech J et al. (1988) Effect of granulocyte colony-stimulating factor on neutropenia induced by cytotoxic chemotherapy. Lancet 1:667
9. Begley CG, Metcalf D, Nicola NA (1987) Purified colony-stimulating factors (G-CSF and GM-CSF) induce differentiation in human HL60 leukemic cells with suppression of clonogenicity. Int J Cancer 39:99
10. Vadhan-Raj S, Keating M, Le maistre A et al. (1987) Effects of recombinant human granulocyte-macrophage colony-stimulating factor in patients with myelodysplastic syndromes. N Engl J Med 317:1545
11. Kobayashi Y, Okabe T, Uzumaki H, Urabe A, Takaku F (1988) Differentiation therapy of myelodysplastic syndrome by granulocyte colony stimulating factor. Clin Res 36:412A

12. Socinski MA, Elias A, Schnipper L, Cannistra SA, Antman KH, Griffin JD (1988) Granulocyte-macrophage colony stimulating factor expands the circulating haemopoietic progenitor cell compartment in man. Lancet 1:1194
13. Nienhuis AW, Donahue RE, Karlson S et al. (1987) Recombinant human granulocyte-macrophage colony stimulating factor (GM-CSF) shortens the period of neutropenia after autologous bone marrow transplantation on a primate model. J Clin Invest 80:573
14. Monsoy RL , Skelly RR, MacVittie TJ, Davis JA, Sarber JJ, Clark SC, Donahue RE (1987) The effect of recombinant GM-CSF on recovery of monkeys transplanted with autologous bone marrow. Blood 70:1690
15. Brandt SJ, Peters WP, Atwater SK, Kurtzberg J, Borowitz MJ, Jones RB, Shpall EJ, Bast JR, Gilbert CJ, Oeete DH (1988) Effect of recombinant human granulocyte-macrophage colony stimulating factor on hematopoietic reconstitution after high dose chemotherapy and autologus bone marrow transplantation. N Engl J Med 318:875

Hematopoietins: New Tools in the Treatment of Hematopoietic Insufficiency

F. Herrmann,[1] A. Lindemann, M. Lübbert, and R. Mertelsmann

The number of circulating blood cells and their function are regulated by a variety of peptide hormones, the so-called hematopoietic growth factors (HGFs) or hematopoietins. In a complex regulatory network of stimulating and inhibiting peptide hormones [1], the number of circulating blood cells is kept at a physiological level. Because many of these blood cells have a relatively short half-life, the bone marrow is in a state of constant active proliferation in order to produce the necessary blood cells. For instance, granulocytes are made at a rate of $5 \times 10^7 - 10 \times 10^7$ cells/s. It is unclear whether additional, hematopoietin-independent regulatory mechanisms exist, which might be responsible for the basic production of blood cells. It is well established, however, that under physical stress, for instance during infections, hematopoietins are essential for an adequate hematopoietic response [1]. The nomenclature which has been chosen for hematopoietins can partly be explained historically, in the sense that these factors have been named according to their most prominent biological activity, e.g., the relatively most granulocyte-specific hematopoietin has been named granulocyte–colony-stimulating factor (G-CSF). For the most recently described hematopoietins, the nomenclature of interleukins has been chosen, which implies that every hematopoietin has not just one target cell, but can act on a broad spectrum of hematopoietic progenitor cells and mature effector cells. The chronological sequence of purification of these proteins is reflected by the numbering system of the interleukins. Hematopoietins have overlapping and partly redundant effects on hematopoietic stem and progenitor cells. Interplay and synergism of these factors are presently a central subject of experimental hematologic research. In addition to their effects on cells of the hematopoietic system, all hematopoietins and other peptide hormones produced by hematopoietic cells have a variety of effects on almost all other cells of the organism. This spectrum of pleiotropic effects explains the variety of biologic phenomena, which can be observed with in vivo application and are only partly predictable. In addition to their direct effects on hematopoietic stem cells, progenitor cells and

---

[1] Department of Hematology, University of Mainz, W-6500 Mainz, FRG

Fleischer (Ed.) Leukemias
© Springer-Verlag Berlin Heidelberg 1993

mature endcells, hematopoietins are indirectly acting on effector cells by triggering the release of secondary cytokines. For instance, activation of monocytes by granulocyte-macrophage–CSF (GM-CSF) leads to the release of tumor necrosis factor-alpha (TNF-α), macrophage–CSF (M-CSF) and other interleukins including IL-1α, IL-1β, and IL-6. The system of indirect and amplifying effects is also called cytokine cascade. Due to pleiotropic effects on nonhematopoietic cells (endothelial cells, fibroblasts, muscle cells, etc.) and due to amplification mechanisms of the cytokine cascade under certain circumstances, the systemic or local overproduction of cytokines can take place. This may bear biologic implications, for instance, systemic overproduction of TNF-α is currently being discussed as a central mediator of septic shock [2].

Factors which stimulate myelopoiesis (GM-CSF, G-CSF) have most broadly been studied in a preclinical setting and will probably be available as standard medication in the therapy of hematopoietic insufficiencies in the near future. Even during stress leading to maximum stimulation of hematopoiesis by endogenous factors, an additional and "supernormal" stimulation of hematopoiesis can be induced with pharmacological doses of these regulators.

It is currently unclear whether, in addition to therapy of hematopoietic insufficiencies, hematopoietins as inducers of a supernormal increase of, e.g., granulocytes during manifest or incipient bacterial infections can be therapeutically effective either alone or in combination with antibiotics. Although above-mentioned hematopoietins have been investigated in clinical trials over the last 2 years, their efficacy could be demonstrated in a number of clinical settings.

Several studies showed that regeneration of neutrophilic granulocytes after cytotoxic anticancer chemotherapy in the presence or absence of autologous bone marrow support could be accelerated dramatically [3–7]. Increase in white blood cell counts with G- or GM-CSF therapy were also demonstrated in other states of hematopoietic insufficiencies such as AIDS, aplastic anemia, myelodysplastic syndrome, and congenital, idiopathic, or cyclic neutropenia [8–11]. Increases in leukocyte number are dependent on dosage and route of administration of hematopoietins. Intravenous continuous infusion or subcutaneous administration are the two forms most likely to be used in routine therapy. In a recently completed study investigating the effect of subcutaneously administered GM-CSF in patients with chemotherapy-induced neutropenia, we could demonstrate that by this regimen, all patients who had been treated with GM-CSF had fewer infectious episodes, therefore needed fewer intravenous antibiotics, and spent about 40% less time in hospital due to a decrease of myelosuppression-related clinical complications [7]. In conclusion, GM-CSF-induced acceleration of leukocyte and monocyte regeneration is not just simply "laboratory cosmetics" but rather is of relevance by decreasing the morbidity of intensive chemotherapy significantly. Similar results have been obtained by others for G-CSF. Although reduced migration of granulocytes exposed to GM-CSF but not to G-CSF has been reported, the clinical relevance of this observation is unclear, particularly since the clinical efficacy of GM-CSF in reducing frequency of infections and days of hospital stay has clearly been demonstrated.

In summary, the enthusiasm accompanying the entering of CSFs into the arena of clinical oncology seems appropriate. Still, there are a number of important questions which have not been fully clarified yet. Side effects of G- and GM-CSFs when given in amounts which seem appropriate for clinical therapy are relatively few. However, one cannot exclude infrequent and possibly idiosyncratic responses by patients, particularly in view of the discussed pleiotropic activities of these molecules on many different non-hematopoietic target cells. Many malignant cells, particularly leukemic blasts, carry receptors for hematopoietins [12]. Therefore, possible stimulation of leukemic cell growth has to be taken into account. This effect of CSFs could clearly be demonstrated in patients with myelodysplastic syndromes with blast excess [12,13]. Since some nonhematopoietic malignant cells such as small-cell lung cancer cells, colon carcinoma, or osteosarcoma cells have been shown to possess receptors for hematopoietins [14–16], the possible growth-stimulatory effect of hematopoietins on these tumor tissues has to be evaluated.

Although it seems to be clear that chemotherapy-associated morbidity can be ameliorated by using hematopoietins as adjuncts, it has still to be determined whether by using hematopoietins one can increase the amounts of cytostatic and/or cytotoxic drugs in a range where therapeutic efficacy and curative rates can be improved significantly. Future studies will show whether nonhematopoietic cytotoxicities will limit further escalation of the currently used chemotherapy protocols. It is likely that GM-CSF- and G-CSF-mediated reduction of hospital stay and of morbidity associated with autologous bone marrow transplantation will widen the indication for the clinical use of hematopoietins for these therapeutic approaches.

Toxicity of long-term administration of CSF in a setting of chronic hematopoietic insufficiencies, e.g., in cyclic neutropenia or congenital neutropenia, remains to be defined. In the transgenic mouse model, introduction of the GM-CSF gene into the germline led to constant oversecretion of GM-CSF with concurrent blindness, muscle loss, exudates, and abdominal fibrosis in these animals. At this point, it is unclear whether, in clinical situations such as aplastic anemias, myelodysplasias, and congenital neutropenias, long-term administration of GM-CSF can induce similar side effects; this seems, however, unlikely considering presently available clinical results. Still, results derived from animal models should continue to define possible caveats in the clinical introduction of hematopoietins.

Future studies will also determine which of the presently tested hematopoietins and other hematopoietins not tested so far will be substances of choice for specific clinical problems. Due to the overall broader effective range of GM-CSF [1], we expect successful application of this factor particularly in hematopoietic insufficiency states which involve not only granulocytes but other hematopoietic cells as well. An increase in erythrocyte and platelet production following in vivo administration of GM-CSF was reported only sporadically, although this effect can reproducibly be seen in vitro. It seems likely that the combination of several hematopoietins will be necessary to utilize these aspects of the effective range of GM-CSF for the clinical application. In clinical conditions which are dominated by granulocytopenia or which necessitate a selective granulocytosis, application of G-CSF, which is relatively granulocyte-specific, seems useful.

Erythropoietin, which has proven greatly successful in the treatment of end-stage renal anemia of dialysis patients in several large studies [17], is presently being tested in phase Ib/II clinical trials in patients with anemia not caused by renal insufficiency (e.g., anemia of chronic disease, erythropoietic insufficiencies such as myelodysplasia, or aplastic anemia). It seems likely that, in those diseases, significantly increased doses (pharmacological doses) of erythropoietin will be necessary. This is in contrast to the application of erythropoietin in the therapy for renal anemia, which is predominantly caused by inadequate production of erythropoietin and can therefore be considered a substitution therapy, similar to therapy for diabetes mellitus with insulin.

If the efficacy of the hematopoietins, either alone or in combination, which up to now has been mostly demonstrated in smaller studies, can be reproduced in large randomized studies, and if no dramatic or side effects not previously observed occur, safety and efficacy of tumor therapy, radiation therapy, and bone marrow transplantation will probably be drastically improved by use of this new family of peptide hormones. Up to now, it has been unclear whether an increase of cytotoxic drugs by 1.5- to 2-fold will increase the curative rate in certain malignancies. Still, reduction of the side effects of myelotoxic therapy regimens in tumor patients will lead to a clear improvement of quality of life in these patients.

References

1. Herrmann F, Mertelsmann R (1989) Polypeptides controlling hematopoietic blood cell development and activation. II. Clinial results. Blut 58:173
2. Tracey KJ, Fong Y, Hesse DG et al. (1987) Anticachectin/TNF monoclonal antibodies prevent septic shock during lethal bacteraemia. Nature 330:662
3. Bronchud MH, Scarffe JH, Thatcher N et al. (1987) Phase I/II study of recombinant human granulocyte colony-stimulating factor in patients receiving intensive chemotherapy for small cell lung cancer. Br J Cancer 56:809
4. Antman KS, Griffin JD, Elisas A et al. (1988) Effect of recombinant human granulocyte-macrophage colony-stimulating factor on chemotherapy-induced myelosuppression. N Engl J Med 319:593
5. Herrmann F, Schulz G, Lindemann A et al. (1989) Hematopoietic responses in patients with advanced malignancy treated with recombinant human granulocyte-macrophage colony-stimulating factor. J Clin Oncol 7:159

6. Gabrilove JL, Jakubowski A, Scher H et al. (1988) Effect of granulocyte colony-stimulating factor on neutropenia and associated morbidity due to chemotherapy for transitional-cell carcinoma of the urothelium. N Engl J Med 318:1414
7. Herrmann F, Schulz G, Wieser M et al. (1989) Effect of GM-CSF on neutropenia and related morbidity induced by myelotoxic chemotherapy. Am J Med (in press)
8. Groopman JE, Misuyasu RT, De Leo MJ et al. (1987) Effects of recombinant human granulocyte-macrophage colony-stimulating factor on myelopoiesis in the acquired immunodeficiency syndrome. N Engl J Med 317:593
9. Vadhan-Raj S, Keating J, Le Maistre A et al. (1987) Effects of recombinant human granulocyte-macrophage colony-stimulating factor in patients with myelodysplastic syndromes. N Engl J Med 317:1547
10. Champlin RE, Nimer SD, Oette D et al. (1988) Granulocyte-macrophage colony-stimulating factor (GM-CSF) treatment for aplastic anemia (AA) or agranulocytosis. Exp Hematol 6:238a
11. Bonilla MA, Gillio AP, Ruggiero M et al. (1988) Correction of neutropenia in patients with congenital agranulocytosis with recombinant human granulocyte colony-stimulating factor. Exp Hematol 5:243a
12. Oster W, Mertelsmann R, Herrmann F (1989) Role of Colony-Stimulating Factors in the Biology of Acute Myelogenous Leukemia. Internal. J Cell Clon 7:13
13. Herrmann F, Schulz G, Klein H (1989) Recombinant human G-CSF in patients with myelodysplastic syndrome. Leukemia (in press)
14. Ruff MR, Farrar WL, Pert CB (1986) Interferon-gamma and granulocyte/macrophage colony-stimulating factor inhibit growth and induce antigens characteristic of myeloid differentiation in small-cell lung cancer cell lines. Proc Natl Acad Sci USA 83:6613
15. Berdel WE, Danhauser-Riedl S, Steinhauser G, Winton EF (1989) Various human hematopoietic growth factors (IL-3, GM-CSF, G-CSF) stimulate clonal growth of nonhematopoietic tumor cells. Blood 73:80
16. Dedhar S, Gaboury L, Galloway P, Eaves C (1988) Human GM-CSF is a growth factor active on a variety of cell types of nonhematopoietic origin. Proc Natl Acad Sci USA 85:9253
17. Eschbach JW, Egrie JC, Downing MR et al. (1987) Correction of the anemia of end-stage renal disease with recombinant human Erythropoietin. N Engl J Med 316:73

Interleukin-1 and Tumor Necrosis Factor Production in Acute Nonlymphoid Leukemia

G. Specchia,[1] E. Erroi, F. Colotta, L. Bersani, N. Pansini, A. Mantovani, and V. Liso

Introduction

Interleukin-1 (IL-1) is a cytokine with an important role in host defense against a number of inflammatory and immunologic challenges. Molecular studies have revealed the existence of two distinct but related species of IL-1, designated IL-1α and IL-1β, which act through a common receptor [6] and appear to have very similar if not identical, biological activities [15]. IL-1 induces the release of other cytokines such as IL-2 [23], inteferon [11], granulocyte-macrophage–colony-stimulating factor (GM-CSF) [25] and granulocyte–colony-stimulating factor (G-CSF) [24]. In vascular endothelium GM-CSF is involved in IL-1-induced colony-stimulating activity (CSA) [22]. Although different cell types have the capacity to produce IL-1, cells of the monocyte-macrophage lineage are a major source of IL-1 [19]. Upon appropriate stimulation, mononuclear phagocytes also release tumor necrosis factor (TNF), a monokine unrelated to IL-1 but with several biological activities [4,18]. IL-1 has been shown to have radioprotective activity in mice [17], an effect that may be related to its direct or indirect action on bone marrow precursors. The capacity of IL-1 to affect hemopoietic precursors together with its action on vessel wall hemostatic properties [14] prompted us to investigate the production of IL-1 in acute nonlymphoid leukemia (ANLL). We report that freshly isolated ANLL cells release considerable amounts of IL-1 upon endotoxin stimulation. Production of IL-1 was maximal in M4-M5 leukemias, but appreciable release of this monokine was also detected in most M1-M3 cases. In contrast, TNF release was restricted to M5 leukemias.

Material and Methods

Leukemic cells. Bone marrow and peripheral blood cell samples were studied at diagnosis. The mononuclear cell fraction was obtained by Ficoll-Hypaque density gradient sedimentation and depleted of monocytes (except

---

[1] Hematology Service, University of Bari, I-70100 Bari, Italy

Fleischer (Ed.) Leukemias
© Springer-Verlag Berlin Heidelberg 1993

for M5 cases) by plastic adherence at 37°C. The diagnosis and classification of ANLL were made by standard criteria according to morphology, cyto-chemical staining [2], and surface marker analysis using a panel of anti-bodies directed against antigens expressed by myelomonocytic cells.

IL-1 Assay. Leukemic cells were resuspended in RPMI 1640 complete medium with 10% fetal bovine serum (FBS). Media and FBS used in the present study were screened for endotoxin contamination using a Limulus assay and found to be negative. Cells (2.5×10^6/ml) were seeded in Petri dishes and cultivated in the presence or absence of lipopolysaccharide (LPS) for 24 h at 37°C. At the end of the incubation, samples were centrifuged at $400\,g$ for 10 min and the supernatants stored at -80°C until used. Supernatants were tested for IL-1 activity by the thymocyte proliferation assay method, as previously described [20], with minor modifications. In order to establish that thymocytes' costimulating activity was indeed to be attributed to IL-1, in a series of tests a specific anti-IL-1 rabbit antiserum was used.

TNF Assay. Mononuclear cells were resuspended in medium at a con-centration of 2.5×10^6 cells/ml and cultivated for 4–5 h at 37°C in the presence or absence of 10 μg/ml LPS. Supernatants were harvested, cen-trifuged at $550\,g$ for 10 min and stored at -20°C until use. To assess the presence of TNF in these supernatants, we used a cytotoxic assay against actinomycin D- (act-D)-treated WEHI 164 sarcoma cells in a 6 h ^{51}Cr-release assay, a system in which drug-treated target cells are highly suscep-tible to TNF-mediated lysis [3]. To ascertain that the lytic activity against act-D-treated WEHI 164 sarcoma cells was indeed to be attributed to TNF, in a series of experiments a specific rabbit anti-TNF antibody was used.

Analysis of mRNA Levels. Northern blot analysis was carried out according to standard procedures [13]. Total RNA was isolated by the guanidine isothiocyanate method [5] and analyzed by electrophoresis through 1% agarose formaldehyde gel, followed by northern blot transfer to gene screen plus membranes. IL-1β cDNA clone [1] was labeled by the random priming method [7]. Membranes were pretreated and hybridized in 50% formamide with 10% dextran sulfate and washed with 2× saline sodium citrate (SSC) and 1% sodium dodecyl sulfate (SDS) at 60°C for 30 min. Membranes were exposed for 4–8 at -80°C using intensifying screens. The IL-1β probe was removed and hybridized to an α-actin probe under the same conditions.

Results

IL-1 and TNF were measured the in the supernatants of ANLL cells cultured for 24 and 4 h, respectively, in the absence of stimulation (spontaneous release) or in the presence of endotoxin. Patients were heterogeneous in

Table 1. Production of IL-1 and TNF in acute nonlymphoid leukemia

Case No.	FAB classification	IL-1 release[a]				TNF release[b]	
		Bone marrow		Blood		Blood	
		− LPS	+ LPS	− LPS	+ LPS	− LPS	+ LPS
1	M1	nt	nt	<0.01	4	<0.1	<0.1
2	M1	11	12	75	52	<0.1	<0.1
3	M1	nt	nt	69	115	<0.1	<0.1
4	M1	<0.01	27	9	66	<0.1	<0.1
5	M1	<0.01	<0.01	13	16	<0.1	<0.1
6	M1	<0.01	<0.01	<0.01	<0.01	<0.1	<0.1
7	M1	<0.01	<0.01	<0.01	<0.01	<0.1	<0.1
8	M1	<0.01	<0.01	<0.01	<0.01	<0.1	<0.1
9	M2	5	5	13	13	<0.1	<0.1
10	M2	<0.01	<0.01	<0.01	4	<0.1	<0.1
11	M2	<0.01	<0.01	10	18	<0.1	<0.1
12	M3	<0.01	<0.01	<0.01	57	<0.1	<0.1
13	M3	<0.01	<0.01	7	6	<0.1	<0.1
14	M3	<0.01	10	<0.01	19	<0.1	<0.1
15	M3	<0.01	<0.01	3	8	<0.1	<0.1
16	M4	69	69	28	43	<0.1	<0.1
17	M4	45	76	15	18	<0.1	<0.1
18	M5a	81	69	69	110	500	1000
19	M5b	<0.01	<0.01	<0.01	43	<0.1	<0.1
20	M5b	60	110	72	156	<0.1	125
21	M5b	240	960	216	960	<0.1	125
22	M5a	80	110	67	125	400	850
23	M5b	60	90	85	97	240	620
24	M5b	120	240	180	420	<0.1	100
25	M5a	65	110	78	220	<0.1	240

[a] Units produced by 2.5×10^6 cells in 24 h. Endotoxin-stimulated normal monocytes ($n = 15$) released 137 ± 40 U/25×10^6 cells of IL-1.
[b] Units produced by 2.5×10^6 cells in 4 h. Normal monocytes ($n = 30$) released 400 ± 250 U/2.5×10^6 cells of TNF.
nt, not tested

their capacity to release IL-1 and TNF (Table 1). In three patients [French-American-British Group classification (FAB) M1] we were unable to demonstrate any IL-1 release using bone marrow or blood cells cultured with or without endotoxin. IL-1 release was detected in 9 of 23 bone marrow samples and in 17 of 25 perioheral blood samples. Comparison of M4−M5 cases with M1−M3 leukemias revealed that, while IL-1 production was not restricted to any specific stage of differentiation, lymphokine release was observed more frequently and at higher levels in the more differentiated M4−M5 cases. All M4−M5 leukemia samples showed IL-1-releasing capacity with 117 U/2.5×10^6 cells (median value range, $18 - 960$ U) released by blood cells in the presence of endotoxin, while three of eight M1 cases had no appreciable IL-1 release, and IL-1 levels for M1−M3 blood cells in the presence of endotoxin ranged from less than 0.01 to 115 U; median value, 17 U/2.5 × 10^6 cells. The different IL-1-releasing capacity of M4–M5 ANLL cases versus M1–M3 leukemias is particularly pronounced when bone marrow samples are considered. The IL-1-producing capacity is shared by ANLL through the FAB classes, but the potential for IL-1 release is found more frequently and at higher levels in the M4–M5 leukemia cases. TNF was evaluated in supernatants from the same ANLL cases. In contrast to IL-1 production, TNF release was restricted to M5 ANLL. No M1-through-M4 ANLL cases showed appreciable levels of TNF release as detected by the bioassay used in the present study. Of the eight M5 patients with TNF-releasing capacity, three showed TNF release in the absence of deliberate stimulation, whereas in seven cases, TNF reactivity was only detected in samples exposed to endotoxin. IL-1 and TNF release by ANLL cells was detected using bioassays. In order to ascertain that thymocyte costimulating activity (IL-1) and cytotoxicity (TNF) were indeed attributable to specific mediators in a number of experiments, ANLL supernatants were treated with appropriate specific antibodies. Anti-IL-1 and anti-TNF antibodies abolished the thymocyte costimulating activity and cytotoxicity of ANLL supernatants. In an effort to investigate whether ANLL cells from some patients indeed had the potential to produce IL-1 constitutively, the presence of IL-1 mRNA was sought immediately after isolation of ANLL cells. Northern blot analysis revealed the existence of appreciable levels of IL-1β transcripts. IL-1β transcript in ANLL was of the same size (1.8 kb) as that detected in endotoxin-stimulated normal monocytes.

Discussion

The results reported here demonstrate that some ANLL leukemias have the capacity to produce IL-1 and TNF, as identified by using appropriate bioassays, blocked by specific antibodies. Moreover, northern blot analysis revealed that ANLL cells express IL-1β and TNF mRNA. Lachmann et al. [12] had already reported that some ANLL cells can be a source of IL-1. The present study demonstrated that IL-1-producing ability is shared by ANLL leukemias of different FAB subtypes. However, IL-1 production was quantitatively greater and more frequently observed in the M4 and M5 ANLL cases. Along the same lines, Furukawa et al. [8] reported that endotoxin-induced costimulatory activity was greater in M4–M5 versus M1–M3 cases. ANLL leukemias of different subtypes were able to produce IL-1. In contrast to IL-1, TNF was only measurable in the culture supernatants of seven or eight M5 cases studied. TNF has been identified as a product of mononuclear phagocytes [4,18]. The present observation raises the interesting possibility that TNF release may help the typing of ANLL leukemias. An intriguing observation made in the present study was that a considerable proportion of ANLL cases released IL-1 culture in the absence of deliberate stimulation. In the absence of in vitro culture, freshly isolated ANLL cells expressed IL-1β mRNA. Griffin et al. [9] have recently demonstrated the presence of IL-1β mRNA in 10 of 17 ANLL patients. The IL-1-producing capacity of ANLL cells could play an important role in the regulation of their proliferative capacity. The hematopoietic growth factor, hemopoietin-1, has been identified as IL-1 [16]. Hemopoietin-1 had been identified as a hematopoietic growth factor capable of synergizing with CSF [16]. Moreover, GM-CSF has been shown to promote the proliferation of leukemic clonogenic cells in ANLL [21]. Along the same line, IL-1 has been shown to stimulate CSF production by widely distributed cell types such as vascular endothelia and fibroblasts [19]. Hoang et al. [10] reported that rIL-1 acts synergistically with GM-CSF or G-CSF in the stimulation of clonogenic cells from many patients with ANLL. Hence, IL-1 produced by leukemic cells may trigger amplifying paracrine circuits in promotion of leukemia proliferation.

References

1. Auron PE, Webb AC, Rosenwasser LJ et al. (1984) Nucleotide sequence of human monocyte interleukin 1 precursor cDNA. Proc Natl Acad Sci USA 81:7907–7911
2. Bennett JM, Katovsky D, Daniel MC et al. (1976) Proposals for the classification of the acute leukemias. Br J Haematol 33:451
3. Bersani L, Colotta F, Mantovani A (1986) Involvement of tumor necrosis factor in monocyte-mediated rapid killing of actinomycin D-pretreated WEHI 164 sarcoma cells. Immunology 59:323–326
4. Beutler B, Cerami A (1986) Cachectin and tumor necrosis factor as two sides of the same biological coin. Nature 320:584–588
5. Chirgwin JM, Przybyla AE, MacDonald RJ, Rutter WJ (1979) Isolation of biologically active ribonucleic acid from sources enriched in ribonuclease. Biochemistry 18: 5294–5299
6. Dower SK, Kronheim SR, Hopp TP, Cantrell M, Deeley M, Gillis S, Henney CS, Urdal DL (1986) The cell surface receptors for interleukin-1α and interleukin-1β are identical. Nature 324:266–268
7. Feinberg AP, Vogelstein B (1983) A technique for radiolabeling DNA restriction endonuclease fragments to high specific activity. Anal Biochem 132:6–13
8. Furukawa Y, Ohta M, Miura Y, Saito M (1987) Interleukin-1 producing ability of leukemia cells and its relationship to morphological diagnosis. Br J Haematol 65: 11–15
9. Griffin JB, Rambaldi A, Vellenga E, Young DC, Ostapovicz D, Cannistra SA (1987) Secretion of interleukin-1 by acute myeloblastic leukemia cells in vitro induces endothelial cells to secrete colony stimulating factors. Blood 70:1218–1221
10. Hoang T, Haman A, Goncalves O, Letendre F, Mathieu M, Wong GG, Clark SC (1988) Interleukin-1 enhances growth factor-dependent proliferation of the clonogenic cells in acute myeloblastic leukemia and of normal human primitive hemopoietic precursors. J Exp Med 168:463
11. Kasahara T, Mukaida N, Hatake K (1985) Interleukin-1 (IL-1) dependent lymphokine production by human leukemic T cell line HSB-2 subclones. J Immunol 134:1682
12. Lachman LB, Moore JO, Metzgar RS (1978) Preparation and characterization of limphocytes-activating factor (LAF) from acute monocytic and myelomonocytic leukemia cells. Cell Immunol 41:199–206

13. Maniatis T (1982) Molecular Cloning. Cold Spring Harbor Laboratory, Cold Spring Harbor
14. Mantovani A, Dejana E (1987) Modulation of endothelial function by interleukin-1. A novel target for pharmacological interventation? Biochem Pharmacol 36:301–305
15. March CJ, Mosley B, Larsen A, Cerretti DP, Braedt G, Price V, Gillis S, Henney CS, Kronheim SR, Grabstein K, Conlon PJ, Hopp TP, Cosman D (1985) Cloning, sequence and expression of two distinct human interleukin-1 complementary cDNAs. Nature 315:641
16. Moore MAS, Warren DJ (1987) IL-1 and CSF synergism: Stimulation of stem cell recovery and hemopoietic regeneration following 5-fluorouracil treatment of mice. Proc Natl Acad Sci USA 84:7134
17. Neta R, Douches S, Oppenheim JJ (1986) Interleukin-1 is a radioprotector. J Immunol 136:2483–2485
18. Old LJ (1985) Tumor necrosis factor (TNF). Science 230:630–632
19. Oppenheim JJ, Kovacs EJ, Matsushima K, Durum SK (1986) There is more than one interleukin-1. Immunol Today 7:45–56
20. Rossi V, Breviario F, Ghezzi P, Dejana E, Mantovani A (1985) Prostacyclin synthesis induced in vascular cells by interleukin-1. Science 229:174–176
21. Sakai K, Hattori T, Matsouka M et al. (1987) Autocrine stimulation of interleukin-1β in acute myelogenous leukemia cells. J Exp Med 166:1597–1602
22. Sieff CA (1987) Hematopoietic growth factors. J Clin Invest 79:1549–1557
23. Smith KA, Lachman LB, Oppenheim JJ, Favata MF (1980) The functional relationship of the interleukins. J Exp Med 151:1551
24. Zsebo KM, Yuschenkoff VN, Schutter S, Chang D, McCall E, Dinarello CA, Altrock B, Bagby GC Jr (1988) Vascular endothelial cells and granulopoiesis: interleukin-1 stimulates release of G-CSF and GM-CSF. Blood 71:99
25. Zucali JR, Dinarello CA, Oblon DJ, Gross MA, Anderson L, Weiner RS (1986) Interleukin-1 stimulates fibroblasts to produce granulocyte-macrophage colony stimulating activity and prostaglandin E2. J Clin Invest 77:1857

Interleukin-2: Biological Activities and Clinical Relevance in Advanced Stage Human Cancer

H. Poliwoda,[1] H. Kirchner, and J. Atzpodien

Interleukin-2 (IL-2), originally described as T cell growth factor by Morgan et al. in 1975 [29], is the first of a new kind of immunotherapeutic agents which work against established tumors through the modulation of host immune functions. Cloning of the human gene for IL-2 and subsequent expression in *E. coli* has allowed for the large scale production and use of IL-2 in laboratory and clinical studies.

Biology of IL-2

IL-2 is naturally produced and secreted by T cells. The biological effects of IL-2 comprise a plethora of immunomodulatory functions, most prominently the induction in natural killer (NK) cells and T lymphocytes of major histocompatibility complex (MHC) nonrestricted cytolytic activity against tumors [2,10,17,26]. IL-2, at concentrations between 100 and 1000 U/ml, is known to be optimal for the ex vivo cytotoxic activation and propagation of peripheral blood lymphocytes [3,44]. In addition, IL-2 has been shown to induce humoral cytotoxicity via induction of interferon-γ, tumor necrosis factor-α and -β (TNF-α and -β), and immunoglobulins in mononuclear cell populations responding to IL-2; besides NK and T cells, macrophages and B cells have been found to exhibit functionally active IL-2 receptors [10,13, 32,48,51,55]. While the relative contributions of cell- vs cytokine-mediated antitumor responses following IL-2 remain to be defined [39], it is believed that the lytic effects of high-dose IL-2 are partly due to the induction of secondary cytotoxic cytokines [14,32,39,53].

Clinical Trials

In most clinical trials involving IL-2, patient follow-up has been short; and only limited data have become available from controlled prospective and

---

[1] Department of Hematology and Oncology, MHH University Medical Center, W-3000 Hannover 61, FRG

Fleischer (Ed.) Leukemias
© Springer-Verlag Berlin Heidelberg 1993

Table 1. Interleukin-2 in the immunotherapy of cancer: overview of clinical trials

Investigator	Trial	Reference No.	No. of patients	Responders (%)
Rosenberg 1988	i.v. IL-2	40	79	17
Mitchell 1988	IL-2 + cyclophosphamide	28	24	25
West 1987	IL-2 + LAK cells	52	40	33
Rosenberg 1988	IL-2 + LAK cells	40	139	21
Fisher 1988	IL-2 + LAK cells	18	32	16
Topalian 1988	IL-2 + TIL	47	12	25
Rosenberg 1988	IL-2 + TIL	41	20	55
Yoshida 1988	IL-2 in malignant glioma	54	23	39
Cortesina 1988	Local IL-2 in head & neck	15	10	60
Eberlein 1988	Low-dose IL-2 + LAK cells	16	29	45
Atzpodien, Kirchner 1990	s.c. IL-2 + IFN-α	6	35	36

Responders include complete and partial remissions.

randomized clinical studies. As yet, IL-2 has shown some promise in the treatment of metastatic renal cell cancer and malignant melanoma.

In December of 1985, Rosenberg and colleagues at the National Cancer Institute, for the first time, reported clinical antitumor responses upon administration of large numbers of cytotoxic lymphocytes, lymphokine-activated killer cells (LAK cells), which had been generated in vitro by incubation with IL-2 of patient-derived peripheral blood mononuclear cells [35].

The first LAK/IL-2 protocol by Rosenberg et al. called for the in vivo application of high dosages of IL-2 (100 000 U/kg as i.v. bolus × 3/day) in conjunction with the harvest, in vitro culturing, and subsequent reinfusion of autologous IL-2-activated killer (LAK) cells [35,37]. Leukapheresis techniques were employed for the separation of large numbers of peripheral blood-derived LAK precursor cells; following the IL-2-mediated induction of autologous killer lymphocytes in vitro, cells were returned into the patient together with bolus dosages of i.v. IL-2, which were administered to augment and prolong the antitumor efficacy of LAK cells in vivo [35,37,38]. In a progress report on the treatment of 106 patients with advanced cancer using LAK cells and IL-2, Rosenberg reported partial and complete antitumor responses in 12 out of 36 patients (33%) with renal cell cancer, 6 out of 26 patients (23%) with melanoma, 3 out of 26 patients (12%) with colorectal cancer, and 2 out of 2 patients presenting with non-Hodgkin's lymphoma. In contrast, no responses were observed in 6 sarcomas, 5 adenocarcinomas of the lung, and 5 other malignancies [37].

Based on these preliminary data, a variety of clinical trials in advanced stage cancer patients (Table 1) have been initiated using IL-2 alone, and in combination with activated cytotoxic lymphocytes, other biological response modifiers, or cytostatic drugs. So far, most centers, including our own institution, have reported clinical results comparable to that observed by Rosenberg and colleagues; however, more work will be needed to define both the frequency and duration of clinical responses.

Toxicity of IL-2

High-dose IL-2 therapy, with and without the adoptive transfer of autologous cytotoxic lymphocytes, is associated with considerable toxicity which may limit both the duration and dosages of treatment [8,18,24,35,37,40,42,52]. The major clinical problems such as severe hypotension and interstitial edema are due to a capillary leak syndrome resulting in intravascular volume depletion upon administration of IL-2; other adverse toxic effects include nausea, vomiting, fever, chills, and malaise [8,18,24,35,37,40,42,52]. Based on these initial observations, attempts have been made to improve the previous treatment protocols and minimize toxicity.

Low-Dose IL-2 in Outpatients

Recently, considerable progress has been made toward lowering the therapeutic dose of IL-2 while concomitantly preserving treatment-induced clinical effects [1,6,16,28]. Preclinical investigations demonstrated the induction of high-affinity IL-2 receptors to enhance responsiveness to lower doses of IL-2. Experimental studies showed fresh, unstimulated peripheral blood lymphocytes (NK cells and a small proportion of T lymphocytes) to respond to IL-2 via an intermediate affinity receptor (β chain; affinity/K_d approx. 5×10^{-10}–$10^{-9}\,M$); activation by high-dose IL-2 was found to induce coexpression of the Tac/α chain (CD25) IL-2 receptor of T lymphocytes, thus resulting in a high-affinity heterodimer receptor molecule (K_d approx. $10^{-11}\,M$) [45,49,51].

As exposure of mononuclear cells to high levels of IL-2 has been demonstrated to both induce non-MHC-restricted lytic activity against tumor and increase mononuclear cell response to IL-2, clinical and biological effects of lower doses of IL-2 are now being investigated [1,6,16,28].

Preclinical and clinical observations by ourselves and others confirm that induction of high-affinity IL-2 receptors allows for a drastic reduction in the dose of IL-2 which will be required for the proliferation and cytotoxic activation of patients' lymphocytes [4].

Based on in vitro data demonstrating the enhancement of IL-2-associated antitumor effects following a dose-reduction of greater than 1 log at our institution, we have now completed a clinical phase II study employing the subcutaneous administration of low-dose IL-2 (starting at 0.15 million U/m^2 twice daily for 6 days per week; EuroCetus, Netherlands) in patients with advanced malignancy. In this clinical trial, while WHO grade 3 and 4

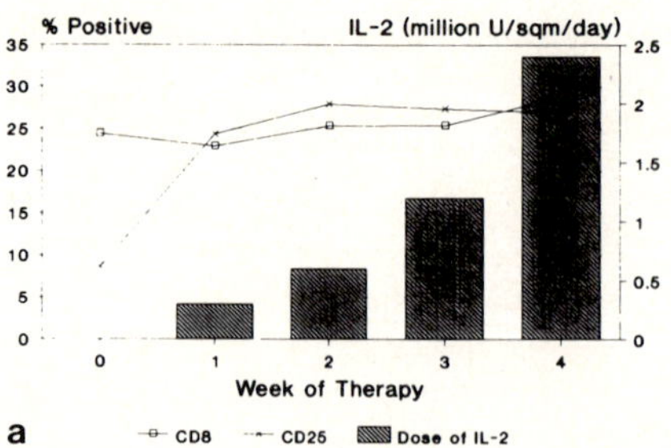

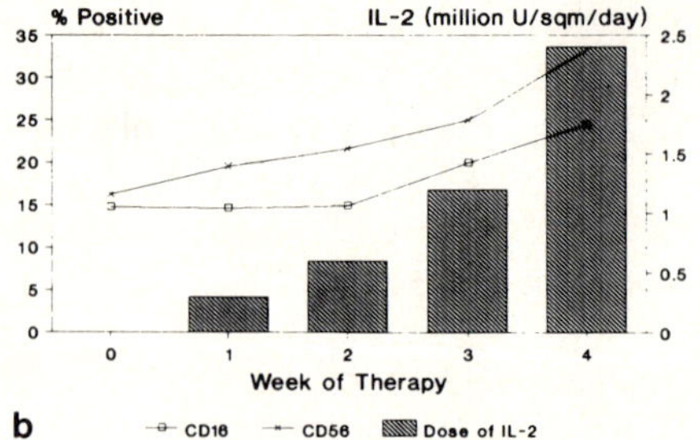

Fig. 1a, b. Peripheral blood lymphocyte subsets in patients receiving subcutaneous IL-2. Patients with advanced malignancy received escalating doses of IL-2, ranging from 0.3 to 2.4 million U/m^2 per day. For phenotypic analyses, peripheral blood lymphocytes were isolated prior to (week 0) and upon therapy (weeks 1 through 4). Lymphocyte subsets were measured by immunofluorescence analysis, whereby cells were separately reacted with monoclonal antibodies against **a** CD8 (T suppressor/cytotoxic cells) and CD25 (Tac α chain IL-2 receptor), and **b** CD16 (Fc receptor) and CD56 (LNK-associated antigen), respectively. Percent positivity was measured using a fluorescence-activated cell sorter (FACS IV; Becton Dickinson, Mountain View, California, USA). All values represent the mean of 11 patients

toxicity was almost totally abrogated when employing low-level subcutaneous IL-2, the immunomodulatory capacity of IL-2 was fully preserved. Thus, preliminary results obtained at our institution show the subcutaneous administration of recombinant IL-2 to produce significant antitumor responses at reduced levels of toxicity. It appears that this novel alternative to the conventional high-dose intravenous IL-2 protocols will introduce antineoplastic immunotherapy to the broader field of ambulatory care [9].

As shown in Fig. 1, the systemic administration of low-dose s.c. IL-2 resulted in a significant expansion in vivo of peripheral blood lymphocyte subsets displaying either CD25, or CD16/CD56 phenotype. Thus, IL-2 at dosages of 0.3–2.4 million U/m^2 per day could induce a three- and twofold increase, respectively, in cells expressing high-affinity IL-2 receptors, and NK-like cells. Concomitantly, a significant increase in cytotoxic activity against standard (K562 and Daudi) tumor targets was noted (data not shown).

IL-2 and Interferon-α

With various alternative modalities of cellular immunotherapy emerging, the combination of recombinant human cytokines has gained increasing relevance for developing new strategies in cancer immunotherapy. Based on animal models, clinical trials are currently under way exploiting the immunomodulatory synergies when combining IL-2 with either interferon-α (IFN-α) [6,12,24,46] or TNF-α [31]. IFN-α is known to upregulate histocompatibility antigens, and also synergize with IL-2 in the activation of cytotoxic effector cells [19]. At our own institution, regressions of advanced stage malignancy are being observed upon the concomitant administration of long-term subcutaneous IL-2 and IFN-α; over a 6-week treatment period, we could achieve partial or complete regression of metastatic disease in 37% of patients presenting with progressive renal cell cancer [6,24].

Tumor-Specific Lymphocytes

With NK and LAK cells providing an unspecific, i.e., non-MHC-restricted, line of defense against tumor, it has been demonstrated that cells other than NK and LAK cells also contribute to IL-2-induced antitumor effects [33].

Cytotoxic T lymphocytes (CTL), by definition, show a productive rearrangement of the α and β chains or γ and δ chains of the CD3-associated T cell receptor (TCR). T cells further exhibit antigen specificity via the TCR-CD3 complex, and recognize tumor only upon expression by target cells of MHC class I (CD3/CD8+ CTL) and MHC class II (CD3/CD4+ cells) antigens, respectively [20,33,43,50]. In contrast, NK cells are defined by their spontaneous and non-MHC-restricted capability to lyse fresh and cultured tumor cells [23,34,55].

Given the considerable controversy on possible mechanisms of target recognition and cell-mediated killing, attempts are being made to define the actual cellular mediators of the antitumor response. While most LAK activity mediated by peripheral blood mononuclear cells in response to IL-2 appears to be attributable to an NK-derived (NKH1/Leu19+ CD3−) cell population, we and others have shown a proportion of T (CD3+) lymphocytes to also account for nonspecific lymphokine-activated killing [2,7,21, 30,34]. When looking at cellular infiltrates of malignant lesions biopsied before and after treatment, a marked increase in the number of CD3+ T lymphocytes (CD4+ or CD8+) was observed; in contrast, there was only little evidence of NKH1/Leu19+ cells mediating direct cytotoxicity at the tumor site, upon activation with IL-2 [14,53].

These findings are consistent with recent observations demonstrating a correlation between MHC class II (HLA-DR) expression on tumor cells and tumor regression following IL-2 therapy [14,25]. Thus, cell-mediated cytotoxicity was observed at increased levels in those tumors displaying a strong expression of MHC antigens. Given this evidence in support of a major role of MHC-restricted T lymphocytes as mediators of IL-2-induced antitumor response, attempts have been made to further isolate and characterize tumor-specific cytotoxic lymphocytes and their progenitors [3,5,11,22,50].

Recently, the selective propagation and subsequent adoptive transfer of tumor-infiltrating lymphocytes (TIL) extracted from freshly resected tumor has been shown to cause significant regression of cancer in patients present-

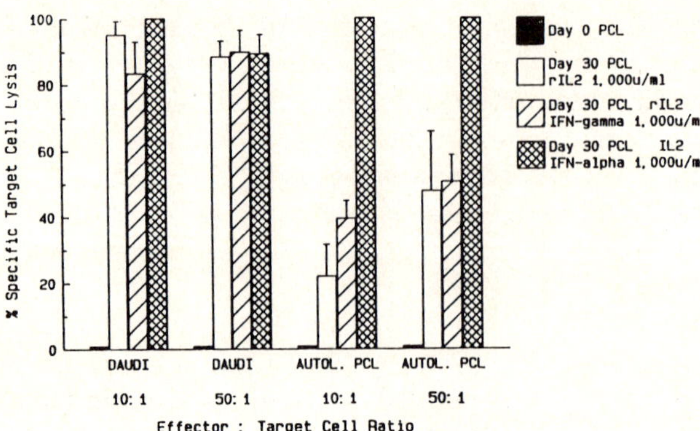

Fig. 2. Effect of IFN-α and -γ on the generation in IL-2-induced plasma cell leukemia (*PCL*) cultures of cell-mediated cytotoxicity against autologous plasma cell leukemia cells (*AUTOL. PCL*) and standard Daudi targets. To assess cytolysis, ^{51}Cr-labeled cells were used as targets in a 4-h radiosotope release assay. Percent-specific target cell lysis by fresh PCL-derived peripheral blood mononuclear cells and PCL peripheral blood mononuclear cells after 4-week culture with IL-2 (1000 U/ml) was compared to percent-specific cytolysis by IL-2-induced PCL peripheral blood mononuclear cells that were preincubated for 18 h in the presence of IFN-α and IFN-γ, respectively. All values represent the mean of three experiments

ing with advanced metastatic malignancy [41,47]. Using an animal model, TIL were found to exhibit cytotoxicity against tumor at levels 50–100 times higher than non-MHC-restricted peripheral blood LAK cells [36]. The overwhelming majority of TIL were found to be CD3+, with varying ratios of CD4+ and CD8+ cells [11,36,41,47]. When employed clinically in patients with metastatic melanoma, cytotoxic TIL could induce objective regression of tumor to the lungs, liver, bone, skin, and subcutaneous sites, respectively, in 11 out of 20 patients treated. Notably, 2 of those patients responding to TIL had previously failed nonadoptive immunotherapy with IL-2 alone [41].

Killer Cells in Leukemia

Among peripheral blood-derived effectors, NK cells constitute a major line of defense against tumor [34]. Thus, the adoptive transfer of autologous LAK cells renders the possibility of enhancing cell-mediated antitumor effects beyond the limits of spontaneous cellular activity in vivo.

Previous studies suggest that cytotoxic activity of NK cells plays an important role in tumor surveillance. Emergence of leukemias and pre-leukemic disorders in humans has been shown to be associated with a decrease of spontaneous NK activity [27]. While the protective potential of both NK and LAK cells against tumor remains to be established, amplification of cellular antitumor functions as employed in clinical adoptive immuno-therapy protocols may circumvent a primary defect of cellular immune functions in cancer [8,18,33,35,37,38,40,52]. Adoptive immunotherapy is likely to restore or augment those antitumor mechanisms that have become ineffective in cancer patients, as reflected by advanced stage disease.

To evaluate the antitumor potential of activated lymphocytes in leukemia, we studied the cell-mediated toxicity against plasma cell leukemia of IL-2 and IL-2 plus IFN-induced killer cells from fresh peripheral blood of patients with plasma cell leukemia. When tested against autologous leukemia cells, patient-derived cytotoxic lymphocytes exhibited significant antileukemic activity (Fig. 2). The generation of specific cytotoxicity in long-term culture of plasma cell leukemia cells with IL-2 was accompanied by a concomitant increase in cytotoxic effector cells from 0% to 40%, coexpress-ing NK (CD56) and T cell (CD3) markers (data not shown). This suggested that the anti-leukemic capacity observed was at least partly due to an NK-like, potentially T-cell-derived effector population [44]. As shown in Fig. 2, a dramatic augmentation of IL-2-induced cytotoxicity could be achieved by preincubating antileukemic effector cells in the presence of IFN-α.

Discussion and Conclusions

Modern immunotherapy of human cancer has evolved as a rapidly expand-ing field of clinical and experimental research. Employing the systemic application of recombinant IL-2 in humans, Rosenberg and colleagues from the National Cancer Institute reported the regression of advanced metastatic tumors in approximately 10%–30% of patients treated. The additional adoptive transfer of autologous patient-derived activated lymphocytes was performed to enhance therapeutic efficacy.

Recently, clinical and experimental studies have been directed toward enhancing both the activation state and the specificity of IL-2-induced killer cells in humans. Considerable toxicity from the use of high-dose IL-2 has prompted attempts to develop low-dose regimens which allow for the broader use of IL-2 in outpatients presenting with poor-prognosis disease.

In summary, at present, the use of biotherapy in cancer is still at an early stage, and much more work will be needed to develop this into an established modality of cancer treatment next to surgery and chemo- and radiotherapy.

The role of biotherapy in multimodality treatment regimens is as yet undefined. Recent studies have demonstrated killer lymphocytes to be among the first immune cells that recur post chemotherapy. Thus, a com-bination or sequential use of chemo- and immunotherapeutic agents may both support restoration of the impaired immune system and contribute to the final cure of minimal residual disease, notably in patients with leukemia.

References

1. Allison MAK, Jones SE, McGuffey P (1989) Phase II trial of outpatient interleukin-2 in malignant lymphoma, chronic lymphocytic leukemia, and selected solid tumors. J Clin Oncol 7:75–80
2. Atzpodien J, Wisniewski D, Gulati SC, Welte K, Knowles RW, Clarkson BD (1987) Interleukin-2- and mitogen-activated NK-like killer cells from highly purified human peripheral blood T cell (CD3+ N901−) cultures. Nat Immun Cell Growth Regul 6:129–140
3. Atzpodien J, Gulati SC, Kwon JH, Kushner BH, Shimazaki C, Bührer C, Öz S, Kolitz JE, Welte K, Clarkson BD (1988) Anti-tumor efficacy of interleukin-2-activated killer cells in human neuroblastoma ex-vivo. Exp Cell Biol 56:236–244
4. Atzpodien J, Kirchner H, Hadam M, Bührer C, Dallmann I, Volgmann TH, Link H, Welte K, Poliwoda H (1988) Lymphokine-activated killing (LAK) and IL-2-receptor expression: perspective for an enhanced therapeutic efficacy. Blut 4 [Suppl] 221
5. Atzpodien J, Shimazaki C, Wisniewski D, Gulati S, Bührer C, Öz S, Link H, Poliwoda H, Welte K, Clarkson B (1989) Interleukin-2 und Interferon-α in der adoptiven Immuntherapie des Plasmozytoms: Ein experimentelles Modell. In: Lutz D, Heinz R, Nowotny H, Stacher A (eds) Leukämien und Lymphome. Forschritte und Hoffnungen. Urban and Schwarzenberg, Munich, pp 211–212
6. Atzpodien J, Körfer A, Franks CR, Poliwoda H, Kirchner H (1990) Outpatient recombinant interleukin-2 and interferon-α_{2b} in advanced human malignancies. Lancet 335:1509–1512
7. Atzopodien J, Bührer C, Gulati SC, Wisniewski D, Öz S, Kirchner H, Benter T, Poliwoda H, Welte K, Clarkson B (1989) Induction of nonspecific cell-mediated cytotoxicity: A multisignal event and its cellular regulation. In: Neth R, Gallo RC (eds) Modern trends in human leukemia VIII. Springer, Berlin Heidelberg New York, pp 273–280
8. Atzpodien J, Link H, Kirchner H, Stahl M, Volgmann TH, Mohr H, Pohl U, Freund M, Schmoll HJ, Poliwoda H (1990) A new, modified protocol for the adoptive immunotherapy of advanced and/or metastatic neoplasms using lymphokine-activated killer (LAK) cells plus natural interleukin-2 (IL-2). In: Jungi WF, Senn HJ (eds) Krebs und Alternativmedizin II. Springer, Berlin Heidelberg New York
9. Atzpodien J, Palmer P, Loriaux E, Hadam M, Schmoll HJ, Poliwoda H, Kirchner H (1989) Biological activities of low-dose interleukin-2 in patients with advanced malignancy. In: Melchers F (ed) Progress in immulogy, vol VII. Springer, Berlin Heidelberg New York
10. Barth NM, Galazka AR, Rudnick SA (1988) Lymphokines and cytokines. In: Oldham RK (ed) Principles of cancer biotherapy. Raven, New York, pp 273–290
11. Belldegrun A, Muul LM, Rosenberg SA (1988) Interleukin-2 expanded tumor infiltrating lymphocytes in human renal cell cancer: isolation, characterization, and antitumor activity. Cancer Res 48:206–214
12. Brunda MJ, Bellantoni D, Sulich V (1987) In vivo anti-tumor activity of combinations of interferon alpha and interleukin-2 in a murine model. Correlation of efficacy with the induction of cells resembling natural killer cells. Int J Cancer 40:3948–3953
13. Carswell EA, Old LJ, Kassel RL (1975) An endotoxin induced serum factor that causes necrosis of tumors. Proc Natl Acad Sci USA 72:3666–3370
14. Cohen PJ, Lotze MT, Roberts JR, Rosenberg SA, Jaffe ES (1987) The immunopathology of sequential tumor biopsies in patients treated with interleukin-2: correlation or response with T-cell infiltration and HLA-DR expression. Am J Pathol 129:208–216
15. Cortesina G, De Stefani A, Giovarelli M, Barioglio MG, Cavallo GV, Jemma C, Forni G (1988) Treatment of recurrent squamous cell carcinoma of the head and neck with low doses of interleukin-2 injected perilymphatically. Cancer 62:2482–2485
16. Eberlein TJ, Schoof DD, Jung SE, Davidson D, Gramolini B, McGrath K, Massaro A, Wilson RE (1988) A new regimen of interleukin 2 and lymphokine-activated killer cells. Arch Intern Med 148:2571–2576

17. Farrar JJ, Benjamin WR, Hilfiker ML, Howard M, Farrar WL, Fuller-Farrar J (1982) The biochemistry, biology, and role of interleukin 2 in the induction of cytotoxic T-cell and antibodyforming B cell responses. Immunol Rev 63:129–166

18. Fisher RI, Coltman CA, Doroshow JH, Rayner AA, Hawkins MJ, Mier JW, Wiernik P, McMannis JD, Weiss GR, Margolin KA, Gemlo BT, Hoth DF, Parkinson DR, Paietta E (1988) Metastatic renal cancer treated with interleukin-2 and lymphokine-activated killer cells. Ann Intern Med 108:518–523

19. Giacomini P, Aguzzi A, Pestha S (1984) Modulation by recombinant DNA leukocyte (α) and fibroblast (β) interferons of the expression and shedding of HLA- and tumor-associated antigens. J Immunol 133:1649–1655

20. Grossman Z, Herberman RB (1986) Natural killer cells and their relationship to T cells: hypothesis on the role of T cell receptor gene rearrangement on the course of adaptive differentiation. Cancer Res 46:2651–2658

21. Herberman RB, Hiserodt J, Vujanovic N, Balch C, Lotzová E, Bolhuis R, Golub S, Lanier LL, Phillips JH, Riccardi C, Ritz J, Santoni A, Schmidt RE, Uchida A (1987) Lymphokine-activated killer cell activity: Characteristics of effector cells and their progenitors in blood and spleen. Immunol Today 8:178–181

22. Hérin M, Lemoine C, Weynants P, Vessière F, Van Pel A, Knuth A, Devos R, Boon T (1987) Production of stable cytolytic T-cell clones directed against autologous human melanoma. Int J Cancer 39:390–396

23. Hersey P, Bolhuis R (1987) "Nonspecific" MHC-unrestricted killer cells and their receptors. Immunol Today 8:233–239

24. Kirchner H, Körfer A, Franks CR, Evers P, Goldmann U, Knüver-Hopf J, Gessner S, Poliwoda H, Atzpodien J (1990) Subcutaneous interleukin-2 and interferon-α in patients with metastatic renal cell cancer: the German outpatient experience. Mol Biother 2:145–154

25. Lobo PI, Spencer CE (1989) Use of anti-HLA antibodies to mask major histocompatibility complex gene products on tumor cells can enhance susceptibility of these cells to lysis by natural killer cells. J Clin Invest 83:278–287

26. Lotze MT, Grimm EA, Mazumder A, Strausser JL, Rosenberg SA (1981) Lysis of fresh and cultured autologous tumor by human lymphocytes cultured in T-cell growth factor. Cancer Res 41:4420–4425

27. Lotzová E, Savary CA, Keating MJ (1982) Studies on the mechanism of defective natural killing in leukemia-diseased patients. Exp Hematol 10:83–88

28. Mitchell MS, Kempf RA, Harel W, Shau H, Boswell WD, Lind S, Bradley EC (1988) Effectiveness and tolerability of low-dose cyclophosphamide and low-dose intravenous interleukin-2 disseminated melanoma. J Clin Oncol 6:409–424

29. Morgan DA, Ruscetti EW, Gallo R (1976) Selective in vitro growth of T-lymphocytes from normal human bone marrow. Science 193:1007–1008

30. Morris DG, Pross HF (1989) Studies of lymphokine-activated killer (LAK) cells. I. Evidence using novel monoclonal antibodies that most human LAK precursor cells share a common surface marker. J Exp Med 169:717–736

31. Nedwin GE, Svedfesky LP, Bringman R (1985) Effect of interleukin 2, interferon-gamma, and mitogens on the production of tumor necrosis factors alpha and beta. J Immunol 135:2492–2497

32. Ortaldo JR, Mason AT, Gerard JP, Henderson LE, Farrar W, Hopkins RF, Herberman RB, Rabin H (1984) Effects of natural and recombinant IL 2 on regulation of IFN production and natural killer activity: Lack of involvement of the Tac antigen for these immunoregulatory effects. J Immunol 133:779–783

33. Ortaldo JR, Longo DL (1988) Human natural lymphocyte effector cells: Definition, analysis of activity, and clinical effectiveness. JNCI 80:999–1010

34. Reynolds CW, Ortaldo JR (1987) Natural killer activity: the definition of a function rather than a cell type. Immunol Today 8:172–174

35. Rosenberg SA, Lotze MT, Muul LM, Leitman S, Chang AE, Ettinghausen SE, Matory YL, Skibber JM, Shilone E, Vetto JT, Seipp CA, Simpson C, Reichert CM (1985) Observations on the systemic administration of autologous lymphokine-activated killer cells and recombinant interleukin-2 to patients with metastatic cancer. N Engl J Med 313:1485–1492

36. Rosenberg SA, Spiess P, Lafreniere R (1986) A new approach to the adoptive immunotherapy of cancer with tumor-infiltrating lymphocytes. Science 233:1318–1321
37. Rosenberg SA, Lotze MT, Muul LM, Chang AE, Avis FP, Leitman S, Linehan WM, Robertson CN, Lee RE, Rubin JT, Seipp CA, Simpson CG, White DE (1987) A progress report on the treatment of 157 patients with advanced cancer using lymphokine-activated killer cells and interleukin-2 or high-dose interleukin-2 alone. N Engl J Med 316:889–897
38. Rosenberg SA (1988) The development of new immunotherapies for the treatment of cancer using interleukin-2. Ann Surg 208:121–135
39. Rosenberg SA (1988) Immunotherapy of cancer using interleukin 2: current status and future prospects. Immunol Today 9:58–62
40. Rosenberg SA, Lotze MT, Mulé JJ (1988) New approaches to the immunotherapy of cancer using interleukin-2. Ann Intern Med 108:853–864
41. Rosenberg SA, Packard BS, Aebersold PM, Solomon D, Topalian SL, Toy ST, Simon P, Lotze MT, Yang JC, Seipp CA, Simpson C, Carter C, Bock S, Schwartzentruber D, Wei JP, White DE (1988) Use of tumor-infiltrating lymphocytes and interleukin-2 in the immunotherapy of patients with metastatic melanoma. N Engl J Med 319:1676–1680
42. Rosenstein M, Ettinghausen SE, Rosenberg SA (1986) Extravasation of intravascular fluid mediated by the systemic administration of recombinant interleukin-2. J Immunol 137:1735–1742
43. Royer HD, Reinherz EL (1987) T lymphocytes: Ontogeny, function, and relevance to clinical disorders. N Engl J Med 317:1136–1142
44. Shimazaki C, Atzpodien J, Wisniewski D, Gulati SC, Kolitz JE, Clark-son BD (1988) Cell-mediated toxicity of interleukin-2-activated lymphocytes against autologous and allogeneic human myeloma calls. Acta Haematol (Basel) 80:203–209
45. Siegel JP, Sharon M, Smith PL, Leonard WJ (1987) The IL-2 receptor β chain (p70): role in mediating signals for LAK, NK, and proliferative activities. Science 238:75–78
46. Spiegel RE (1987) The alpha interferons: clinical overview. Semin Oncol 14:1–12
47. Topalian SL, Solomon D, Avis FP, Chang AE, Freersen DL, Linehan WM, Lotze MT, Robertson CN, Seipp CA, Simon P, Simpson CG, Rosenberg SA (1988) Immunotherapy of patients with advanced cancer using tumor-infiltrating lymphocytes and recombinant interleukin-2: a pilot study. J Clin Oncol 6:839–853
48. Trinchieri G, Perussia B (1985) Immune interferon: a pleiotropic lymphokine with multiple effects. Immunol Today 6:131–136
49. Tsudo M, Goldman CK, Bongiovanni KF, Chan WC, Winton EF, Yagita M, Grimm EA, Waldmann TA (1987) The p75 peptide is the receptor for interleukin 2 expressed on large granular lymphocytes and is responsible for the interleukin 2 activation of these cells. Proc Natl Acad Sci USA 84:5394–5398
50. Uchida A, Moore M, Klein E (1988) Autologous mixed lymphocyte-tumor reaction and autologous mixed lymphocyte reaction. II. Generation of specific and non-specific killer T cells capable of lysing autologous tumor. Int J Cancer 41:651–656
51. Wang HM, Smith KA (1987) The interleukin 2 receptors. J Exp Med 166:1055–1069
52. West WH, Tauer KW, Yannelli JR, Marshall GD, Orr DW, Thurman GB, Old-ham RK (1987) Constant-infusion recombinant interleukin-2 in adoptive immunotherapy of advanced cancer. N Engl J Med 316:898–905
53. Yamamura T, Fujitani Y, Kawauchi T, Wada E, Kobayashi Y, Yoshikawa K, Owaga H, Sugiyama H, Ohsawa M, Aozasa K (1989) Histological evidence of natural killer cell aggregation against malignant melanoma induced by adoptive immunotherapy with lymphokine-activated killer cells. J Pathol 157:201–204
54. Yoshida S, Tanaka R, Takai N, Ono K (1988) Local administration of autologous lymphokine-activated killer cells and recombinant interleukin 2 to patients with malignant brain tumors. Cancer Res 48:5011–5016
55. Young JDE, Liu CC (1988) Multiple mechanisms of lymphocyte-mediated killing. Immunol Today 9:140–144

Interleukin-2 in the Treatment of Cancer Disease: Introduction of a Therapeutic Model and some Immunological Data*

E. Weidmann,[1] L. Bergmann, P. Hechler, U. Schwulera, H. Grieser, and P.S. Mitrou

Introduction

Therapeutic administration of interleukin-2 (IL-2) in patients with metastatic cancer disease has been shown to lead to tumor regression [1]. This therapeutic approach is associated with the activation of cytotoxic cell populations [2], proliferation of various lymphocyte subsets [3], and induction of secondary cytokines released by different effectors of the human immunes system [4].

Although many studies of the physiology of IL-2 were undertaken, some questions related to the antitumor activity and to the mediation of side effects are unsolved. From in vitro studies it is increasingly evident that the lymphokine-activated killer (LAK) cell population is heterogeneous. Cells expressing T-cell or natural killer (NK) cell antigens have been shown to mediate lysis of tumor cells [5,6]. In vivo LAK cells were described to demonstrate a $CD3^-$ $CD56^+$ phenotype [7]. After bolus administration of IL-2 the release of tumor necrosis factor- (TNF)-alpha and interferon-gamma (IFN-γ) could be detected [4]. The importance of these cytokines for antitumor efficacy is unclear.

The present study was undertaken to identify the changes of antigen expression on T-cells and NK cells and to characterize cytotoxic lymphocyte populations after discontinuation of IL-2 therapy. Since the release of secondary cytokines was described after bolus injection of IL-2 [4], we looked for serum levels of TNF-α, IFN-γ, and soluble IL-2 recptors during continuous infusion of IL-2.

Patients and Methods

Patients. All immunologic investigations were performed in patients with advanced renal cell cancer or malignant melanoma, undergoing a period of

---

* This work was supported by the Bundesministerium für Forschung und Technologie (Grant 01GA8802), Cilly-Weilstiftung, Riese-Stiftung and the Paul and Ursula Klein Stiftung.

[1] Division of Hematology, Department of Internal Medicine, J.W. Goethe-University, W-6000 Frankfurt, FRG

Fleischer (Ed.) Leukemias
© Springer-Verlag Berlin Heidelberg 1993

continuous intravenous infusion of 3×10^6 U recombinant IL-2/m^2 per day (rIL-2, EuroCetus, Amsterdam, Netherlands) for 5 days.

Analyses and Isolation of Lymphocyte Subsets. Peripheral lymphocytes were stained with fluorescein isothiocyanate (FITC) or plycoerythrin (PE) labeled monoclonal antibodies (CD2, CD3, CD4, CD8, CD19, CD25, CD56, and anti-HLA-DR; Becton Dickinson, Heidelberg, FRG) before and 24–36 h after IL-2 therapy. Quantitative analyses and separation of lymphocyte subsets were performed by double fluorescent technic using a flow cytometer (FACStar, Becton Dickinson).

Cytotoxic assays. The cytotoxic activity of isolated lymphocyte subsets were tested against K562 and Daudi tumor target cell lines using the standard chromium-51-release assay as described elsewhere [8]. Effector to target ratio was 5:1. Lysis of tumor targets was calculated by the determination of chromium-51-release in the supernatants of the test cultures.

TNF-α, IFN-γ, and Free IL-2-Receptor Assays. Serum levels of TNF-α and IFN-γ were determined with immunoradiometric assays (IRMA: TNF IRMA and IFN-γ IRMA; Medgenix Fleurus, Belgium) and of soluble IL-2 receptors with an enzyme-linked immunosorbent assay (ELISA: IL-2r ELISA; T-Cell Sciences, Cambridge, MA, USA).

Results

A rebound lymphocytosis in the peripheral blood of the patients was observed 24–36 h after discontinuation of continuous IL-2 infusion for 5 days. This lymphocytosis implied a significant increase of the total counts of all lymphocyte populations (T-, B-, and NK cells and their subsets).

As shown in Fig. 1a, the percentage of HLA-DR antigens and Tac receptors (CD25) was highly expressed on T-cells. Whereas DR antigen was expressecd on both CD4$^+$ and CD8$^+$ populations, allmost all of the Tac receptor positive cells were CD4$^+$. Looking for expression of DR antigen and Tac receptors on CD56$^+$ (Leu 19, NKH1) cells an increasing amount of DR but not of Tac receptors (CD25) could be detected on this population after cessation of IL-2 administration (Fig. 1b). The coexpression of T-cell receptor-associated antigen (CD3) on CD56$^+$ cells slighty increased following IL-2 therapy. This increase was predominantly connected with an augmented CD8 antigen expression, but coexpression of CD4 antigen slightly increased, too (Fig. 1b). In some patients different lymphocyte populations were isolated after completion of IL-2 therapy, and tested for cytotoxic activity (Table 1).

High cytotoxic activity was detected within the non-T–non-B cells, the CD3$^-$ CD56$^+$ cells, the CD3$^-$ CD2$^+$ cells, the CD2$^+$ CD56$^+$, and the

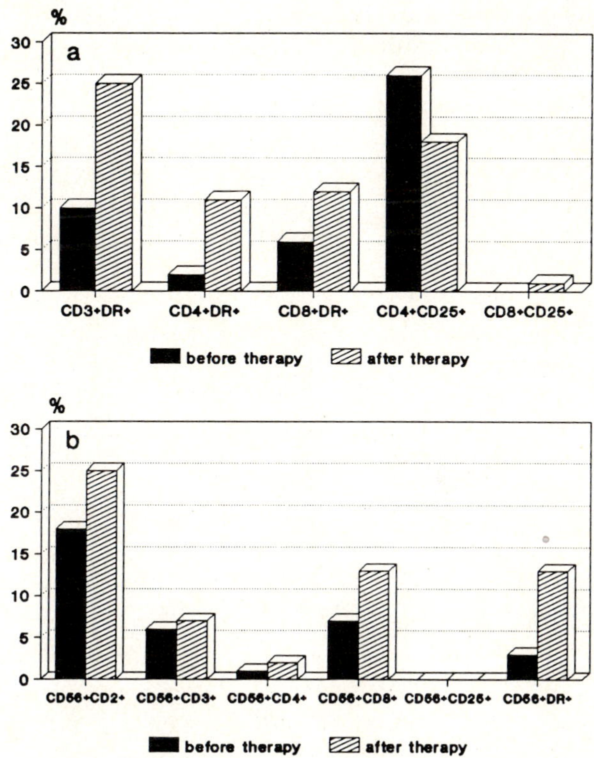

Fig. 1a, b. Percentage of Tac (CD25) and HLA-DR expression on T-cell subsets (**a**) and coexpression of T-cell antigens, Tac, and HLA-DR on CD56$^+$ (NKH1) cells (**b**) before and after continuous intravenous infusion of IL-2 (mean of 8 treatment cycles)

CD3$^+$ CD56$^+$ cells. Within the total T-cell population, which also mediated considerable cytotoxic activity in some patients, the CD8$^+$ lymphocytes were identified to contain cells with lytic capability compared to lower effects of the CD4$^+$ population. CD3$^+$ CD56$^-$ lymphocytes did not show lytic activity (Table 1).

Low amounts of 10–35 U IL-2/ml in the serum of the patients (data not shown) were able to induce considerable release of TNF-α into the serum of patients. TNF serum levels, reaching maxima of 56–120 pg/ml during IL-2 administration remained elevated some days after discontinuation of IL-2 therapy (Fig. 2). In one out of five patients investigated so far for cytokine release during IL-2 therapy, IFN-γ serum levels rising up to 9 U/ml were detectable (data not shown). In all patients high amounts of soluble IL-2 receptors with maximal levels of 10 000–16 000 U/ml were added into the serum (data not shown).

Table 1. Cytotoxic activity of lymphocyte subsets, isolated 24–36 h after IL-2 continuous i.v. infusion

	Lymphocyte subset	Lysis (%)	
		K562	Daudi
Patient 1	CD3+ CD19−	29	40
	CD3− CD19−	n.d.	62
	CD3− CD56+	n.d.	23
	CD3+ CD56−	4	6
	CD3+ CD56+	62	61
Patient 2	CD3+ CD19−	24	4
	CD3− CD19−	52	26
	CD3− CD56+	52	33
	CD3+ CD56−	2	0
	CD3+ CD56+	30	7
Patient 3	CD3+ CD19	22	20
	CD3− CD19−	65	68
	CD3− CD56+	60	58
	CD3− CD56−	14	12
	CD3+ CD56+		
Patient 4	CD2+ CD3−	14	0
	CD2+ CD3−	54	0
	CD4+ CD8−	2	0
	CD8+ CD4−	56	0
Patient 5	CD2+ CD3−	16	1
	CD2+ CD3+	66	24
	CD4+ CD8−	35	7
	CD8+ CD4−	54	26
Patient 6	CD2+ CD56+	n.d.	82

Effector: target ratio = 5 : 1
n.d., no data

Discussion

The current opinion on the source for the antitumor efficacy of IL-2 and the treatment-related side effects is that IL-2 leads to an activation of various lymphocyte populations (including cytotoxic cells) followed by the release of secondary cytokines [9]. Since those complex immunologic responses to the administration of IL-2 in vivo are not finally clarified, the present study was addressed to the questions of how surface antigen expression of T-cell subsets and NK cells changes after continuous infusion of IL-2, which cell populations contain mediators of cytotoxicity, and which further cytokines are released following IL-2. The findings obtained from our investigations are the results of maximal IL-2 serum levels ranging from 10–35 U/ml, measured during a 5-day period of continous IL-2 infusion.

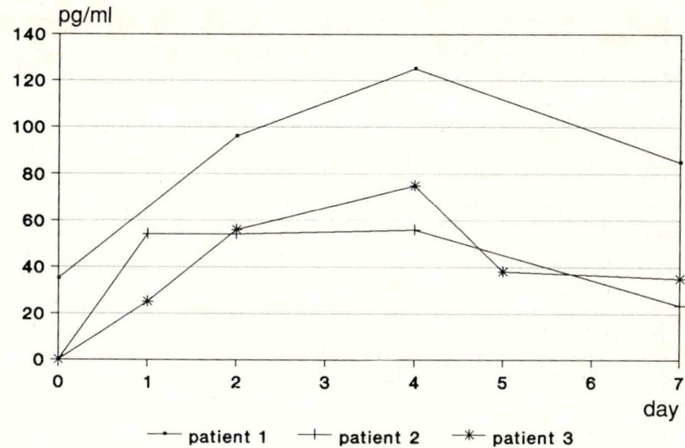

Fig. 2. TNF-alpha release during and after IL-2 continuous intravenous infusion in three patients with renal cell cancer

To get more detailed information about the immunologic phenotypes of T and NK cells, we analysed the expression of HLA-DR antigen and the Tac receptor on $CD4^+$, $CD8^+$, and $CD56^+$ as well as the expression of T-cell-associated antigens on cells with NK phenotype ($CD56^+$). An increased expression of DR antigen was noticed on $CD4^+$, $CD8^+$, and on $CD56^+$ cells. Since the expression of this antigen, which is known to be related to activation of cells, was low before therapy, a rise of DR^+ cells might be a correlate for the activation of both T- and NK cells. IL-2 (Tac) receptors were almost exclusively detected on $CD4^+$ cells. Despite a certain influence of IL-2 on the properties even of $CD8^+$ and $CD56^+$ lymphocytes the importance of this phenomenon remains unclear. One mechanism may be the activation of these Tac receptor negative populations by another IL-2 receptor. As described by Lotze et al. [4] and as confirmed by our investigations, high levels of free IL-2 receptors are measurable during IL-2 therapy. Possibly the $CD8^+$ and $CD56^+$ cells shed Tac receptors before they are detectable with our methods. It has been found that cytotoxic cells, isolated ex vivo after discontinuation of IL-2 therapy, possess the phenotype $CD56^+$ $CD3^-$ [7]. That might be relevant for patients with predominantly $CD3^-$ NK cells. As shown in Fig. 1b, an increase of $CD3^-$ and $CD8^-$ antigens on $CD56^+$ cells could be detected after IL-2 therapy. From in vitro studies it is known that $CD56^+$ cells express a broad variety of cell surface antigens [10]. Therefore we separated different populations of lymphocytes (Table 1) 24–36 h after IL-2 administration and tested them for cytotoxic activity. High cytotoxic activities were detected in $CD3^-$ $CD19^-$, $CD3^-$ $CD2^+$, and $CD56^+$ cells, positive or negative for markers such as CD2, CD3, and CD8.

It remains unclear whether T cells acquire the capability to lyse tumor cells in an NK-like non-MHC-restricted manner, or whether NK cells express

T-cell antigens (CD3, CD8) during maturation and activation. From the results described so far, it seems to be obvious that IL-2 in vivo is a pluripotent activator of functionally different lymphocyte populations. Additionally, IL-2 continuous infusion regularly induces the release of TNF-α and occasionally of IFN-γ, cytokines, which are both involved in the immune system [4]. These secondary cytokines may contribute to immunological changes, to the mediation of side effects, and to antitumor activity connected with IL-2 administration in vivo [9]. Further trials of all these events are necessary to detect the therapeutically expedient mechanisms of IL-2 with the aim to obtain optimal treatment strategies and to avoid abundant side effects.

Acknowledgments. The authors thank Mrs. S. Christ, Mrs. C. Heller, and Mrs. S. Fuck for expert technical assistance.

References

1. Rosenberg SA, Lotze MT, Muul LM, Chang AE, Avis FP, Leitmann S, Linehan M, Robertson CN, Lee RE, Rubin JT, Seipp CA, Simpson CG, White DE (1987) A progress report on the treatment of 157 patients with advanced cancer using lymphokine-activated killer cells and interleukin-2 or high-dose interleukin-2 alone. N Engl J Med 316:889–897
2. Bergmann L, Mitrou PS, Weidmann E, Schmidt-Matthiesen A, Hanke P, Hoelzer D (1989) In vitro and in vivo induction of lymphokine activated killer (LAK) cells in patients with gastric cancer and other solid tumors. In: Koldovsky et al. (eds) Lymphocytes in immunotherapy of cancer. Springer, Berlin Heidelberg New York, pp 32–43
3. Weidmann E, Bergmann L, Christ S, Mitrou PS, Bank H (1988) Follow-up of lymphocyte subsets after in vitro and in vivo application of recmobinant interleukin-2 (rIL-2) and the induction of LAK-activity within different lymphocyte subsets. Blut 57:259
4. Lotze MT, Matory YL, Ettinghausen SE, Rayner AA, Sharrow SO, Seipp CA, Custer MC, Rosenberg SA (1985) In vivo administration of purified Interleukin-2. II. Half-life immunologic effects and expansion of peripheral lymphoid cells in vivo with recombinant IL-2. J Immunol 135:2865–2875
5. Ferrini S, Miescher S, Zocchi MR, von Fliedner V, Moretta A (1987) Phenotypic and functional characterization of recombinant Interleukin-2 (rIL-2) induced activated killer cells: analyses at the population and clonal levels. J Immunol 138:1297–1302
6. Tilden AB, Itoh K, Balch CM (1987) Human lymphokine-activated killer (LAK) cells: identification of two types of effector cells. J Immunol 138:1068–1073
7. Phillips JH, Gemlo BT, Myers WW, Rayner AA, Lanier LL (1987) In vivo and in vitro activation of natural killer cells in advanced cancer patients undergoing combined Interleukin-2 and LAK-cell therapy. J Clin Oncol 139:1933–1941
8. Bol SJ, Rosendorf HS, Rontelap CP, Hennen LA (1986) Cellular cytotoxicity, assessed by the Cr51-release assay. J Immunol Methods 90:15–23
9. Parkinson DR (1988) Interleukin-2 in cancer therapy. Semin Oncol 316:10–26
10. Ritz J, Schmidt RE, Michon J, Hercend T, Schlossman SF (1988) Characterization of functional surface structures on human natural killer cells. Adv Immunol 42:181–211

Enhancement of Growth of Murine Colony-Forming Units-Granulocyte-Macrophage at Suboptimal Colony-Stimulating Factor-Granulocyte-Macrophage Concentrations by Nucleosides, Nucleobases and Their Analogues, and the Dimer of the Hemoregulatory Pentapeptide

P. Langen,[1] H. Schunck, B. Hunger, M. Schütt, and O.D. Laerum

As reported earlier, deoxycytidine (dC) antagonizes the effect of a natural growth inhibitor, isolated from bovine mammary gland, on mouse Ehrlich ascites carcinoma cells in the same way as the polypeptide growth factors insulin and epidermal growth-factor (EGF) do [6]. Bhalla et al. [1] found that this nucleoside is able to overcome the inhibitory effect of acidic isoferritin, prostaglandin E_1 and leukemia inhibitory factor on colony-forming unit–granulocyte macrophage (CFU-GM). Moreover, these authors found that dC stimulates the growth of CFU-GM. We demonstrated [8] that dC antagonizes the effect of the hemoregulatory pentapeptide, described by Kreja et al. [3], and of an inhibitor of colony-forming unit–spleen (CFU-S), described by Lord et al. [7]. Again, dC effects were identical to those of insulin and EGF in these systems.

We now studied the effect of dC and other nucleosides, nucleobases and analogues of these compounds as dependent on colony-stimulating factor–granulocyte macrophage (CSF-GM) concentration. They proved to be co-stimulators in the same way as the dimer of the hemoregulatory peptide [4].

The effect is demonstrated with CSF from lung-conditioned medium as well as with recombinant murine CSF-GM.

Materials and Methods

McCoy's 5A medium and the natural nucleosides and nucleobases were obtained commercially. 5′-Deoxy-5′-fluorothymidine was synthesized according to Langen and Kowollik [5]. Recombinant murine CSF-GM was obtained commercially, the dimer of the hemoregulatory pentapeptide, from Nycomed, Oslo, Norway.

For the preparation of CSF-GM in lung-conditioned media, mice were injected with 0.05 mg endotoxin (lipopolysaccharide from *Salmonella*

[1] Central Institute of Molecular Biology, Academy of Sciences, O-1115 Berlin, FRG

Fleischer (Ed.) Leukemias
© Springer-Verlag Berlin Heidelberg 1993

Table 1. Stimulation of CFU-GM proliferation by $10^{-5}M$ dC or $10^{-7}M$ pentapeptide dimer at CSF-GM (lung-conditioned medium) concentrations increasing from very low to saturating levels

Additions	CSF (%)					
	0.5	1.0	2.0	3.0	4.0	5.0
None	196	238	331	409	405	401
dC	339	369	404	390	381	420
Dimer	316	416	405	424	443	438

Numbers = colonies + clusters. Assays were run in duplicate; deviations from the mean value, no more than 10%.

typhosa), sacrificed 3 h later and their lungs (after washings) incubated in McCoy's 5A medium containing 1.2 g/liter LiCl for 2 days at 37°C. After removal of the lungs the medium was directly used. It was stored in the frozen state.

Cell cultures. Mouse bone marrow cells were obtained from 8–12-weeks-old DBA/2 mice by flushing the femora with phosphate buffered saline and gently aspirating the cell plug with a syringe. 5×10^4 cells were incubated in 35-mm Petri dishes in 1 ml McCoy's 5A medium containing 0.3% agar and 20% fetal calf serum and CSF-GM as indicated. Incubation time was between 4 and 6 days. Aggregates of more than 40 cells were counted as colonies, from 5 to 40 cells as clusters. For each experimental point two or three dishes were evaluated and the numbers shown in the Tables.

Results

From Table 1 it follows that dC and the pentapeptide dimer strongly stimulate aggregate (colonies plus clusters) formation at suboptimal concentrations of CSF-GM (lung-conditioned medium). The effects of the peptide dimer and the nucleoside are not distinguishable. As CSF concentrations approach optimal ones, stimulation becomes lower. Finally the compounds no longer stimulate and the combined effect of nucleoside or pentapeptide dimer and suboptimal concentrations of CSF-GM never exceeds that of optimal concentrations of CSF-GM alone (also, not at other nucleoside or pentapeptide dimer concentrations, results not shown). This is most convincingly shown by results from different experiments (i.e., different bone marrow) with different response to CSF-GM (Table 2). It may be due to the fact that the maximal number of aggregates found corresponds to all cells of a given bone marrow able to respond to CFU-GM or that the maximal number per dish is limited by other factors not analyzed. The stimulatory

Table 2. Stimulation of CFU-GM proliferation by dC or the pentapeptide dimer in different experiments with bone marrow cells responding differently to CSF-GM concentrations

CSF (%)	Aggregates	Dimer		dC	
0.5	197	310	1.6	340	1.7
	17	–		210	12.4
	18	170	9.5	–	
1.0	240	422	1.7	367	1.5
	78	–		265	3.4
	51	206	4.0	–	
4.0 (optimal	411	441	1.1	382	
concentration)	328	–		293	
	214	228	1.1	–	

Table 3. Effect of dC and pentapeptide dimer with murine recombinant CSF-GM. In addition, uracil and 5′-deoxy-5′-fluorthymidine were studied

	mU					
Additions	0.015	0.15	1.5	15	150	1500
None	18	19	73	171	302	318
dC	76	102	162	205	302	n.d.
Dimer	68	84	138	179	313	n.d.
Uracil	67	109	186	207	322	n.d.
5′-FTdR	52	91	136	179	277	n.d.

Evaluation as in Table 1.
5′-FTdR, 5′-deoxy-5′-fluorthymidiue

effect of dC or the dimer pentapeptide is higher, the lower the response of CFU-GM to a given suboptimal CSF-GM concentration is (Table 2). The stimulatory effects of dC and the pentapeptide dimer become lower at CSF-GM concentrations below 0.1% and are not found in the absence of this factor.

From Table 3 it follows that similar effects are obtained also with recombinant murine CSF-GM. However, while stimulation at suboptimal concentrations of CSF-GM from lung-conditioned medium is so high that the same aggregate number is obtained as with optimal concentrations, the one in the presence of recombinant CSF-GM is lower.

In these experiments the thymidine analogue 5′-deoxy-5′-fluorothymidine and the nucleobase uracil were also investigated. Both were as effective as dC and the pentapeptide dimer (they were also effective with CSF-GM from lung-conditioned medium, as was thymidine; results not shown).

Preliminary experiments, not shown, revealed that also thymine and uracil or thymine analogues, such as 6-aminothymine and 6-methyluracil, are effective. These compounds differ from uracil in that they serve only poorly for nucleic acid synthesis or not at all.

Discussion

It can be reasonably assumed that CSF-GM induces in its target cells a pleiotropic response as other growth factors do. Nucleosides and nucleobases as well as the pentapeptide dimer seem to mediate in the cell within this response process, which can be brought about by high concentrations of CSF-GM alone but not by lower ones. In our earlier papers on the dC effect [6] we proposed that the key enzyme of cell proliferation, ribonucleotide reductase, might be involved. It provides the substrates for DNA synthesis, the formation of dC being correlated to the rate of this process [9]. However, the fact that nucleobases such as uracil and even nucleoside or nucleobase analogues are effective does not fit (well) into this theory. Since there is no effect in the complete absence of CSF-GM and because of the similarity of the effect with that of the pentapeptide dimer one might speculate that all these compounds induce the appearance of a greater number of receptors for CSF-GM or a higher receptor occupancy. Possibly, there are special types of receptors for nucleobases and nucleosides, as already described for adenosine in vegetative regulation [2,10]. Studies are under way to find optimal nucleoside or nucleobase structures and their way of action.

If nucleosides or nucleobases are also effective in vivo, they might be of practical value for modulation of CSF-GM effects in patients.

References

1. Bhalla K, Cole J, MacLanghlin W, Baker M, Arlin Z, Graham G, Grant S (1986) Deoxycytidine stimulates the in vitro growth of normal CFU-GM and reverses the negative regulatory effects of acidic isoferritin and prostaglandin E_1. Blood 68: 1136–1141
2. Collis MG (1989) The vasodilatator role of adenosine. Pharmacol Ther 41:143–162
3. Kreja L, Haga P, Müller-Berat N, Laerum OD, Sletvold O, Pankovits WR (1986) Effecs of a hemoregulatory pentapeptide (HP5b) on erythroid and myelopoietic colony formation in vitro. Scand J Haematol 37:79–86
4. Laerum OD, Slevold O, Bjerkness R, Eriksen JA, Johansen JH, Schanche JS, Tveterås T, Pankovits WR (1988) The dimer of hemoregulatory peptide (HP5b) stimulates mouse and human myelopoiesis in vitro. Exp Haematol 16:274–280
5. Langen P, Kowollik G (1968) 5′-Deoxy-5′-fluorothymidine, a biochemical analogue of thymidylate selectively inhibiting DNA synthesis. Eur J Biochem 6:344–351
6. Langen P, Lehmann W, Graetz H, Grosse R (1984) Is ribonucleotide reductase in Ehrlich ascites mammary tumour cells the target of a growth inhibitor purified from bovine mammary gland? Biomed Biochim Acta 43:1377–1383

7. Lord BI, Mori KJ, Wright EG, Lajtha LG (1976) An inhibitor of stem cell proliferation in normal bone marrow cells. Br J Haematol 34:441–445
8. Schunck H, Schütt M, Langen P, Lord B, Laerum OD (1988) Deoxycytidine, insulin and epidermal growth factor overcome the effect of two natural inhibitors of the hemopoietic system. Acta Pathol Microbiol Immunol Scand 96 [Suppl 2]:120–129
9. Skook LK, Nordenskjöld BA, Bjursell KG (1973) Deoxyribonucleoside triphosphate pools and DNA synthesis in synchronized hamster cells. Eur J Biochem 33:428–432
10. White TD (1988) Role of adenine compounds in automatec neurotransmission. Pharmacol Ther 38:129–168

Induction of Lymphokine-Activated Killer Cells from Human Leukemic T Cells by Interleukin-2

M. Hartwig,[1] I.J. Körner, M. Schöntube, and B. Voigt

When cultured with interleukin-2 (IL-2), human peripheral blood lymphocytes acquire the ability to lyse in a selective manner a wide range of tumor cells. Such lymphokine-activated killer cells (LAK cells) appear to develop from phenotypically quite heterogenous precursors, but in short-term cultures predominantly from natural killer cells [4]. This phenomenon has attracted great interest as a promising approach to cancer therapy. Clinical trials have indicated that adoptive immunotherapy with autologous LAK cells along with IL-2 in humans may be effective in reducing established metastatic cancer of several histological forms [6]. The available data relate preferentially to experimental and clinical studies of solid tumors, while only little is known about the effect of LAK cells against human leukemia. We report here on our studies aimed at inducing LAK cells in vitro among the peripheral lymphoid cells from childhood T-cell leukemia. Our conclusion is that LAK cells under the action of IL-2 can develop from leukemic T cells and may be cytolytic against the autologous leukemic cells.

Peripheral blood lymphoid cells from childhood T-cell leukemia were separated by density gradient centrifugation [1]. The percentage of atypical cells ranged from 60% to 95%. Recombinant human IL-2 (rIL-2) was added in various concentrations in order to induce LAK cell activity. Cytotoxicity (% C) of LAK cells was measured in a 4-h ^{51}Cr-releasing assay, mixing various numbers of effector cells with 10^4 labeled target cells.

Peripheral blood lymphoid cells from T-cell leukemias can be induced by rIL-2 to manifest significant cytotoxicity both against the commonly used target cells of the leukemic cell line K562, but also against the autologous leukemia target cells. There is no effect without IL-2 (Fig. 1).

Cytotoxicity induced in the peripheral blood lymphoid cells from T-cell leukemia is dependent on the effector (E) to target (T) ratio and on the concentration of IL-2 used for activation (Fig. 2). In our investigation we mostly worked with an E to T ratio of 20:1 and an IL-2 concentration of 250 U/ml, both at the beginning of a plateau.

Cytotoxicity as measured here could result from residual normal lymphocytes or from leukemic T cells. However, normal lymphocytes

[1] Zentralinstitut für Molekularbiologie der Akademie der Wissenschaften, O-1115 Berlin, FRG

Fleischer (Ed.) Leukemias
© Springer-Verlag Berlin Heidelberg 1993

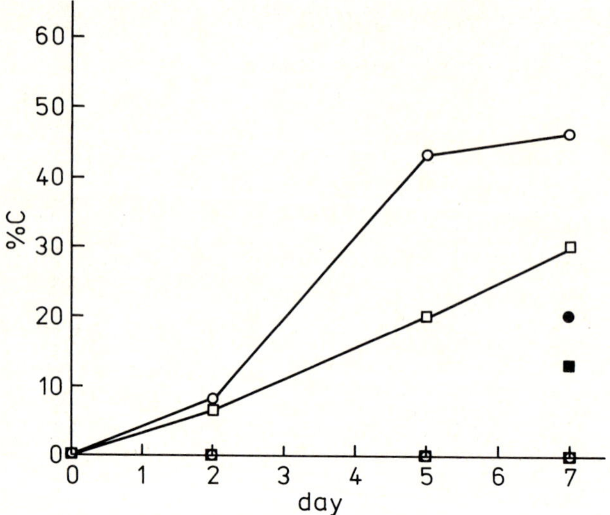

Fig. 1. Kinetics of LAK cell induction in peripheral blood lymphoid cells from two T-cell leukemias by IL-2 (*open symbols*: cytotoxicity against K562 target cells; *closed symbols*: cytotoxicity against autologous leukemia target cells; 250 U/ml rIL-2, E:T ratio = 20:1). Cytotoxicity after incubation without IL-2 remains zero

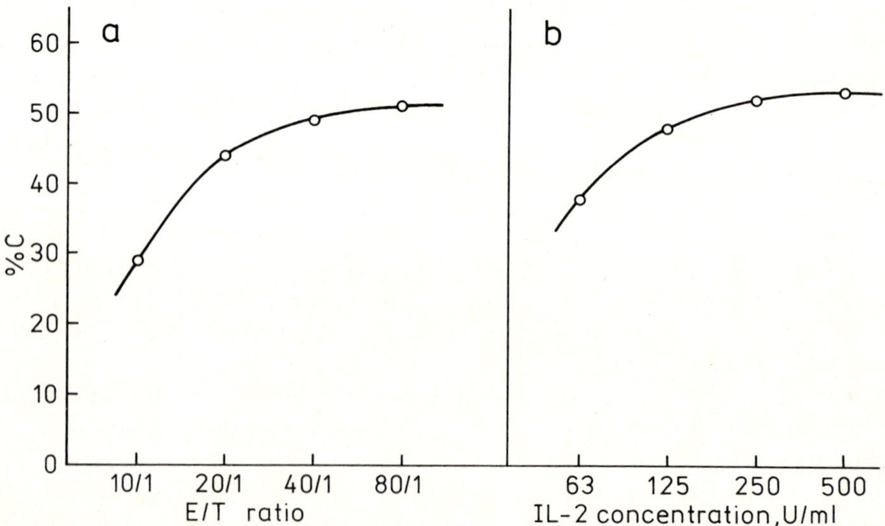

Fig. 2a, b. LAK cell cytotoxicity induced in the peripheral blood lymphoid cells from a T-cell leukemia against K562 target cells in dependence on **a** E to T ratio (250 U/ml rIL-2; day 5) and **b** IL-2 concentration (E:T ratio = 20:1; day 7)

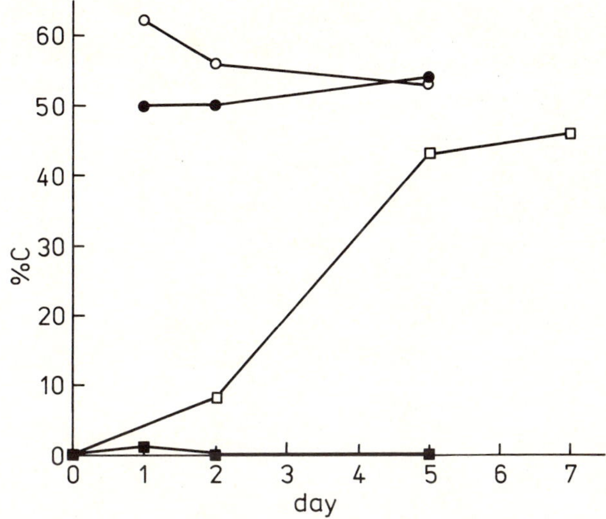

Fig. 3. Kinetics of LAK cell induction in normal peripheral blood lymphocytes (*open circles*: nonirradiated cells; *closed circles*: irradiated cells) and in peripheral blood lymphoid cells from a T-cell leukemia (*open squares*: non-irradiated cells; *closed squares*: irradiated cells) against K562 target cells (250 U/ml rIL-2, E:T ratio = 20:1)

appear functionally suppressed in leukemia and require generally long-term cultivation for killer cell activation [3]. On the other hand, it has been shown that immature T cells such as thymocytes can be induced to manifest LAK cell activity [5], suggesting that even immature leukemic T cells can do so. Our study favors the latter possibility.

First, as shown in model experiments, because of the high amount of atypical cells, cytotoxicity from normal lymphocytes would, in our assay, be not only very small due to a low, real E to T ratio, but would actually be zero due to the competing presence of a high excess of leukemic T cells. Second, while normal lymphocytes retain their cytotoxicity after an X-irradiation with 1 krad, our cells responsible for cytotoxicity do not (Fig. 3). Our results are in accord with those of Kaufmann [2], but additionally demonstrate LAK activity against autologous leukemic cells. A possible clinical significance remains to be investigated.

References

1. Böyum A (1986) Isolation of mononuclear cells and granulocytes from human blood. Scand J Clin Lab Invest 21 [Suppl 97]:77
2. Kaufmann Y et al. (1987) Interleukin 2 induces human acute lymphocytic leukemia cells to manifest lymphokine-activated-killer (LAK) cytotoxicity. J Immunol 139:977

3. Lotzová E (1987) Interleukin-2-generated killer cells, their characterization and role in cancer therapy. Cancer Bull 39:30
4. Phillips JH, Lanier LL (1986) Dissection of the lymphokine-activated killer phenomenon. J Exp Med 164:814
5. Ramsdell FJ, Golub SH (1987) Generation of lymphokine-activated killer cell activity from human thymocytes. J Immunol 139:1446
6. Rosenberg SA et al. (1987) A progress report on the treatment of 157 patients with advanced cancer using lymphokine-activated killer cells and interleukin-2 or high-dose interleukin-2 alone. N Engl J Med 316:889

The Influence of Recombinant Human Granulocyte-Monocyte-Colony-Stimulating Factor on Stroma Formation by Normal Human Bone Marrow Cells In Vitro

M. WÄCHTER,[1] E. ELSTNER, J. MACIEJEWSKI, H.D. VOLK, and R. IHLE

Introduction

Granulocyte-monocyte–colony-stimulating factor (GM-CSF) is a glyco-protein that plays a key role as a humoral mediator in the induction and regulation of hemopoiesis both in vitro and in vivo. In vitro recombinant human (rh) GM-CSF proved to be active on hemopoietic precursor as well as on mature cells [5,18].

At present the phenomenon of communication and interaction between the stromal cells and hemopoietic stem cells is in the focus of interest. The question of which role CSFs play in this respect and whether there is the possibility to manipulate this process is important for the development of new therapeutic strategies. The Dexter liquid culture is a good in vitro model to study stromal cells and their function. In this culture system an adherent layer of stromal cells develops, including reticular cells, macrophages, fibroblasts, and endothelial cells, which is the in vitro equivalent of the hemopoietic microenvironment [2,3]. Active hemopoiesis is supported in this system for several weeks.

There are indications for defects of the hemopoietic stroma in diseases such as leukemias, aplastic anemias, myelodysplastic syndromes [1,9,10,15,19], and chemotherapy [8,12]. Up to now little was known about the influence of CSFs on stromal precursors. The aim of our study is to test the influence of exogenous rhGM-CSF on the establishment of the stromal layer, its supportive function for hemopoiesis, and the composition of the resulting cell population after 10 days in Dexter liquid culture.

Material and Methods

Mononuclear cells were isolated from iliac bone marrow aspirates (1:1 diluted with Iscove's modified Dulbecco's medium (IMDM) containing preservative-free heparin (Gedeon Richter, Hungary) by Ficoll-Visotrast gradient separation at a density of 1.077 g/ml.

[1] Hematological Division of Clinic for Internal Medicine, School of Medicine (Charité), Humboldt University Berlin, Schumannstraße 20–21, O-1040 Berlin, FRG

Fleischer (Ed.) Leukemias
© Springer-Verlag Berlin Heidelberg 1993

The cells were tested for colony-forming unit–GM (CFU-GM) growth, cytomorphological composition (staining according to Pappenheim), and expression of HLA-DR and CD14 antigens [fluorescence-activated cell sorter (FACS) analysis after incubation with the monoclonal antibodies L234 (HLA-DR) derived from hybridomas (ATCC, Rockeville, CA, USA), and LeuM3 (CD14) from Becton Dickinson, Heidelberg, FRG].

The Dexter liquid culture [2,4] introduced for human bone marrow cells [11] was slightly modified [10]. Briefly, 5×10^5 cells/ml culture medium (70% IMDM, 10% horse serum, 10% fetal calf serum, 10% autologous bone marrow plasma, $10^{-6}M$ hydrocortisone sodium succinate) were incubated in 7.5% CO_2 at 37°C. At the beginning of the culture 100 IU rhGM-CSF/ml (Behring, FRG), and 10 IU recombinant human interferon-γ (rhIFN-γ)/ml (Boehringer, FRG) were added alone or in combination. After 10 days in Dexter liquid culture the stromal formation was evaluated by the expansion of the adherent cell layer (stromal grade 1–4 corresponds to an area covered from 25% to 100% by adherent cells). The establishment of active hemopoiesis was evaluated by the presence of hemopoietic islands.

Adherent cells were removed from the culture dishes with a cell scraper. After washing twice, the whole cell population (adherent plus nonadherent cells) was tested again for CFU-GM growth, cytomorphology, and expression of HLA-DR and CD14.

CFU-GM Assay. The estimation of CFU-GM counts was performed in a monolayer system with soft agar, IMDM supplemented with 20% fetal calf serum, 20% mixed culture conditioned medium, and $5 \times 10^{-5}M$ mercaptoethanol.

Preparation of Mixed Culture Conditioned Medium. Peripheral buffy coat cell suspension (1×10^6 cells/ml) from a healthy donor, and the suspension of normal, allogeneic mononuclear bone marrow cells (1×10^5 cells/ml) were made in IMDM with 20% fetal calf serum, mixed in a 1:1 ratio, and incubated in 7.5% CO_2 at 37°C for 6 days. The supernatant of the culture was removed after centrifugation, and stored at 4°C. The same batch was used for all CFU-GM tests.

Results and Discussion

Exogenous rhGM-CSF caused an increase in stromal grade (Fig. 1) as well as in activity of hemopoiesis (number and size of hemopoietic islands). Cultures with 10 IU rhIFN-γ/ml showed nearly the same degree of stromal formation as the control cultures. The combination of 100 IU rhGM-CSF/ml with 10 IU rhIFN-γ/ml caused a slight increase in the stromal grade.

The composition of hemopoietic cells was influenced by the factors added (Fig. 2). 10 IU rhIFN-γ/ml caused a switch of the differentiation of

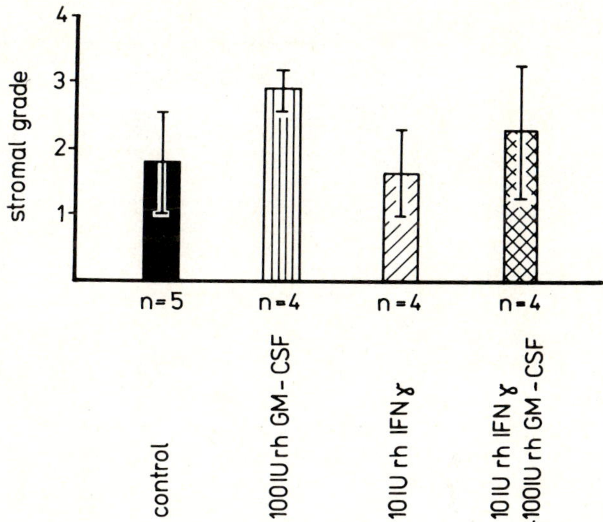

Fig. 1. Stromal formation of normal human bone marrow cells after 10 days in Dexter liquid culture

hemopoietic cells to monocytes and macrophages. There was an elevation in immature cells in cultures with rhGM-CSF both alone and in combination with rhIFN-γ.

The CFU-GM derived from the Dexter cultures were elevated as compared to the controls without precultivation in suspension (Fig. 3). An additional increase in CFU-GM count was seen in all Dexter cultures with rhGM-CSF both alone and in combination with rhIFN-γ. This elevation in CFU-GM count was mainly due to an increase in the number of small compact aggregates. This is expressed by an elevated cluster to colony ratio (see Fig. 3).

Our preliminary data seem to indicate that exogenous rhGM-CSF has activities on CFU-GM as well as on stromal precursor cells in Dexter liquid culture.

GM-CSF, added to a preestablished Dexter culture, had no effect [6, 7,20]. In our study, however, we examined the important early period of the process of establishing the microenvironment. Exogenous rhGM-CSF accelerates the maturation of monocytes to macrophages and, therefore, shortens the time which these cells need to acquire the ability to function within the network of stromal cells.

Another humoral mediator for hemopoietic regulation is IFN-γ; it exerts an inhibitory action on CFU-GM growth [13,14,17], and is able to induce myeloid progenitor cells to differentiate toward the monocytic lineage [16].

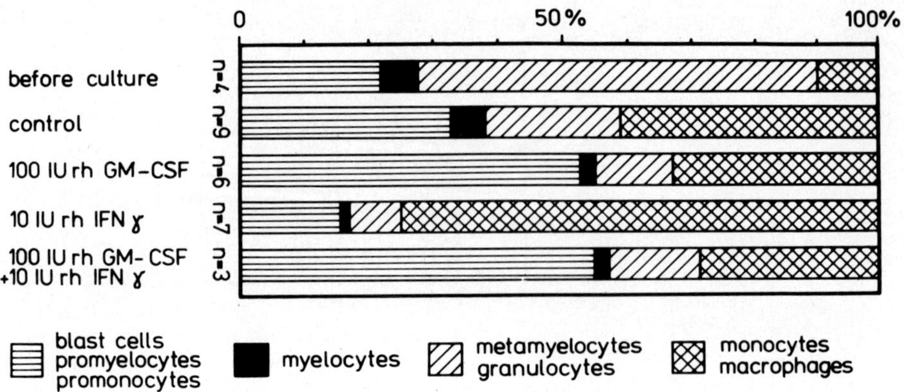

Fig. 2. Distribution of cytomorphologically differentiated subpopulations of hemopoietic cells derived from Dexter cultures after 10 days of cultivation

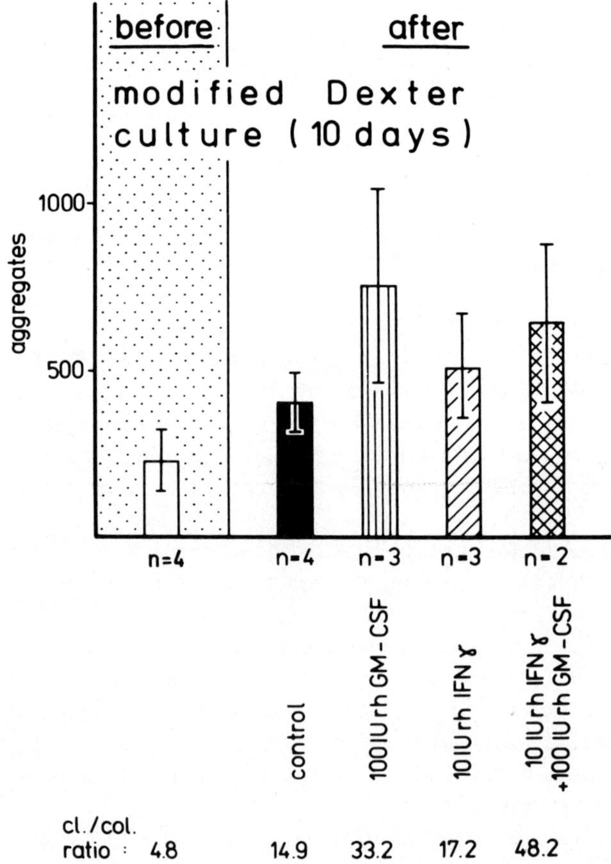

Fig. 3. CFU-GM counts derived from Dexter cultures after 10 days of cultivation

Table 1. The influence of rhGM-CSF and rhIFN-γ on the expression of the CD14 and DR antigen on bone marrow cells derived from 10-day Dexter liquid cultures

Marker	Control (%)	GM-CSF (%)	IFN-γ (%)	GM-CSF + IFN-γ (%)
HLA-DR	18	33	21	37
CD14	6	12	11	20

In our cultures there was no effect of 10 IU rhIFN-γ/ml on stromal formation, and a minimal enhancing effect on the CFU-GM count. Combination of rhIFN-γ and rhGM-CSF had the same stimulatory effect on CFU-GM derived from Dexter cultures as rhGM-CSF alone. Simultaneously, an expansion of immature cells (blasts, promyelocytes, promonocytes) was observed, which correlated with an elevated HLA-DR expression (activation marker). It is of special interest that further specification of the cells by FACS analysis revealed an elevated expression of the monocytic marker CD14 by the combined application of rhGM-CSF and rhIFN-γ but not by rhGM-CSF alone (see Table 1). We assume that after addition of both factors, GM-CSF caused proliferation of stem cells whereas IFN-γ determined its commitment in Dexter liquid culture.

References

1. Ben-Ishay Z, Prindull G, Borenstein A, Sharon S (1984) Bone marrow stromal deficiency in acute myeloid leukemia in mice. Leuk Res 8:1057–1064
2. Dexter TM, Allen TD, Lajtha LG (1977) Conditions controlling the proliferation of haemopoietic stem cells in vitro. J Cell Physiol 91:335–344
3. Dexter TM, Spooncer E, Toksoz D, Lajtha LG (1980) The role of cells and their products in the regulation of in vitro stem cell proliferation and granulocyte development. J Supramol Struct 13:512–524
4. Dexter TM, Testa NG (1976) Differentiation and proliferation of hemopoietic cells in culture. Methods Cell Biol 14:387–405
5. Clark SC, Kamen R (1987) The human hematopoietic colony stimulating factors. Science 236:1229–1237
6. Eaves AC, Eaves CJ (1988) Maintenance and proliferation control of primitive hemopoietic progenitors in long-term cultures of human marrow cells. Blood Cells 14:355–361
7. Eliason JF, Thorens B, Kindler V, Vasalli P (1988) The roles of granulocyte-macrophage colony-stimulating factor and interluekin 3 in stromal cell-mediated hemopoiesis in vitro. Exp Hematol 16:307–312
8. Elstner E, Goldschmidt H, Wächter M, Ihle R (1987) Sensitivity of stromal elements from human bone marrow cells to cytosine arabinoside in vitro. In: Neth R, Gallo RC, Greaves M, Kabisch H (eds) Modern trends in human leukemia VII. Springer, Berling Heidelberg New York, pp 177–180
9. Elstner E, Schulze E, Ihle R, Stobbe H, Grunze S (1985) Stromal progenitor cells in bone marrow of patients with aplastic anemia. In: Neth R, Gallo RC, Greaves M, Janka G (eds) Modern trends in human leukemia VI. Springer, Berlin Heidelberg New York, pp 168–171

10. Elstner E, Wächter M, Ihle R (1989) Bone marrow stromal culture from patients with myelodysplastic sydromes and patients at different stages of acute nonlymphocytic leukemia. Folia Haematol 116:167–174
11. Gartner S, Kaplan HS (1980) Long-term culture of human bone marrow cells. Proc Natl Acad Sci USA 77:4756–4759
12. Hays E, Hale L, Villareal B, Fitchen JH (1982) "Stromal" and hemo-poietic stem cell abnormalities in long-term cultures of marrow from busulfan-treated mice. Exp Hematol 10:383–392
13. Hosoi T, Ozawa K, Urabe A, Takaku F (1985) Effects of recombinant interferons on the clonogenic growth of leukemic cells and normal hemopoietic progenitors. Int J Cell Cloning 3:304–312
14. Krumwieh D, Hermann R, Kurrle R, Seiler FR (1986) Effect of recombinant human interferon gamma and interleukin 2 on CFU-GM. Behring Inst Mitt 80:59–63
15. Nagao T, Komatsuda M, Yamanchi K, Arimori S (1981) Fibroblast colonies in monolayer cultures of human leukemia. J Cell Physiol 108:155–161
16. Perussia B, Dayton ET (1983) Fanning V, Thiagarajan P, Hoxie J, Trinchieri G (1983) Immune interferon and leukocyte-conditioned medium induce normal and leukemic myeloid cells to differentiate along the monocytic pathway. J Exp Med 158:2058–2080
17. Raefsky EL, Platanias LC, Zoumbos NC, Young NS (1985) Studies of interferon as a regulator of hematopoietic cell proliferation. J Immunol 135:2507–2512
18. Sieff CA (1987) Hematopoietic growth factors. J Clin Invest 79:1549–1557
19. Singer JW, Keating A, Cuttner J, Gown AM, Jacobson R, Killen PD, Moohr JW, Najfeld V, Powell J, Sanders J, Striker GE, Fialkow PJ (1984) Evidence for a stem cell common to hematopoiesis and its in vitro microenvironment: studies of patients with clonal hematopoietic neoplasia. Leuk Res 8:535–543
20. Williams N, Burgess AW (1980) The effect of mouse lung granulocyte-macrophage colony-stimulating factor and other colony-stimulating activities on the proliferation of murine bone marrow cells in long-term cultures. J Cell Physiol 102:287–295

Adoptive Transfer of Autologous Cytotoxic Macrophages Grown from Blood Monocytes. A New Approach to Cancer Immunotherapy*

R. Andreesen,[1] C. Scheibenbogen, W. Brugger, and G.W. Löhr

Introduction

Clinical trials to evaluate the potential of adoptive immunotherapy in cancer patients have been restricted to the use of lymphoid effector cells [1,2]. Of the other probably even more important host defense system against tumor growth, the mononuclear phagocyte system [3], only monocytes (mo) have been reinfused [4] which, however, represent immature precursor cells and acquire full functional competence only upon further maturation. This might at least in part be due to the many technical problems associated with the generation of human mature macrophages (MO).

Here we report on a pilot phase I trial of adoptive immunotherapy with tumorcytotoxic MO derived from circulating blood mo by suspension culture on hydrophobic Teflon membranes [5] and subsequent activation with human recombinant interferon-γ (rhIFN-γ). It could be shown that large scale generation of cytotoxic MO is technically feasible [6] and their reinfusion into patients is tolerated without major clinical side effects observed.

Material and Methods

Patient Population. Seven patients with advanced metastasized cancer were treated according to a protocol that had been approved by the local ethical committee on human experimentation. Four patients had bronchiogenic non-small-cell carcinoma of the lung, two had malignant melanoma, and one had squamous cell carcinoma of the tongue. Signed informed consent was obtained from all patients prior to entry in the study.

Leukapheresis, Cell Isolation, and Culture. Large numbers of mononuclear cells (MNC) were obtained by leukapheresis with a continuous-flow cell

* Supported by a grant from the Bundesminister für Forschung und Technologie of the FRG
[1] Medizinische Klinik der Albert-Ludwigs-Universität, Hugstetter Straße 55, D-7800 Freiburg, FRG

separator (CS3000, Baxter, Munich, FRG). MNC were further separated from red cells and contaminating granulocytes by Ficoll gradient centrifugation. The separated cells were washed at least three times, then resuspended in RPMI 1640 supplemented with 2% autologous serum. They were seeded into bags made of hydrophobic Teflon (Biofolie 25, Heraeus GmbH, Biberach, FRG) at 5×10^6/ml and incubated for 7 days [11]. Eighteen hours prior to harvest rhIFN-γ (Dr. Karl Thomae GmbH, Biberach, FRG) was added to give a final concentration of 200 IU/ml. On day 7 of culture, cells were harvested and resuspended in Hank's balanced salt solution (HBSS) with 2% human albumin. They were elutriated (Beckman JE5-0, standard elutriation chamber) at 2500 rpm and a flow rate of 30 ml/min. They were resuspended in 5% human albumin for infusion into patients.

Administration of MO. The mo-derived MO were administered i.v. over a period of 10 min using an infusion set for blood products (Baxter, Munich, FRG).

Trafficking of Radiolabeled MO In Vivo. Macrophages (10^8) were labeled with a total of 2 mCi [^{111}In]indium oxine (Amersham and Buchler, Braunschweig, FRG). Following infusion of the labeled cells, gamma camera imaging was performed and radioactivity was measured in blood samples taken at regular intervals.

Determination of a Biological Response in Patients Receiving MO Autografts. Blood samples were collected as indicated and assayed for tumor necrosis factor-alpha (TNF-α) (sensitivity >10 pg/ml) and microglobulin (β2M; normal value <3 µg/ml) by enzyme-linked immunosorbent assay (ELISA), neopterin by radioimmuno-assay (RIA) (normal values <2.5 ng/ml), and IL-6 with a bioassay (normal values <8 U/ml).

Results

In this pilot phase I study, autologous, in vitro-generated tumorcytotoxic MO were reinfused into patients at escalating cell doses: three patients were treated at each dose level with 10^8 MO (dose level 1), 2×10^8 MO (2), 4×10^8 MO (3), the maximal number of MO obtained through one isolation or culture (4), and twice the maximal MO number given on alternate days (5). Dose escalation was done intraindividually, i.e., patients were treated at the higher dose level if no major side effects were observed. Seven patients with advanced metastasized cancer were accepted into the protocol who received a total of 26 MO autografts. On average, 1.5×10^9 mo were collected from the peripheral blood, of which an average of 6.7×10^8 MO (42% of mo initially seeded) could be recovered from the Teflon bag cultures as mo-derived MO and were purified by elutriation up to 96%. These MO proved to be mature by the expression of maturation-associated MAX antigens [7] and were active as cytotoxic and secretory cells [6]. At no cell dose level were any clinical side effects observed except low-grade fever (<38°C) in six out of seven patients. Fever was transient with the maximum being at 1 to 8 h post-therapy and its magnitude did not correlate with the number of MO infused. No evidence for pulmonary embolisms was observed by physical examination, echo- and electrocardiography, and radiography. From the laboratory parameters tested, the only pathological finding was the detection of circulating fibrin monomers shortly after the MO transfusion. However, no corresponding decrease in fibrinogen or in platelet counts was noted. The infusion of these ex vivo-manipulated MO also did not induce autoimmune reactivity as tests for antinuclear antibodies remained negative 2 months after therapy.

The tumor progressed during therapy in three out of five patients studied two patients showed stable disease. When serum parameters were analyzed which could indicate a biological response to MO therapy or which may directly reflect the functional activity of the autografted MO, in four out of seven patients neopterin could be demonstrated to increase. Serum concentrations of IL-6, TNF-α, β2M, and lysozyme showed no changes following MO therapy. Following infusion of [^{111}In]indium-oxine-labeled MO, only a slow increase in blood radioactivity with a maximum peak at 7 h was observed. Even 7 days after MO infusion, cell-associated radiolabel could be measured in the peripheral blood and by sensitive immunostaining technique circulating MAX.1$^+$ MO could be detected. In addition, bio-distribution was detected by gamma camera imaging and showed that cells first appeared in the lungs and then accumulated in the liver and spleen. Labeling of tumor sites could not be observed. The lung transit time for adoptively transferred MO was significantly longer in patients with lung cancer than in others.

Discussion

For the adoptive transfer of immune cells with antitumor reactivity, lymphokine-activated killer (LAK) cells and tumor-infiltrating lymphocyte (TIL) cells have been used as effector cells so far [1,2]. Though strong experimental evidence suggests the important role MO play in host defense against tumor development and spread, and though murine tumors have been successfully treated with MO adoptive immunotherapy [8,9] there is only one preliminary report in the literature on how to use cells of the MO lineage for therapy in cancer patients [4]. Our approach to MO immuno-therapy is based on findings that circulating blood mo represent precursor cells which acquire their full functional competence only upon further dif-ferentiation to mature MO. It has been shown that MO derived in vitro from blood mo have a higher spontaneous tumorcytotoxicity [10,11], respond to IFN-γ more efficiently [12], and release higher amounts of TNF-α than blood mo. In addition, MO but not blood mo, express Fc receptors of low affinity (CD16) which are important to mediate antibody-dependent cellular cytotoxicity of MO against malignant and other cells [12,13]. Furthermore, blood mo are only short-lived intermediate cells of the MO lineage. When reinfused they may rapidly develop, along their physiological pathway of differentiation, into the many different phenotypes of resident and inflammatory MO subpopulations [3]. In tumors, they are subjected to site-specific differentiative signals which could modulate the development into mature MO that actually support tumor growth and expansion. In contrast, in vitro-generated, terminally differentiated MO of proven cytotoxic potential may be "frozen" in their developmental state and be of stable phenotype when retransfused.

In this report we have described the result of a pilot phase I study to test the feasibility and possible toxicity of the infusion into humans of rhIFN-γ-activated MO grown in vitro from the peripheral blood. It is demonstrated that large-scale cell isolation, suspension culture technology on hydrophobic Teflon, activation by rhIFN-γ, and MO purification by elutriation can be technically performed and that the reinfusion of these MO into cancer patients is well tolerated.

No clinical response could be observed so far. Further studies will include systemic administration of rhIFN-γ along with the adoptive cell therapy in order to achieve a constant level of in situ activation of the transferred cells. The increase in serum neopterin, however, which is similar to that seen after rhIFN-γ treatment [14], might indicate the functional activity of the autografted MO. Especial attention will be paid in further studies to improve the affinity of the infused cells to tumor sites.

In conclusion, MO adoptive immunotherapy is technically feasible and clinically safe. The ex vivo manipulation of the MO system, and especially the fact that MO autografts can be safely stored in liquid nitrogen [15], offers the possibility of using this treatment modality not only in malignancy. As MO are potent microbicidal cells and secrete a number of hematopoietic factors [16], their adoptive transfer may also be used as a prophylactic or therapeutic measure in the management of infectious diseases or as supportive care during the reconstitution after bone marrow ablative chemotherapy. In the setting of bone marrow transplantation, MO autografts may be especially of benefit: to cure minimal residual disease (analogous to graft-versus-leukemia effect), to accelerate hematopoietic recovery, and to prevent opportunistic infections.

References

1. Rosenberg SA (1984) Adoptive immunotherapy of cancer: accomplishments and prospects. Cancer Treat Rep 68:233–255

2. Rosenberg SA, Packard BS, Aebersold PM et al. (1988) Use of tumor-infiltrating lymphocytes and interleukin-2 in the immunotherapy of patients with metastatic melanoma. N Engl J Med 319:1676–1680
3. van Furth R (1985) Current view on the mononuclear phagocyte system. Immunobiology 161:178–185
4. Stevenson HC, Lacarna LV, Sugarbaker PH (1988) Ex vivo activation of killer monocytes (AKM) and their application to the treatment of human cancer. J Clin Apheresis 4:118–121
5. Andreesen R, Picht J, Löhr GW (1983) Primary cultures of human blood-born macrophages grown on hydrophobic teflon membranes. J Immunol Methods 56:295–304
6. Brugger W, Scheibenbogen S, Krause S, Andreesen R (1991) Large scale production of human tumorcytotoxic macrophages grown from blood monocytes for the use in adoptive immunotherapy trials. Cancer Detect Prev (in press)
7. Andreesen R, Bross KJ, Osterholz J, Emmrich F (1986) Human macrophage maturation and heterogeneity: analysis with a newly generated set of monoclonal antibodies to differentiation antigens. Blood 67:1257–1264
8. Fidler IJ (1974) Inhibition of pulmonary metastasis by intravenous injection of specifically activated macrophages. Cancer Res 34:1074–1078
9. Wang BS, Lumanglas AL, Durr FE (1986) Immunotherapy of a murine lymphoma by adoptive transfer of syngeneic macrophages activated with bisantrene. Cancer Res 46:503–506
10. Andreesen R, Osterholz J, Bross KJ, Schulz A, Löhr GW (1983) Cytotoxic effector cell function at different stages of human monocyte-macrophage maturation. Cancer Res 43:5931–5936
11. Rinehart JJ, Vessella R, Lange P, Kaplan ME (1979) Characterization and comparison of human monocyte- and macrophage-induced tumor cell cytotoxicity. J Lab Clin Med 93:361–369
12. Andreesen R, Brugger W, Gadd S, Löhr GW, Atkins RC (1988) Activation of human monocyte-derived macrophages cultured on teflon: response to interferon-gamma during terminal maturation in vitro. Immunobiology 177:186–198
13. Clarkson SB, Ory PA (1988) Developmentally regulated IgG Fc receptors on cultured human monocytes. J Exp Med 167:408–417
14. Aulitzky W, Gastl G, Aulitzky WE et al. (1987) Interferon-gamma for the treatment of metastatic renal cancer: dose-dependent stimulation and downregulation of beta-2 microglobulin and neopterin responses. Immunobiology 176:85–95
15. Brugger W, Scheibenbogen S, Krause S, Andreesen R (1989) Production of large amounts of human tumorcytotoxic macrophages grown from the peripheral blood of cancer patients for use in adoptive immunotherapy trials. Exp Cell Biol 57:88 (abstract)
16. Nathan CF (1987) Secretory products of macrophages. J Clin Invest 79:319–326

Interferon Therapy

Strategies for Optimizing Cytokine Treatment of Malignancies: Determination of Interferon Sensitivity in Chronic Myelocytic Leukemia*

G. Gastl,[1] D. Geissler, E. Leiter, B. Eibl, J. Drach, I. Lüttichau, M. Berger, and C. Huber

Interferons (IFNs) comprise a heterogenous group of cytokines with pleiotropic activities. The mode of action of IFNs in human disease is still poorly understood. In particular it is not established whether IFNs exert their antineoplastic activity by direct interaction with tumor cells or indirectly by enhancing host antitumor responses. Nor is it known which biological features of a tumor and which host factors determine the sensitivity of malignant diseases to IFN therapy. In order to select IFN-α-sensitive tumor patients we have chosen Philadelphia chromosome- (Ph[1])-positive chronic myelocytic leukemia (CML) as a model disease.

In the past five years several clinical studies have shown that the majority of patients with Ph[1]-positive CML are responsive to IFN-alpha during the chronic phase of their disease [6,12,14]. Even after long-term IFN-α treatment, however, only about 20%–40% of chronic phase CML patients achieve durable cytogenetic responses. Preliminary data of Talpaz et al. suggest that complete responders bear a favourable prognosis and that only these patients might benefit from IFN-α treatment [15]. Thus from the clinical point of view, the early selection of such optimally responding CML patients is most desirable. This contribution deals with the clinical evaluation of two assays for predicting clinical responsiveness of Ph[1]-positive CML patients to treatment with recombinant IFN-α_{2c}.

Material and Methods

Patients. A total of 31 patients with Ph[1]-positive CML were investigated. None of the patients showed signs of disease acceleration or blastic crisis at study entry. Twenty patients were previously untreated, the remainder had received busulfan (eight patients), hydroxyurea (two patients), or both agents (one patient) for a median of 17 months (range, 2–128 months). Chemotherapy was discontinued 1–3 months before testing and IFN treatment.

* This work was financially supported by the Austrian Funds *Zur Förderung der wissenschaflichen Forschung*, project no. 6526.
[1] Department of Internal Medicine, University Hospital, A-6020 Innsbruck, Austria

Study Design. Before entering a clinical phase II study for treatment with recombinant IFN-α_{2c}, all patients were pretested in vitro or in vivo for IFN-α sensitivity. In 14 patients the IFN-α sensitivity of leukemic bone marrow progenitor cells was assessed in vitro by means of a microagar colony-forming assay. In the remainder the in vivo effect of a single therapeutic dose of recombinant IFN-α_{2c} (3.5 MU; Böhringer-Ingelheim International, FRG) on the expression of the protooncogene c-*myc* in leukemic blood cells was determined. Subsequent to testing, all patients were treated with 3.5 MU of recombinant IFN-α_{2c} daily s.c. for a median time of 9 months (range, 1–40 months).

Response Criteria. The criteria for response evaluation were those defined by Talpaz et al. [15].

Laboratory Investigations

Colony-Forming Assay. Microagar cultures were performed as described previously [7]. Briefly, low-dense bone marrow mononuclear cells prepared from 14 CML patients were plated in 0.3% agar with various concentrations of recombinant IFN-α_{2c} ranging from 0 to 10^5 U. For induction of colony growth of burst-forming units–erythrocytic (BFU-E) and colony-forming units–megakaryocytic (CFU-Meg), the solidified agar was overlayered with alpha medium containing 20% serum obtained from a patient with severe aplastic anemia. Colony-forming units–granulo-monocytic (CFU-GM) growth was stimulated with conditioned medium of the GCT cell line. Staining and scoring was done as described previously [10]. The patients' results were compared with those of healthy controls.

Northern Blot Analysis. After informed consent 17 previously untreated CML patients were treated with a single dose of 3.5 MU recombinant IFN-α_{2c} s.c. and heparinized blood samples were drawn before and 6, 10, 24, and 48 h after IFN administration. Northern blot analysis was performed according to the procedures previously described by Maniatis et al. [11]: In brief, mononuclear blood cells from patients and healthy controls were separated by density gradient centrifugation and total RNA was extracted using guanidine-thiocyanate buffer. 10 µg total RNA was glyoxylated and electrophoresed in a 1.0% agarose gel containing 0.66 M formaldehyde. After transfer to nylon membranes (Hybond-N, Amersham, UK), they were hybridized to a ^{32}P-labeled *Eco*I-*Eco*I fragment (1800 bp) of human c-*myc* (third exon) cDNA (Oncor, Gaithersburg, USA) or a ^{32}P-labeled *Nca*I-*Taq*I fragment (770 bp) of chicken actin cDNA (Oncor) as probes. Probes were labeled with ^{32}P and nick translated to a specific activity of 10^8 cpm/µg using a commercially available nick-translation kit (Amersham, UK). The size of c-*myc* and actin transcripts was estimated using 28S- and 18S-ribosomal RNA as markers. Quantitation of the levels of RNA was carried out

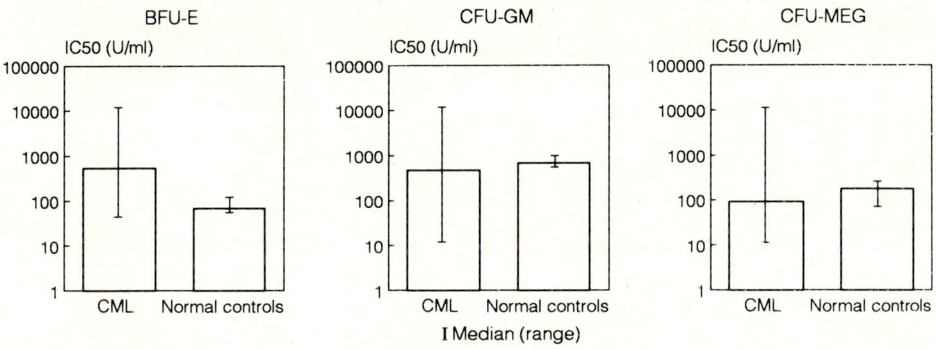

Fig. 1. Comparison of recombinant IFN-α_{2c} IC$_{50}$ values (median and range) for BFU-E, CFU-GM, and CFU-Meg in 14 CML patients and 5 healthy controls

directly on the autoradiograms of the blots, using a soft-laser densitometer. Densitometer scans of actin RNA levels were used to correct c-*myc* scan values for slight loading inequalities. c-*myc* RNA blots of normal blood mononuclear cells and K562 cells were taken as controls.

Statistical Analysis. The colony numbers in normal controls and CML patients were analyzed for significant differences by the Wilcoxon signed-ranks test. The Fisher's exact test was applied to analyze the relationship of in vitro IFN sensitivity and IFN-induced changes of c-*myc* RNA with clinical response.

Results

In Vitro Effect of IFN-α on Colony Formation of Bone Marrow Progenitor Cells and Its Relation to the Clinical Response. The IFN-α sensitivity of normal and leukemic hematopoietic bone marrow progenitor cells was assessed in 14 CML patients and 5 healthy controls. Results are depicted in Fig. 1. Similar to "normals", colony formation of leukemic BFU-E, CFU-GM and CFU-Meg were inhibited in a dose-dependent manner. The median recombinant IFN-α_{2c} concentrations that produced 50% inhibition of colony formation (IC$_{50}$) were 460 U/ml (range, 4–10^4) for BFU-E, 400 U/ml (range, 10–10^4) for CFU-GM, and 85 U/ml (range, 10–10^4) for CFU-Meg. Individual patients greatly differed in their sensitivity to the inhibitory effect of recombinant IFN-α_{2c}. In 3 of the 14 patients BFU-E, CFU-GM and/or CFU-Meg growth were almost unaffected by IFN with less than 50% suppression of colony formation even at the highest IFN concentration tested. This finding was arbitrarily designated as "in vitro resistance". On the other hand, four CML patients proved to be extremely sensitive to IFN-α with IC$_{50}$ values below the 95% confidence limits of normal controls.

Table 1. Correlation of in vitro recombinant IFN-α_{2c} responsiveness in 14 patients with Ph[1]-positive CML

	No. of patients	
	Remission[b]	Therapy failure
IC_{50}[a] $\geq$ 10 000 U/ml IFN-α	0	3
IC_{50}[a] $<$ 10 000 U/ml IFN-α	10	1

$p < 0.01$ (Fisher's exact test)
[a] 50% inhibitory concentration for BFU-E, CFU-GM, and/or CFU-Meg.
[b] Response according to the criteria of Talpaz et al. [15].

The results of in vitro testing were also compared with clinical responses of CML patients to recombinant IFN-α_{2c}. The relationship of in vitro sensitivity testing to in vivo responsiveness is summarized in Table 1. A statistically significant correlation was found between the inability of IFN-α to inhibit colony formation in vitro ($IC_{50} > 10^4$ U/ml) and treatment failure ($p < 0.01$). Furthermore, in three cases, in vitro IFN resistance was closely associated with rapid disease progression.

In Vivo Effect of IFN-α on c-myc Expression of Leukemic Blood Cells and Its Relationship to Clinical Responsiveness. In order to exclude carryover effects of chemotherapy the short-term in vivo effect of a single dose of recombinant IFN-α_{2c} given s.c. was exclusively assessed in previously untreated CML patients. In 17 patients three different response patterns of c-*myc* expression were observed: In 6 patients c-*myc* RNA was reduced by more than 50% from pretreatment values, whereas in 8 patients c-*myc* expression was enhanced by more than 50% from baseline values (Fig. 2). In three patients c-*myc* expression remained more or less unaffected by IFN-alpha with less than 50% changes of baseline values. This short-term in vivo effect of recombinant IFN-alpha on c-*myc* expression was closely related to clinical responsiveness and disease course (Table 2).

Discussion

The purpose of our study was to develop predictive assays for IFN-α sensitivity in Ph[1]-positive CML. Several aspects of this hematological malignancy prompted us to choose CML as a model disease for optimizing cytokine treatment: IFN-α can induce hematological remissions, and more importantly, cytogenetic responses in Ph[1]-positive CML patients [6,12,14]. However, preliminary data suggest that only a minority of patients achieving complete hematological remission and cytogenetic improvement might

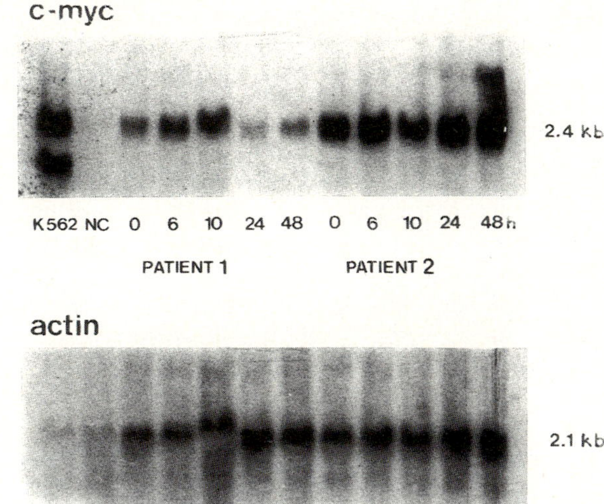

Fig. 2. IFN-α-induced modulation of c-*myc* RNA expression in leukemic blood mononuclear cells of two previously untreated Ph[1]-positive CML cases: c-*myc* RNA expression before (timepoint 0) and after s.c. injection of a single dose of 3.5 MU of recombinant IFN-α_{2c}

Table 2. Correlation of IFN-alpha-induced changes of c-*myc* expression in leukemic blood cells to clinical responsiveness and disease course of 17 previously untreated patients with Ph[1]-positive CML

Clinical responsiveness	Non-progressive disease[a] ($n = 13$)	Blastic crisis ($n = 4$)
c-*myc* RNA reduction <50%	7	4
c-*myc* RNA reduction ≥50%	6	–

Disease course	Remission ($n = 9$)	Therapy failure ($n = 8$)
c-*myc* RNA downregulation	9	4[b]
No c-*myc* RNA downregulation	–	4[c]

BC, blastic crisis
$p < 0.01$ Median duration of treatment, 9 months (range, 3–18 months)
[a] "Non-progressive disease" refers to patients without symptoms of disease acceleration or blastic transformation.
[b] 1 BC.
[c] 3 BC.

benefit from long-term treatment with IFN-α [15]. Therefore, the selection of presumably "good responders" is most desirable. Moreover, the mode of action of IFNs in CML is still poorly understood. In particular it is not established whether in CML IFN-α exerts its antileukemic effect by direct interaction with tumor cells [1] or indirectly by enhancing host antitumor mechanisms [16]. Taking into account the profound direct antiproliferative effect on CML cells in vitro, we have chosen two proliferation assays for determining IFN-α sensitivity of CML in vitro and in vivo.

Along with others we have found that in Ph[1]-positive CML the growth of leukemic commited progenitor cells was supressed by IFN-α in a dose-dependent fashion [3,13]. However, in contrast to previous reports demonstrating an equal or even higher sensitivity of the leukemic clone to IFN-α [8,13], we found a marked heterogeneity of IFN sensitivity among patients with chronic phase Ph[1]-positive CML. In vitro sensitivity to IFN-α was closely related to in vivo responsiveness following therapeutic administration of recombinant IFN-α_{2c}. Although our sample size is still small, these findings suggest that (a) in Ph[1]-positive CML in vitro resistance to IFN-α by bone marrow progenitors implies an unfavorable prognosis, and (b) the microagar assay may be a useful in vitro tool to identify patients who may best benefit from IFN-α therapy. We further assessed the in vivo effect of recombinant IFN-α_{2c} on the expression of the c-*myc* proto-oncogene. Accumulated data suggest c-*myc* to be a key regulator of normal and malignant cell growth and differentiation [5,9]. It has been shown previously that in normal and malignant human myeloid cells c-*myc* is expressed in a cell cycle-dependent manner [2,5]. Moreover, in Daudi cells downregulation of c-*myc* expression by IFN-α was found to be closely linked to cell growth inhibition [4]. In malignant blood cells of the majority of 17 CML patients a profound effect of a single therapeutic dose of IFN-α on the steady state expression of c-*myc* was seen. This effect was closely related to clinical responsiveness to IFN-α and the disease course.

Based on these results we assume that at a given stage of Ph[1]-positive CML IFN-α sensitivity of the leukemic cell pool varies considerably. The heterogenous response rates found in several clinical IFN trials, which comprise mainly of CML patients in the benign phase of their disease, would support this assumption [6,12,14,15]. Duration and stage of disease, pretreatment modalities, and risk factors may further influence IFN responsiveness of individual CML cases. Although the cellular basis of the heterogenous response to IFN-α remains largely unknown, the correlation of IFN-mediated inhibition of colony formation and downregulation of c-*myc* expression in leukemic cells with clinical responsiveness to IFN-α provides further evidence for a profound direct antiproliferative effect of IFN-α on the leukemic clone. Thus the application of sensitivity assays in individual CML patients may provide a novel strategy for optimizing IFN treatment of CML.

References

1. Broxmeyer HE, Lu L, Platzer E, Feit C, Juliano L, Rubin BY (1983) Comparative analysis of the influences of human gamma, alpha and beta-interferons on human multipotential (CFU-GEMM), erythroid (BFU-E) and granulocyte-macrophage (CFU-GM) progenitor cells. J Immunol 131:1300–1305
2. Calabretta B, Venturetti D, Kaczmarek L, Narni F, Talpaz M, Anderson B, Beran M, Baserga R (1986) Altered expression of G1-specific genes in human malignant myeloid cells. Proc Natl Acad Sci USA 83:1495–1498
3. Carlo-Stella C, Cazzola M, Ganser A, Bergamaschi G, Pedrazzoli P, Hoelzer D, Ascari E (1988) Synergistic antiproliferative effect of recombinant interferon-gamma with recombinant interferon-alpha on chronic myelogenous progenitor cells (CFU-GEMM, CFU-Mk, BFU-E, and CFU-GM). Blood 72:1293–1299
4. Einat M, Resnitzky D, Kimchi A (1985) Close link between reduction of c-*myc* expression by interferon and Go/G1 arrest. Nature 313:597–600
5. Ferrari S, Narni F, Mars W, Kaczmarek L, Venturetti D, Anderson B, Calabretta B (1986) Expression of growth-regulated genes in human acute leukemias. Cancer Res 46:5162–5166
6. Gastl G, Aulitzky W, Tilg H, Huber H, Hausmaninger H, Seewann HL, Coser C, Prinoth P, Huber C (1987) Dose-related effectiveness of alpha-interferon in chronic myelogenous leukemia. Blut 54:251–252
7. Geissler D, Lu L, Bruno E, Yang HH, Broxmeyer HE, Hoffman R (1986) The influence of T lymphocyte subsets and humoral factors on colony formation by human bone marrow and blood megakaryocyte progenitor cells in vitro. J Immunol 137:2508–2513
8. Greenberg PL, Mosney SA (1987) Cytotoxic effect of interferon in vitro on granulocytic progenitor cells. Cancer Res 37:1794–1799
9. Kelly K, Siebenlist U (1985) The role of c-*myc* in the proliferation of normal and malignant cells. J Clin Immunol 5:65–77
10. Konwalinka G, Geissler D, Peschel Ch, Tomaschek B, Schmalzl F, Huber H, Odavic R, Braunsteiner H (1982) A microagar culture system for cloning human erythropoietic progenitors. Exp Hematol 10:71–76
11. Sambrook J, Fritsch EF, Maniatis T (1989) Molecular cloning. A laboratory manual, 2nd edn. Cold Spring Harbor Laboratory Press, Cold Spring Harbor
12. Niederle N, Kloke O, Osieka R, Wandl U, Opalka B, Schmidt CG (1987) Interferon-alpha2b in the treatment of chronic myelogenous leukemia. Semin Oncol 14 (Suppl 2):29–35
13. Oladipupo-Williams CK, Svet-Moldavskaya I, Vilcek J, Ohnuma T, Holland JF (1981) Inhibitory effects of human leukocyte and fibroblast interferons on normal and chronic myelogenous leukemia granulocytic progenitor cells. Oncology 38:356–360
14. Talpaz M, Kantarjian HM, McCredie K, Trujillo JM, Keating MJ, Gutterman JU (1986) Hematologic remission and cytogenetic improvement induced by recombinant human interferon-alpha in chronic myelogenous leukemia. N Engl J Med 314:1065–1069
15. Talpaz M, Kantarjian HM, McCredie KB, Keating MJ, Trujillo J, Gutterman (1987) Clinical investigation of human alpha interferon in chronic myelogenous leukemia. Blood 69:1280–1288
16. Zarling JM, Eskra L, Borden EC, Horoszewicz J, Carter WA (1979) Activation of human natural killer cells cytotoxic for human leukemic cells by purified interferon. J Immunol 123:63–70

Clinical Study with Human Recombinant Interferon-α_{2a} in Chronic Myeloid Leukemia. Protocol of the Italian Cooperative Study Group on Chronic Myeloid Leukemia: Preliminary Analysis of Results

S. Tura,[1] for the Italian Cooperative Study Group on CML

Introduction

Chronic myeloid leukemia (CML) is a neoplastic disease of the multi-potential hematopoietic stem cell which develops through three phases: the chronic phase, characterized by uncontrolled proliferation of granulopoietic cells which mature to neutrophils; the accelerated phase, characterized by a progressive defect of cellular maturation; and lastly, the blastic phase [1].

The course of disease seems to be tightly linked with a cytogenetic abnormality which is the Philadelphia chromosome (Ph), consisting of the reciprocal translocation of a genic portion between chromosomes 9 and 22 [2,3].

CML was left untreated until the beginning of the century; busulfan (BUS) or other drugs were introduced in the 1950s [4,5]. The conventional chemotherapy (BUS, hydroxyurea (HU), dibromomannitol, etc.) provided a good control of leukemic mass and an improvement in quality of life, but it did not prevent or delay the evolution of the disease from chronic to accelerated or blastic phase [6–8].

Also, the intensive chemotherapy protocols performed in CML did not modify the length of survival, but showed the possibility of suppressing the Ph-positive (Ph+) cells and to restore, partially, the normal hemopoiesis [9,10]. The allogeneic bone marrow transplant (BMT) can be considered the only therapy which allows eradication of the Ph+ leukemic clone and is likely to cure the patients [11]. However, allogeneic BMT can be applied only to a minority of CML patients and for these reasons it cannot have a major impact on the overall survival.

Interferon-α (IFN-α) is the most important experimental drug for therapy of CML. IFN-α was found to induce a clinical and hematological remission in about 80% of the patients and a partial and sometimes complete karyotypic remission in about 40%–50% of the responders [12–17]. However, the clinical effects of prolonged use of IFN-α on survival and on the duration of the chronic phase are unknown. Moreover, the incidence and the significance of karyotypic conversion is yet to be determined.

---

[1] Institute of Hematology "L. e A. Seràgnoli," University of Bologna, I-40100 Bologna, Italy

Fleischer (Ed.) Leukemias
© Springer-Verlag Berlin Heidelberg 1993

Protocol Study of the Italian Cooperative Study Group on CML

In June 1986 the Italian Cooperative Study Group on CML designed a protocol study to evaluate the effects of recombinant human IFN-α_{2a} (Roferon-A) on untreated patients with Ph+ CML. The main objectives of this study are the following: To evaluate the frequency and duration of karyotypic conversion; and to compare the duration of chronic phase and survival rate of patients treated with IFN-α versus patients treated with conventional chemotherapy (CHT).

To be eligible for this study, patients had to be 70 years old, or younger, with nonblastic Ph+ CML and not more than 6 months from diagnosis. They also had to be untreated or treated only with small doses of BUS or HU.

At entry into the trial, patients were randomized, with a ratio of 2:1, to receive Roferon-A or CHT. During the first month, Roferon-A was administered at dosages of 3–6 MU/day, then, during the second and third month, the IFN dose was escalated to 9 MU/day. At the end of the third month, the clinical-hematologic response was checked for the first time.

From the fourth to the eighth month the Roferon-A dose of 9 MU/day was maintained and CHT was added in case of no response or disease progression. At the end of the eighth month the first karyotypic response was evaluated and IFN treatment was modulated according to karyotypic response.

In case of complete karyotypic response (100% Ph-negative (Ph-) metaphases) IFN-α was administered at the same maximum tolerated dose; while in case of partial (any reduction of Ph+ metaphases) and negative (same percentage of Ph+ metaphases) karyotypic response, IFN dosage was increased by 25% and 50% respectively.

At the end of the 14th month, a second evaluation of karyotypic response was made, and Roferon-A dosage was adjusted again according to karyotypic response.

However, in this case, if there was no karyotypic response Roferon-A was given at a dose of 3 MU/3 times a week. During all the time of treatment the Roferon-A dosage was adjusted according to toxicity.

Results

From June 1986 to July 1988, 346 patients entered the study and 316 of them were analyzed.

Of these, 219 (69%) patients were randomized to receive Roferon-A and 97 (31%) patients to receive conventional CHT.

After 3 months of therapy, the hematologic response rate (response grade I + II + III) was similar in both groups of patients (84% in the IFN group versus 94% in the CHT group).

The overall clinical-hematologic response after 8 and 14 months was similar in both groups of patients, but the patients treated with Roferon-A showed a higher percentage of good response (grade I) (35% and 34%) than patients treated with conventional CHT (20% and 15%).

At the end of the eighth month, a partial karyotypic response was observed in 43% of evaluable patients treated with Roferon-A and two patients achieved a complete karyotypic response. The percentage of Ph− metaphases ranged from 1% to 100% with a median of 30%. Of patients treated with conventional CHT, 20% obtained a partial karyotypic conversion, but the percentage of Ph− metaphases was significantly lower than that of Roferon-A patients (range, 2%−79%; median, 14%).

At the end of 14th month, the results of karyotypic conversion were confirmed. A partial karyotypic conversion was obtained in 46% of Roferon-A patients and 21% of CHT patients. One of the Roferon-A patients achieved a complete karyotypic response.

The patients showed a good tolerance to the Roferon-A treatment. Most side effects were observed during the first 3 months but they were not severe. A temporary discontinuation of treatment was necessary in about 20% of the patients and only 12 patients had to discontinue Roferon-A permanently because of severe toxicity (fatigue, headache, pain, fever).

The majority of patients received the fixed dose of Roferon-A during the first 2 months of treatment. A reduction of Roferon-A was necessary in about 30% of patients during the 3rd month, to coincide with the higher incidence of side effects.

These preliminary results confirm that IFN-α is able to provide hematologic control of CML and karyotypic conversion in about 50% of patients. However, considering the short follow-up it is still too early to establish the effects of IFN-α therapy on the duration of chronic phase and survival rate.

References

1. Tura S, Baccarani M, Zaccaria A (1986) Chronic myeloid leukemia. Editorial. Haematologica 71:169−176
2. Nowell PC, Hungerford DA (1960) Chromosome studies on normal and leukemic human leukocytes. J N C I 25:85−109
3. Fialkow PL, Martin PL, Najfeld V et al. (1983) Evidence for a multistep pathogenesis of chronic myelogenous leukemia. Blood 58:158−163
4. Senn N (1903) NY Med J 77: 665 cited in Minot (1924) JAMA 82:1489−1494
5. Haut A, Abbot WS, Wintrobe MM, Cartwright GE (1961) Busulfan in the treatment of chronic myelocytic leukemia. The effect of long-term intermittent therapy. Blood 17:1−19
6. Tura S, Baccarani M (1967) Il Dibromomannitolo nella terapia delle emoblastosi. Haematologica 52 [Suppl 12]:1039−1062
7. Medical Research Council's Working Party for Therapeutic Trials in leukemia (1968) Chronic granulocytic leukemia: comparison of radiotherapy and busulfan therapy. Br Med J 1:201−208

 8. Schwarzenberg L, Mathé G, Pouillard P et al. (1973) Chemotherapy with hydroxyurea leukopheresis and splenectomy in chronic granulocytic leukemia at the problastic phase. Br Med J 1:700–703
 9. Cunningham I, Gee T, Dowling M et al. (1979) Results of treatment of Ph1+ chronic myelogenous leukemia with an intensive treatment regime (L5-protocol). Blood 53:375–393
10. Kantarjian HM, Vellekoop L, McCredie KB et al. (1985) Intensive combination chemotherapy (ROAP-10) and splenectomy in the management of chronic myelogenous leukemia. J Clin Oncol 3:192–200
11. Goldman JM, Apperley JF, Jones et al. (1986) Bone marrow transplantation for patients with chronic myeloid leukemia. N Engl J Med 314:202–207
12. Talpaz M, McCredie KB, Mavlight GM, Gutterman JU (1983) Leukocyte interferon induced myeloid cytoreduction in chronic myelogenous leukemia. Blood 62:689–692
13. Talpaz M, Kantarjian HM, McCredie KB, Keating MJ, Gutterman JU (1986) Chronic myelogenous leukemia: hematologic remission and cytogenetic improvement induced by recombinant alpha A interferon. N Engl J Med 314:1065–1069
14. Bersagel DR, Haas RH, Messner HA (1986) Interferon alpha 2b in the treatment of chronic granulocytic leukemia. Semin Oncol 13:29–34
15. Talpaz M, Kantarjian HM, McCredie KB, Keating MJ, Trujillo J, Gutterman JU (1987) Clinical investigation of human alpha interferon in chronic myelogenous leukemia. Blood 69:1280–1288
16. Alimena G, Morra E, Lazzarino M, Liberati AM et al. (1988) Interferon alpha 2b as therapy for Ph-positive chronic myelogenous leukemia: a study of 82 patients treated with intermittent or daily administration. Blood 72:642–647
17. Russo D per il Gruppo Cooperatore Italiano per lo Studio della Leucemia Mieloide Cronica (LMC) (1989) Protocollo del Gruppo Cooperatore Italiano e analisi preliminare dei risultati. XXXII Congresso della Società Italiana di Ematologia, Rome 8–12 October, p 51

Alpha-Interferon in Hematological Disorders with Special Emphasis on Chronic Myeloid Leukemia

P. Stryckmans,[1] C. Dorval, K. Huygen, B. Vandenplas, C. Vanhaelen, I. Clauss, G. Huez, A. Delforge, and the EORTC Leukemia Group

A phase II European Organisation for Research on Treatment of Cancer (EORTC) study was started in 1985 to assess the activity of recombinant interferon-α_{2c} (rIFN-α_{2c}). Sixty-two chronic myeloid leukemia (CML) patients were studied. A dose of 3×10^6 units (3 MU) was given once daily i.m. It was progressively increased up to 5, 10, or 15 MU according to response and tolerance. Induction treatment lasted 6–16 weeks. Patients reaching hematological response (HR) received maintenance IFN-α for 3 years or until progression of the disease. Our results in general confirm those of others [1]. IFN-α produced HR in 75% of previously untreated patients. Chemotherapy prior to IFN-α had a negative impact. Indeed, the response rate to IFN-α decreased to 58% in 27 patients still responsive to chemotherapy and to 44% in 9 treated but resistant. A decrease of percentage Philadelphia chromosome-positive (%Ph+) mitosis as a consequence of IFN-α was seen in 40% of the previously untreated patients and was virtually absent in previously treated patients. The survival from start of IFN-α therapy also was significantly better in patients receiving IFN-α as first treatment ($n = 25$). In the group of patients below 45 years of age, never treated before and responding to INF-α ($n = 5$), the survival is still 100%. This group of patients with an average follow-up of 139 weeks in the age range suitable for allogeneic bone marrow (BM) transplantation deserves special attention since IFN-α in these patients could be the best alternative when no BM donor is available.

Our in vitro studies [2] of the effect of IFN-α on the peripheral blood myeloid progenitors (colony-forming unit–granulo-monocytic, CFU-GM) of normal control ($n = 13$) and CML patients ($n = 11$) have shown that IFN-α during the 14 days of culture is usually exerting a dose-dependent inhibitory effect on these cells. Resistance to this inhibitory effect however was observed in both normal and CML subjects but was more frequent in CML (5 out of 11) than in normal (1 out of 13). When excluding the cases resistant to IFN-α in vitro, the mean inhibitory effect of IFN-α was exactly the same on normal CFU-GM and on CML CFU-GM (Fig. 1). This observation

---

[1] Institut J. Bordet, Rhode St Genèse, Belgium

Fleischer (Ed.) Leukemias
© Springer-Verlag Berlin Heidelberg 1993

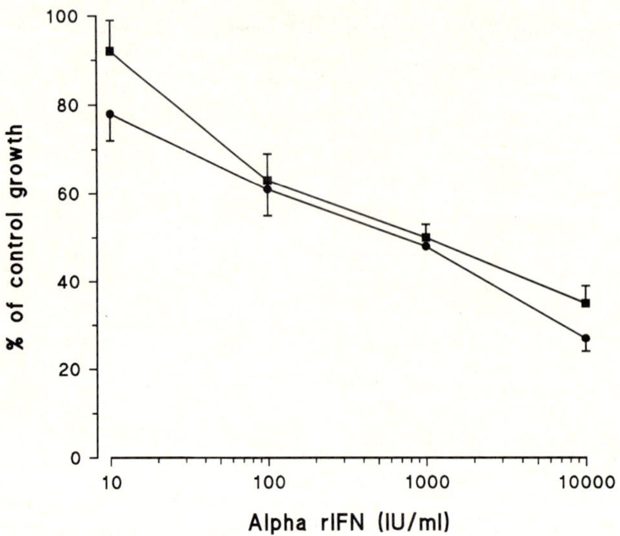

Fig. 1. Influence of human recombinant alpha- interferon on GFU-GM from 13 normal subjects (●——●) and 11 patients with CML (■——■)

suggests that the selective inhibitory effect of IFN-α on the malignant clone sometimes observed in CML in vivo (the patients showing partial or total cytogenetic conversion during IFN-α therapy) is not taking place at the CFU-GM level but probably at a more ancestral, stem cell level.

In vitro studies were also conducted in order to compare the production of IFN-α and -γ by peripheral blood cells in normal controls ($n = 22$) and patients with CML ($n = 18$) [3]. These cells were stimulated in vitro either by Newcastle disease virus (NDV) or *Corynebacterium parvum* (CP) for IFN-α or by phytohemagglutinin (PHA) for IFN-γ. The production of IFN-α by peripheral blood cells of CML patients was found to be significantly decreased in comparison to normal. This was observed whatever the method used for dosage of IFN-α (RIA or bioassay), and therefore excludes the possibility of the production of an abnormal IFN-α. The production of IFN-γ, on the other hand, was found to be normal. The mechanism of this abnormality and its possible role in the pathogenesis of the disease remain to be elucidated. A recent publication having indicated IFN-α gene deletion on chromosome 9 in several human malignant cell lines, including K562 cells, our CML patients are now investigated at the level of IFN-α genes.

The mechanism of resistance to IFN-α observed in some CML patients was also examined [4]. Ten cellular genes induced by IFN-α and probably mediating various of its biological activities were tested by northern blot analysis of RNA in marrow and in blood cells. Normal controls ($n = 6$), IFN-α-sensitive CML patients ($n = 2$), and CML patients clinically resistant to IFN-α ($n = 3$; two acquired and one initial resistance) were studied. The ten IFN-α-inducible genes were induced similarly in all the cases examined. The cells of one resistant case were studied after addition of IFN-α either in vivo or in vitro; the results were similar for the two administration modalities. We conclude that the resistance to IFN-α treatment of the CML patients we studied is not due to (a) the absence of induction of any of the ten IFN-inducible genes we studied, including the low molecular weight $2'-5'$-oligoadenylate synthetase, (b) the presence of an antagonist of IFN-α in the peripheral blood or bone marrow cells, (c) or the presence of neutralizing anti-IFN-α antibodies.

It is concluded: (a) that rIFN-α_{2c} in CML is therapeutically as active as -α_{2a} and -α_{2b} types in terms of HR, cytogenetic conversion, and survival; (b) that in vitro resistance of CFU-GM to IFN-α is observed in some cases of CML but that greater sensitivity in CML than in normal CFU-GM was not encountered; (c) that the fractional endogenous production of IFN-α by peripheral blood cells is decreased in CML and that this could possibly give an explanation for the efficacy of therapy of CML with IFN-α, and (d) at least in the three IFN-α-resistant CML cases tested, resistance to IFN-α therapy could not be explained by the absence of induction of the ten IFN-α-inducible genes studied.

References

1. Talpaz M, Kantarjian HM, Kurzrock R, Gutterman J (1988) Therapy of chronic myelogenous leukemia: chemotherapy and interferons. Semin Hematol 25:62–73
2. Delforge A, Vandenplas B, Lagneaux L, Loos M, Bron D, Debusscher L, Stryckmans P (1990) Influence of recombinant alpha and gamma interferons on the in vitro proliferation of myeloid and leukemic progenitors. Eur J Haematol 44:307–311
3. Stryckmans P, Dorval C, Clauss I, Vandenplas B, Huygen K, Fruhling J, Delforge A, Huez G (1989) Decreased production of alpha interferon (A-IFN) by peripheral blood cells of patients with chronic myeloid leukemia (CML). Blood 74(7):277 a [Suppl 1]
4. Claus I, Vandenplas B, Wathelet M, Dorval C, Delforge A, Content J, Stryckmans P, Huez G (1991) Analysis of interferon-inducible genes in cells of chronic myeloid leukemia patients responsive or resistant to an interferon-alpha treatment. Blood (in press)

Long-Term Treatment with Alpha-Interferon of Excessive Thrombocytosis in Myeloproliferative Disorders

H. Gisslinger,[1] W. Linkesch, A. Chott, and H. Ludwig

Long-term alpha-interferon (IFN-α) treatment was initiated in 31 patients with excessive thrombocytosis due to myeloproliferative disorders: 9 with essential thrombocythemia (ET); 12, polycythemia vera (PV); 5 with idiopathic myelofibrosis (IMF); and 5 with chronic myeloid leukemia (CML). After 12 months of IFN treatment 22 patients were randomized either to continuation or withdrawal of the treatment.

Normalization of platelet counts was achieved in 80% of patients after a median treatment duration of 6 weeks (range, 1–39 weeks). The platelet counts of the other patients decreased by more than 25% of the pretreatment values. Disease-associated circulation disturbances and bleeding events normalized or improved in all patients.

The beneficial effects of IFN treatment could be maintained for as long as three years. However, withdrawal of treatment resulted in relapse of thrombocytosis and reoccurrence of disease-associated symptoms. After discontinuation of IFN, 4 patients were reinduced and all of them responded. Serial bone marrow biopsies showed a significant reduction of bone marrow megakaryocytosis. IFN-related side effects were tolerable in the majority of patients.

Long-term IFN therapy is feasible in most patients with symptomatic excessive thrombocytosis and results in a reduction or normalization of thrombocytosis and a marked improvement of clinical symptoms.

[1] Second Department of Medicine, University of Vienna, A-1090 Vienna, Austria

Fleischer (Ed.) Leukemias
© Springer-Verlag Berlin Heidelberg 1993

Sustained Remission After Interferon Treatment for Essential Thrombocythemia

D. Lutz,[1] H. Kasparu, M. Bernhart, and O. Krieger

Introduction

Essential thrombocythemia (ET) is a myeloproliferative disorder of clonal origin [1] resulting in excessive production of platelets [2,3] and in an increased risk of thrombohemorrhagic complications. The Polycythemia Vera Study Group (PVSG) has proposed a number of diagnostic criteria to exclude the remaining chronic myeloproliferative disorders with elevated platelet counts and other conditions potentially causing thrombocytosis [4]. The aim of treatment for patients with ET is the prevention of thrombotic and/or hemorrhagic complications. Control of thrombocytosis and attributable symptoms is obtained in the majority of patients by myelosuppressive therapy, e.g., radioactive phosphorus, busulphan, chlorambucil, melphalan, pipobroman, and hydroxyurea [5–11]. Rapid and prolonged remission has been frequently achieved but continuous treatment for maintaining remission, as well as treatment complications such as induction of unwarranted bone marrow aplasia or secondary malignancy, limit the usefulness of these cytotoxic drugs. Interferon-α (IFN-α) is effective in cases of ET and excessive thrombocytosis in myeloproliferative diseases [12–15]. We report results from studies of 12 patients with ET receiving recombinant IFN-α_{2b} (rIFN-α_{2b}), some of whom have achieved an unmaintained remission for more than one year.

Patients and Treatment

Twelve patients below the age of 65 years (9 female, 3 male; age, 36–65 years) with essential thrombocythemia developed various clinical symptoms concomitant with excessive thrombocytosis ($777–2104 \times 10^9$/l) requiring therapy.

ET was diagnosed between 1 and 84 months (median, 11 months) before treatment was initiated following the criteria of the PVSG [4]. Bone

[1] 3rd Medical Department and Ludwig Boltzmann Institute for Leukemia Research and Hematology, Hanusch Hospital, Vienna, Austria and 1st Int. Dept., Elisabethinen Hospital, Linz, Austria

Fleischer (Ed.) Leukemias
© Springer-Verlag Berlin Heidelberg 1993

marrow aspiration and biopsy were performed in all patients. None of the patients showed a Philadelphia chromosome. Leukocyte alkaline phosphatase (LAP) scores were within the normal range (25–100) in all patients.

Two patients showed a slightly enlarged spleen (<+5 cm in diameter) on ultrasonic assessment. All except one of the patients (with thrombophlebitis) were free of infectious episodes during the 3 months before IFN therapy was initiated.

rIFN-α_{2b} (5 × 10^6 U) was administered s.c. once a day throughout the study. Induction therapy was given daily until relief of disease-related symptoms was obtained and platelet counts dropped to below 450 × 10^9/l (phase I). Thereafter, IFN therapy was continued every other day for 3–6 months, followed by further tapering to twice and once weekly (phase II). The aim of this schedule is to determine whether a platelet count held within the normal range (<450 × 10^9/l) for at least 1 year may be followed by a period of sustained hematological and clinical remission without further treatment. All patients were managed on an outpatient basis. Most patients administered IFN injections by themselves. Oral paracetamol up to 2 g/day was given to control side effects of IFN treatment. Whenever platelet counts increased for more than 4 weeks to above 450 × 10^9/l during phase II, IFN therapy was reinforced with daily administration for another 4 months before treatment reduction was repeated. Clinical examination and routine blood tests were carried out at least three times a week during phase I; thereafter frequency was reduced to once a week and later to once a month.

Results

Interferon-α_{2b} (5 × 10^6 U) s.c. daily resulted in a decrease in platelet count and a relief of clinical symptoms in all 12 patients within 7–10 days. However, only 10 achieved remission (platelets, <450 × 10^9/l) after a treatment period of between 14 and 75 days. In addition, WBC count dropped in response to induction treatment (median, 9.8 × 10^9/l vs. 4.7 × 10^9/l) but values for hemoglobin did not change. Early remission (within 5 weeks) was usually obtained in younger patients and in those with lower initial platelet counts.

Six patients remained in remission throughout the maintenance treatment when the frequency of IFN therapy was reduced (phase II). One of these patients receiving IFN every other day suddenly developed an ischemic cerebral stroke without preceding clinical symptoms. Of the remaining five patients one is still on maintenance therapy whereas four had come off treatment after a period of 9–18 months.

Four of ten patients in remission relapsed within 3 months during IFN administration every second day and reached platelet values greater than 700 × 10^9/l without developing any clinical symptoms attributed to thrombocytosis.

Four patients terminated phase II and remained off further treatment. Until now, one patient has relapsed after 19 months, whereas three patients have been without IFN treatment for 2, 13, and 30 months, respectively. They still remain free of any clinical symptoms and continue to have normal or only slightly elevated platelet counts.

Adverse side effects to initial IFN treatment have been observed with an incidence comparable with other reports (12–15): "Flu-like" symptoms for a median of 5 days (fever, 83%; chills, 17%; fatigue and malaise, 26%, headache, 17%; myalgia and arthralgia, 17%); anorexia/nausea, 9%; and itching, 9%. All subjective and objective side effects disappeared within 14 days and were controlled by repeated doses of oral paracetamol.

Discussion

Of 12 patients with ET according to the PVSG criteria (4), 10 under the age of 65 years achieved remission within 75 days of starting induction treatment administering 5×10^6 U IFN-α s.c. daily which is comparable with results reported earlier (12–15). Stepwise reduction in the frequency of IFN administration was successfull for 60% of those in remission. However, these patients had lower initial platelet counts and responded early to induction treatment. Relapses during maintenance (four patients) were observed in elderly patients achieving late remission (after more than 5 weeks of induction therapy). Reinforced IFN treatment was finally withdrawn in these patients due to unacceptable side effects or patients' lack of compliance. Therefore, the group of ET patients who benefited from IFN maintenance therapy may be recognized by an initial platelet count below 1600×10^9/liter and/or by the time taken to respond to induction therapy (within 5 weeks).

Half of the initially treated patients remained in continuous remission during maintenance therapy for 9–18 months; four of them came off treatment. Despite the fact that the median observation time is short, three patients have been free of treatment for 2, 13, and 30+ months which is in part equal to or even longer than the duration of IFN treatment. This implies that IFN may induce prolonged unmaintained remission in ET such as has been observed with alkylating agents [6,7] and radioactive phosphorus but seldom with hydroxyurea [16]. Regarding the risk of inducing secondary malignancies with these cytotoxic drugs, our data support the use of IFN for frontline therapy in younger patients with ET, especially for those in which early treatment is taken into consideration [17–18].

References

1. Fialkow PJ, Faguet GB, Jacobson RJ, Vaidya K, Murphy S (1981) Evidence that essential thrombocythemia is a clonal disorder with origin in a multipotent stem cell. Blood 58:916–919
2. Harker LA, Finch CA (1969) Thrombokinetics in man. J Clin Invest 48:963–968
3. Pareti FJ, Gugliotta L, Mannucci L, Guarini A, Mannucci PM (1982) Biochemical and metabolic aspects of platelet dysfunction in chronic myeloproliferative disorders. Thromb Haemost 47:84–89
4. Murphy S, Iiand H, Rosenthal D, Laszlo J (1986) Essential thrombocythemia: an interim report from the Polycythemia Vera Study Group. Semin Hematol 23:177–182
5. Hehlmann R, Jahn M, Baumann B, Köpcke W (1988) Essential thrombocythemia: Clinical characteristics and course of 61 cases. Cancer 61:2487–2496
6. Case DC Jr (1984) Therapy of essential thrombocythemia with thiotepa and chlorambucil. Blood 63:51–54
7. Pauw BE de (1985) Bergen ANL van, Haanen C, Steenbergen J (1985) Intermittent melphalan in the treatment of essential thrombocytosis with haemorrhage or thrombosis. Scand J Haematol 35:448–450
8. Gunz F (1980) Hemorrhagic thrombocythemia: a critical review. Blood 15:706–723
9. Murphy S (1983) Thromobocytosis and thrombocythemia. Clin Hematol 12:89–106
10. Mazzucconi M, Francesconi M, Chistolini E et al. (1986) Pipobroman therapy of essential thrombocythemia. Scand J Haematol 37:306–309
11. Löfvenberg E, Wahlin A (1988) Management of polycythemia vera, essential thrombocythemia and myelofibrosis with hydroxyurea. Eur J Haematol 41:375–381
12. Bellucci S, Harousseau JL, Brice P, Tobelem G (1988) Treatment of essential thrombocythemia by α-2a interferon. Lancet II:960–961
13. Giles FJ, Gray AG, Brozovic M et al. (1988) Alpha-Interferon therapy for essential thrombocythaemia. Lancet II:70–72
14. Talpaz M, Mavligit G, Keating M, Walters RS, Gutterman JU (1983) Human leucocyte interferon to control thrombocytosis in chronic myelogenous leukemia. Ann Intern Med 99:789–792
15. Gisslinger H, Linkesch W, Fritz E, Ludwig H, Chott A, Radaszkiewicz T (1989) Long-term interferon therapy for thrombocytosis in myeloproliferative diseases. Lancet I:634–637
16. Fernaux P, Simon M, Caulier MT, Lai JL, Goudemand J, Bauters F (1990) Clinical course of essential thrombocythemia in 147 cases. Cancer 66:549–556
17. Mitus AJ, Barbi T, Schulman LN et al. (1989) Hemostatic complications in young patients with essential thrombocythaemia. Blood 74 [Suppl 1]:274
18. Lichtman S, Allen SL, Schulman P et al. (1989) Essential thrombocythaemia in young adults. Blood 74 [Suppl 1]:402

Treatment of Chronic Myeloproliferative Disorders with Interferon-α

H.L. Seewann[1]

Chronic myeloproliferative disorders (CMPD) are not curable except when it is possible to carry out allogeneic bone marrow transplantation. Therapeutic modalities vary according to the subtype and course of CMPD. In most cases of advanced disease chemotherapeutic agents have been standard therapy for decades. During the last few years trials with interferon-α (IFN-α) have been designed to influence the course of disease. Beneficial effects have been reported in chronic myeloid leukemia (CML) [1,6,8] and thrombocytosis [2,3,5], and controversial results were observed in myelofibrosis [4,7].

The aim of this paper is to report our experience with IFN-α in respect to therapeutic approach, side effects, dosage modifications and remission rates in CMPD subtypes.

Material and Methods

A total of 45 patients with CMPD have been treated with IFN-α. Patients fell into three groups:

1. CML, Philadelphia chromosome-positive, 21 (juvenile CML, Philadelphia chromosome-negative, 1)
2. CMPD, Philadelphia chromosome-negative with thrombocytosis, 15
   a) Chronic megakaryocytic granulocytic myelosis (CMGM), 4
   b) Essential thrombocythemia (ETH), 9
   c) Polycythemia vera (PV), 2
3. Idiopathic myelofibrosis, 5

Characteristics of Patients

The Philadelphia chromosome-positive CML patients were aged 26–66 years (median, 49 years); male to female ratio was 13:8. The duration of disease prior to IFN therapy was 0–44 months (median, 5 months);

[1] Medizinische Abteilung III des Landeskrankenhauses, A-8036 Graz, Austria

Fleischer (Ed.) Leukemias
© Springer-Verlag Berlin Heidelberg 1993

17 patients were in chronic phase, and 4 patients were in accelerated phase. Patients in chronic phase were all, except one, previously untreated. Performance status was 90%–100%; patients presenting with symptoms (weight loss, and night sweats with or without fever), 7 out of 17; spleen size was 0–19 cm (median, 4 cm) below the costal margin; leucocytes, 30×10^3–345×10^3 cells/mm³ (median, 81×10^3/mm³). Patients with promyelocytes and/or myeloblasts of more than 10% in peripheral blood (PB), 3 out of 17; patients with basophils of more than 10% in PB, 2 out of 17; with haemoglobin less than 100 g/liter, 3 out of 17.

Three out of four patients in accelerated phase were pretreated and resistant to hydroxyurea and/or busulfan. Performance status was 90%–100%. Two patients showed myelofibrosis at bone marrow biopsy; all patients presented with symptoms. Promyelocytes and blasts in PB in all cases were found to be between 14% and 20%.

The age of patients with CMPD and thrombocytosis was 26–73 years (median, 62 years); male to female ratio, 5:10. Performance status was 90%–100%. Thrombocytosis was designated as mild (450–700), moderate (700–1000) and excessive (more than 1000×10^3 thrombocytes/mm³). According to this designation, one CMGM patient showed mild thrombocytosis, two, moderate and one, excessive. One PV patient showed mild thrombocytosis and one, moderate; and one ETH patient showed mild thrombocytosis, one, moderate and there were seven excessive cases.

Patients with myelofibrosis were aged 43–74 years (median, 64 years); male to female ratio was 4:1. All patients were regularly transfusion-dependent. White blood cell count was 2.2–26×10^3/mm³; platelet count was 25–181×10^3/mm³. Spleen size was 7.5–13 cm below the costal margin.

Treatment Strategies

In CML, IFN-α_2c 5 MU were given daily sc until complete peripheral haematological remission (CPHR). After gaining remission, the lowest IFN dosage to maintain remission was administered.

In CMPD with thrombocytosis, IFN-α_{2b} 3 MU daily sc were given until normalisation of thrombocyte count, but in no case longer than 10 weeks. After this time, or earlier after normalisation of platelet count, IFN dosage was reduced to 3 MU 3 × weekly and effect of this low dosage on platelet count was studied.

In idiopathic myelofibrosis, IFN-α_{2c} was given in low dosage (0.5–2 MU daily) according to low leucocyte and platelet counts. The effect was estimated by reduction in transfusion requirements.

Results

Philadelphia chromosome-positive CML patients in chronic phase ($n = 17$) showed CPHR in 9, partial remission or stable disease in 5 and progression in 3 cases. CPHR was gained 1–16 months (median, 2 months) after onset of treatment. Progression occurred after 6, 9 and 38 months respectively. Therapeutic effects were maintained in patients with CPHR from over 1 month to over 25 months and in patients with partial remission or stable disease, respectively, over 4 months–over 15 months. In patients with accelerated phase, stable disease was observed for 3–9 months. IFN treatment had to be disrupted because of blast crisis in three patients and excessive myelofibrosis in one patient.

Side effects of IFN therapy were: fever in 90%; weakness, 67%; arthralgias, 57%; hairloss, 24%; malaise, 24%; hyperhidrosis, 19%; dyspnoea, 19%; headache, 19%; diarrhoea, 14%; loss of taste, 10%; paraesthesia, 10%; and aphthosis, 10%.

In seven out of nine patients with chronic phase gaining CPHR, dosage reduction was possible (5 MU IFN-α 4 × weekly in one patient, 5 MU 3 × weekly in four patients, 2 MU 3 × weekly in one patient and one patient was without any therapy for more than 6 months).

In patients with CMPD with thrombocytosis, median platelet nadir within 10 weeks after onset of IFN-α treatment varied between 48% and 56% of pretherapeutic values. Platelet normalisation was found in all cases with CMGM and PV. In ETH only three out of nine patients showed a decline towards normal platelet counts. After dosis reduction to 3 MU 3 × weekly, however, half of the patients with CMGM and PV and all patients with ETH showed increase in platelets. Side effects did not significantly differ compared with those seen in CML.

In patients with myelofibrosis improvement in respect of decreased transfusion requirements was seen only in one of the five patients. In two patients cessation of treatment was necessary because of thrombocytopenia and neutropenia respectively.

Discussion

It could be shown that IFN-α is an effective treatment modality in patients with CML and CMPD with thrombocytosis. CPHR was reached in 53% of patients with CML chronic phase, and platelet normalisation was seen in 60% of patients with thrombocytosis. After gaining CPHR in patients with CML, dosage reduction was possible without loss of CPHR in 78% of patients. In CMPD with thrombocytosis, however, dosage reduction was followed by increasing platelet counts in most of the cases. In a few patients reexamined by bone marrow biopsy it was seen that IFN could not prevent progression of marrow fibrosis. The spectrum of side effects was similar in both conditions; however, side effects seemed to be felt more severely in patients with thrombocytosis, which was thought to be due to the advanced age of these patients.

At the present time, IFN-α seems to be an adequate treatment regimen for CML in chronic phase. In CMPD with thrombocytosis, decrease in elevated thrombocyte counts was obtained and thromboses or haemorrhages were prevented, but benefits of long-term treatment are not yet recognized.

References

1. Gastl G, Aulitzky Q, Tilg H, Huber H, Hausmaninger H, Seewann HL, Coser C, Prinoth P, Huber C (1987) Dose related effectiveness of alpha interferon in chronic myelogenous leukemia. Blut 54:251–252
2. Giles FJ, Gray AG, Brozovic M, et al. (1988) Alpha-interferon therapy for essential thrombocythaemia. Lancet 2(8602):70–72
3. Gisslinger H, Ludwig H, Linkesch W, et al. (1989) Long-term interferon therapy for thrombocytosis in myeloproliferative diseases. Lancet 1(8639):634–637
4. Gilbert HS (1988) Remission of myeloid metaplasia induced by recombinant alpha interferon. Clin Res 36(3):613A
5. Ludwig H, Linkesch W, Gisslinger H, Fritz E, Sinzinger H, Radaszkiewicz T, Chott A, Flener R, Micksche M (1987) Interferon-alpha corrects thrombocytosis in patients with myeloproliferative disorders. Cancer Immunol Immunother 25:266–273
6. Niederle N, Kloke O, Doberauer C, Becher R, Beelen DW, Schmidt CG (1986) Alpha$_2$-Interferon: erste Behandlungsergebnisse bei der chronischen myeloischen Leukämie. Dtsch Med Wochenschr 111:767–772
7. Seewann HL, Gastl G, Lang A, Abbrederis K, Thaler J, Flener R, Huber C (1988) Interferon-alpha-2 in the treatment of idiopathic myelofibrosis. Blut 56:161–163
8. Talpaz M, Kantarijan HM, McCredie K, Trujillo JM, Keating MJ, Gutterman JU (1986) Hematologic remission and cytogenetic improvement induced by recombinant human interferon Alpha$_A$ in chronic myelogenous leukemia. N Engl J Med 314: 1065–1069

Interferon-α and Hairy Cell Leukemia

J.D. Schwarzmeier[1] and G.C. Ihra

The excellent therapeutic response of hairy cell leukemia (HCL) to natural interferon-α (IFN-α) reported for the first time by Quesada et al. [1] and subsequently confirmed by numerous studies using recombinant IFN-α (e.g. [2]), has prompted a broad array of clinical trials with this substance. Among the diseases investigated so far, HCL is still the most sensitive disorder and has become a model system for the investigation of the anti-tumor effects of IFN-α.

In this article we summarize clinical data from a multicenter study on HCL and present results of in vitro studies on the mechanism of action of IFN-α in this disease.

Multicenter Study

216 HCL patients were treated with IFN-α_{2b} (Schering-Plough) at a dose of $2 \times 10^6 \, \mathrm{IU/m^2}$ s.c. thrice weekly.

The *diagnosis* of HCL was made using standard criteria. Parameters studied were progression of the disease, anemia, thrombocytopenia or leukopenia, and bone marrow involvement. Life expectancy had to be at least 3 months and the Karnofsky index at least 3. The dose of IFN-α was increased to $5 \times 10^6 \, \mathrm{IU/m^2}$ in patients who did not respond to therapy after 3 months.

A complete remission (CR) was defined as absence of hairy cells in the peripheral blood and bone marrow and restoration of hemoglobin levels to >12 g/dl, platelet counts to >100 000/µl and absolute granulocyte counts to >1500/µl. A partial remission (PR) was defined by restoration of peripheral blood values as indicated above and the occurrence of >5% of hairy cells in bone marrow aspirate. Minor responses (MR) were defined by normalization of one or more hematologic indices, but without recovery of all hematologic values.

The results indicate that 79% of the 216 patients studied entered remission (Table 1), 75% in PR and 3.8% in CR. 10% of the patients failed

---

[1] 1st Medical University Clinic, AKH-Wien, A-1090 Vienna, Austria

Fleischer (Ed.) Leukemias
© Springer-Verlag Berlin Heidelberg 1993

Table 1. Clinical response to IFN-α (open label study, SCH 30500)

	(*n*)	Patients (%)
Complete remission	8	3.8
Partial remission	162	75
Minor responses	23	10.6
No responses	23	10.6
Total	216	100

to respond to IFN-α therapy, either due to primary resistance or after termination of IFN-α treatment because of side effects. Most patients had undergone splenectomy before IFN-α therapy. Thus, evaluation of regression of splenomegaly was performed in nonsplenectomized individuals: 50% showed a substantial decrease in spleen sizes.

Initial side effects like transient fever, headache, and myalgia occurred in most patients, but only 19% suffered from severe symptoms (up to WHO grade III). Side effects included urticaria and pruritus, gastrointestinal symptoms (nausea, vomiting, diarrhea), and symptoms of the central nervous system (dizziness, depression). Symptoms were reversible in most patients.

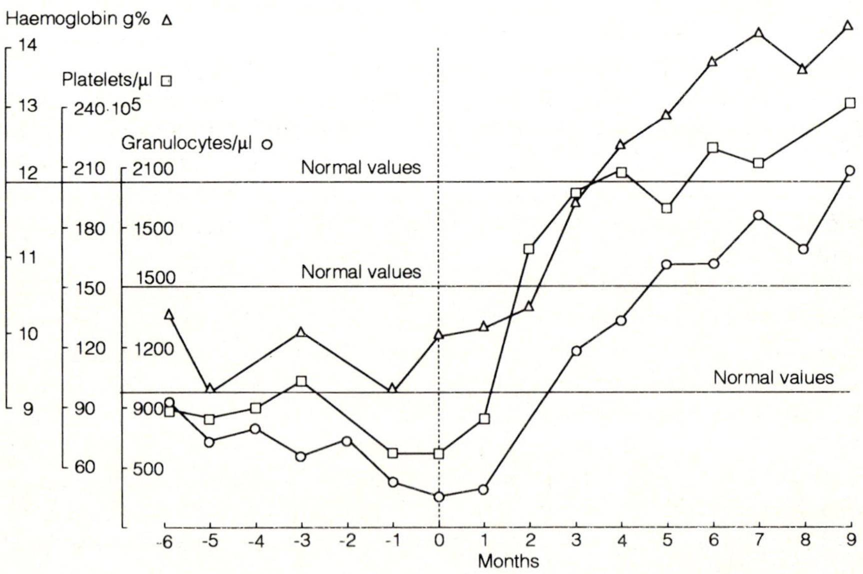

Fig. 1. Course of blood parameters in HCL patients during IFN-α therapy (multicenter study)

Figure 1 demonstrates the course of hemoglobin values and of granulocyte and platelet counts during therapy. The vertical line indicates the start of IFN-α administration. Platelets were the first hematologic parameter to normalize (within 1 month), followed by restoration of hemoglobin (after 3 months) and granulocyte counts (after 5 months). Simultaneously, bone marrow infiltration by hairy cells was reduced.

In summary, the study indicates that: (1) an optimal clinical response to IFN-α therapy requires at least 4–6 months of continuous treatment with IFN-α; (2) maximal improvement in bone marrow occurs at 9 months, while continued treatment beyond this point does not appear to produce a greater decline in hairy cell infiltration; (3) the low-dose IFN-α regimen described is well tolerated; (4) the majority of patients experience a striking improvement of hematologic parameters with no need for blood transfusions, and infections are reduced to a minimum. However, CR, characterized by complete clearance of hairy cells from the bone marrow, is achieved in only 3% of cases. Discontinuation of IFN-α therapy leads to reappearance of hairy cells but can be reversed by renewed IFN-α administration.

In Vitro Studies

The mechanism of action of IFN-α in HCL remains an enigma. It seems unlikely that DNA synthesis and hence the proliferation kinetics of hairy cells are a prime target of IFN-α. In previous studies we were unable to demonstrate a significant inhibition of [^{3}H]-thymidine incorporation into hairy cells by IFN-α [3]. Furthermore, the cytokine did not alter antigenic determinants in vitro, thus making a cell differentiating effect on hairy cells highly unlikely. We also did not find a consistent correlation between activation of natural killer cells in vivo and the response to therapy. Likewise, others were unable to demonstrate a direct cytolytic action of natural killer cells on hairy cells [4]. Therefore, natural killer cells probably play no major role in the regression of hairy cells during IFN-α therapy.

An attractive hypothesis is that IFN-α regulates the differentiation of malignant multilineage stem cells in HCL [5]. It was postulated that IFN-α causes a change in the composition of multilineage colonies obtained from HCL patients by induction of differentiation of "malignant lymphoid stem cells" into myelomonocytic cells. To test this idea we performed colony-forming assays from peripheral mononuclear cells of HCL patients. However, even over a wide range of IFN-α concentrations we could detect no differentiating effect of the cytokine in these colonies. This was true for colonies containing hairy cells and B-cells, as well as colonies without them (hairy cells and B-cells having been eliminated by complement-mediated lysis). In fact, colony formation was severely reduced in HCL and it was very difficult to detect a possible stimulatory effect.

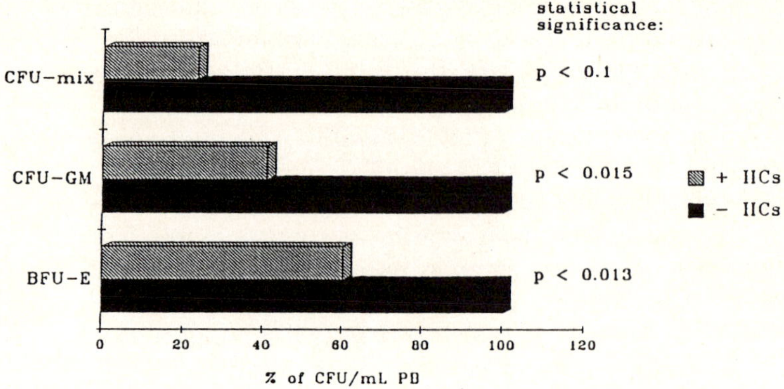

Fig. 2. Inhibition of colony formation (CFU-mixed CFU-GM, BFU-E) by hairy cells

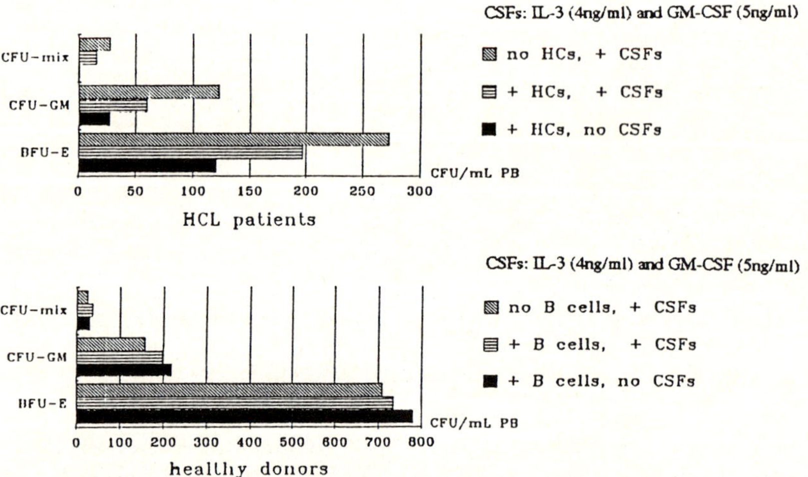

Fig. 3. Improvement of colony growth with interleukin-3 and GM-CSF

It has been speculated that inhibitory factors released by hairy cells play a causative role in the reduced colony formation [6] and hence in the development of hematopoietic failure in HCL patients. Our findings support this assumption, since the removal of hairy cells from the peripheral blood mononuclear cell fraction obtained from the patients resulted in a significant improvement of colony formation (Fig. 2). Supplementation of the culture medium with haemopoietic growth factors (recombinant interleukin-3 and recombinant GM-CSF) led to a further increase in colony number [7] and in some cases to levels comparable to those from healthy donors (Fig. 3). This points to a deficiency of growth factors in HCL. Indirect evidence for such a deficiency has also been provided by the observation that treatment with recombinant G-CSF increases neutrophil counts in HCL patients [8]. IFN-α in some way seems to improve this deficiency and to restore normal hematopoiesis. It is as yet unclear whether this is achieved by interacting with the production or action of inhibitory factors (e.g. IFN-α) or by restoration of a cell compartment (monocytes?) known to be essential for the supply of hematopoietic growth factors. It is tempting to speculate that monocytopenia, which is one of the most frequent findings in HCL, is causally related to the inadequate supply of cytokines. Preliminary data from our laboratory indicate that IFN-α has in fact a regulatory effect on the impaired cytokine production in HCL.

References

1. Quesada JR, Reuben J, Manning JT, Hersh EM, Gutterman JU (1984) Alpha interferon for induction of remission in hairy cell leukemia. N Engl J Med 310:15
2. Hofmann V, Scheel A, Schwarzmeier J, et al. (1985) Wirksamkeit von Interferon-α2 bei der Haarzell Leukämie. Schweiz Med Wochenschrift 115:235
3. Schwarzmeier JD, Schwabe M, Prischl F, Wagner L, Lion T, Micksche M, Köller U (1987) Interferon-alpha-2 for hairy cell leukemia: Evidence for induction of RNA synthesis in hairy cells and failure to corrlate enhancement of natural killer cells with elimination of hairy cells. Eur J Haematol 39:418
4. Griffiths SD, Cawley JC (1990) The effect of cytokines, including IL-1, IL-4, and IL-6, in hairy cell proliferation/differentiation. Leukemia 4:337
5. Michalewiz R, Revel M (1987) Interferons regulate the in vitro differentiation of multilineage lymphomyeloid stem cells in hairy cell leukemia. Proc Natl Acad Sci USA 84:2307
6. Taniguchi N, Karatsune H, Kanamaru A, Tokumine Y, Tagawa S, Machii T, Kitani T (1989) Inhibition against CFU-C and CFU-E colony formation by soluble factors derived from hairy cells. Blood 73:907
7. Gasché C, Reinisch W, Winkler K, Schwarzmeier JD (1992) Myelosuppression in hairy cell leukemia: role of hairy cells, haemopoietic growth factors, and tumor necrosis factor-α/β. (submitted)
8. Glaspy JA, Baldwin GC, Robertson PA, Souza L, Vincent M, Ambersley J, Golde DW (1988) Therapy for neutropenia in hairy cell leukemia with recombinant human granulocyte colony-stimulating factor. Ann Int Med 109:789

Bone Marrow Transplantation

Allogeneic Marrow Transplantation for Acute Leukemia*

R. STORB,[1] for the Seattle Bone Marrow Transplant Team

Introduction

Remarkable advances in marrow transplantation for acute leukemia have been made since the early 1970s when treatment was restricted to patients with advanced disease, and long-term survival was only on the order of 15% [1]. In the mid-1970s marrow grafting was applied earlier, during the first remission in patients with acute nonlymphoblastic leukemia (ANL) and during second or subsequent remission in patients with acute lymphoblastic leukemia (ALL) [2,3]. Patients with ANL grafted in first remission have survived better than those given chemotherapy (50% versus 20% actuarial survival, with the longest survivors currently at 11 years in continued remission) [4]. Thirty-five percent of patients with ALL given grafts in second or subsequent remission have survived, whereas similar patients undergoing chemotherapy all died of recurrent disease within $3\frac{1}{2}$ years of the initiation of therapy [5]. Patients with ANL grafted in early first relapse, incurable by chemotherapy, have shown 5-year disease-free survivals on the order of 30%, which is equal to or better than that seen in patients transplanted in second remission of ANL [6].

Despite improvements in the results of marrow transplantation for acute leukemia, major problems and complications remain [1–8]; these are shown in Table 1. Relapse of leukemia accounts for 22%–75% of treatment failures. Significant acute graft-versus-host disease (GVHD) is seen in 30%–45% of patients and is responsible for 10%–25% of treatment failures. Conditioning regimen-related toxicity and bacterial or fungal infections during the early period of pancytopenia result in 5%–10% of deaths. Fatal interstitial pneumonias may accompany acute GVHD or be the result of drug and radiation toxicity. For results of marrow grafting to improve, progress in each of these problem areas is needed.

* Supported in part by grants CA31787, CA18105, CA18221, CA15704, and CA18029, awarded by the National Cancer Institute of the National Institutes of Health, DHHS
[1] Division of Clinical Research of the Fred Hutchinson Cancer Research Center and the Department of Medicine, University of Washington School of Medicine, Seattle, Washington, USA

Table 1. HLA-identical marrow transplantation: complications and survival

	Disease						
	Acute lymphoblastic leukemia				Acute nonlymphoblastic leukemia		
Disease phase	1st CR	2nd CR	2nd+ Rel	3rd CR	1st CR	1st Rel	2nd+ CR
5-year disease-free survival (%)	54	35	18	30	50	30	25
Relapse (%)	35	45	75	58	22	31	45
Interstitial pneumonia[a] (%)			15			15–35	
Grades II-IV acute GvHD (%)			35			30–45	
Chronic GvHD (%)			25			25–35	
VOD (%)			7			28	
Failure to engraft (%)				<1			
Secondary malignancies (%)				5			
Infections (bacterial + fungal)							
During first 3 months, before engraftment (%)				20			
During first 3 months, after engraftment (%)				12			
After first 3 months (%)				20			

CR, complete remission; Rel, relapse; GvHD, graft-versus-host disease; VOD, veno-occlusive disease of the liver
[a] Includes both idiopathic and cytomegalovirus interstitial pneumonia.

Conditioning Regimens

The ideal conditioning program for marrow grafting both destroys the underlying malignant disease and suppresses host immunity sufficiently for acceptance of allogeneic grafts without fatal toxicity. Such a regimen, unfortunately, does not exist. Commonly used regimens in Seattle include cyclophosphamide (Cy) and 12–15.75 Gy fractionated total body irradiation (TBI) [1–8]. As shown in Table 1, however, these regimens are not sufficient to eradicate leukemia in all cases. Furthermore, there is a high incidence of graft failure in patients given T-depleted HLA-identical or non-T-depleted HLA-nonidentical marrow grafts [9,10]. Finally, while inadequately serving their purpose, the regimens have a 5%–10% mortality from associated toxicities. Results of recent studies have suggested advantages with newer programs. We have combined additional chemotherapy with TBI and also tried to optimize TBI itself. In one regimen, busulfan (6.9–8.7 mg/kg over 4 days) and Cy (49–67 mg/kg over 2 days) were combined with 12 Gy fractionated TBI [11]. This has resulted in 40% disease-free survival at 18 months among 33 patients with advanced leukemia. In another regimen, high-dose cytosine arabinoside (3 g/m^2 every 12 h for 12 doses) was combined with 12 Gy fractionated TBI with or without 60 mg/kg

Cy in 29 patients with advanced leukemia [12]. Despite considerable early toxicity with this regimen, 40% disease-free survival at 2 years was seen. Results of these early studies are sufficiently encouraging to warrant formal phase III studies comparing these regimens to more established regimens for efficacy. Conventional Cy also can be combined with 16 Gy TBI given as 200 cGy in two daily fractions or 14.4 Gy TBI given as 120 cGy in three daily fractions [unpublished]. However, for all approaches involving systemic chemotherapy and TBI, the limits of nonhemopoietic toxicity have been reached and, barring the development of new drugs, no quantum improvements can be anticipated from these approaches.

The most effective way to eradicate leukemia would be to use agents which interact specifically with leukemic cells. A method approaching this ideal most closely is the use of monoclonal antibodies directed against antigens expressed on leukemic cells. Monoclonal antibodies injected in vivo are known to concentrate on leukemic cells; however, the antileukemic effect is limited, in part because some leukemic cells may lack target antigens, and in part because some cells, though coated by antibody, may not be killed by it. Antibodies linked to toxins such as the ricin A chain may provide more effective tumor cell kill; however, there have been problems with this approach. Another approach involves attaching monoclonal antibodies to short-lived–high-energy radioactive isotopes which deposit most of their energy within a 1- to 2-mm radius. This way, leukemic cells expressing the target antigens would be killed, as would be neighboring antigen-negative cells. Because this approach would ablate normal marrow cells, subsequent marrow "rescue" would be needed. Initial studies in a canine model have shown appropriate antibody isotope conjugates to localize preferentially in marrow and spleen and, to a lesser extent, in lymph nodes [13,14,15]. The amount of isotope in the marrow compared to other organs has shown ratios of 20:1 or better. The otherwise fatal marrow aplasia caused by radiolabeled antibodies is reversible through infusion of cryopreserved autologous marrow 8 days after isotope injection, at a time when very little radioactivity is left. Combinations of chemotherapy, TBI, and radiolabeled antibodies are being explored for their ability to prepare dogs for T cell-depleted marrow grafts. Refinements of this approach, particularly the use of high-energy–beta-emitting isotopes with short linear energy transfers, are likely to result in less toxic but more efficient conditioning programs, not only providing better elimination of leukemia but also improving the problem of graft failure in patients with T cell-depleted HLA-identical or HLA-nonidentical marrow grafts.

Prevention of GVHD

A critical issue of successful transplantation is the prevention of GVHD without simultaneously increasing the risk of graft failure and of recurrent leukemia. Prevention has customarily involved postgrafting immunosuppression for a period of 3–6 months. Controlled randomized trials have shown the drugs methotrexate and cyclosporine to be equivalent in preventing acute GVHD [16]. A combination of methotrexate and cyclosporine is significantly better than either drug alone in preventing acute GVHD [17]. Another way to reduce the incidence of acute GVHD has been to remove T cells from the marrow by immunological or mechanical means. Nearly all clinical studies to date have shown a significant reduction in acute GVHD, providing convincing evidence for a favorable effect of T cell depletion on GVHD [10,18]. However, the reduction in acute GVHD was achieved at the price of substantial increases in graft rejection and leukemic relapse.

Prevention or Treatment of Interstitial Pneumonia

Pneumocystis carinii infection, formerly the cause of about 10% of all interstitial pneumonias, is now being prevented by prophylactic trimethoprim sulfamethoxazole. By far the most serious infection is due to cytomegalovirus (CMV). CMV activation can develop into pneumonia which has a case fatality rate of approximately 85%. Patients who are seronegative before transplant can be protected by the use of CMV-negative blood products after transplant. The use of CMV immunoglobulin has been controversial. Interferon, acyclovir, adenine arabinoside, and an acyclovir derivative, dihydroxymethylethoxymethylguanine (DHPG), are not effective in treating CMV pneumonias. However, the use of DHPG reduces the amount of virus in the lungs. DHPG may be beneficial, when given along with CMV immunoglobulin, in treating established CMV pneumonia. Idiopathic interstitial pneumonia was seen in approximately 13% of patients given single-dose TBI, but only in 3% of patients given fractionated TBI. [Reviewed in 19.]

Conditioning-Related Toxicity and Early Infections

Conditioning regimen-related toxicity may be reduced with the use of more directed therapy, such as the radiolabeled monoclonal antibodies described above. Certain recombinant human hematopoietic growth factors such as granulocyte–colony-stimulating factor (G-CSF) and granulocyte-macrophage–CSF (GM-CSF) may shorten the period of granulocytopenia after grafting, and this may reduce the incidence of early infections and result in a modest improvement in survival, on the order of 5%.

References

1. Thomas ED, et al. (1975) Bone-marrow transplantation. N Engl J Med 292:832–843, 895–902
2. Thomas ED, et al. (1979) Marrow transplantation for acute nonlymphoblastic leukemia in first remission. N Engl J Med 301:597–599

3. Thomas ED, et al. (1979) Marrow transplantation for patients with acute lymphoblastic leukemia in remission. Blood 54:468–476
4. Appelbaum FR et al. (1984) Bone marrow transplantation or chemotherapy after remission induction for adults with acute nonlymphoblastic leukemia – a prospective comparison. Ann Intern Med 101:581–588
5. Johnson FL, et al. (1981) A comparison of marrow transplantation with chemotherapy for children with acute lymphoblastic leukemia in second or subsequent remission. N Engl J Med 305:846–851
6. Clift RA, et al. (1987) The treatment of acute non-lymphoblastic leukemia by allogeneic marrow transplantation. Bone Marrow Transplant 2:243–258
7. Sanders JE, et al. (1988) Allogeneic marrow transplantation for children with juvenile chronic myelogenous leukemia. Concise Report. Blood 71:1144–1146
8. Storb R (1989) Bone marrow transplantation. In: DeVita VT Jr, Hellman S, Rosenberg SA (eds) Cancer: principles and practice of oncology, 3rd edn. Lippincott, Philadelphia, pp 2474–2489
9. Anasetti C, et al. (1989) Effect of HLA compatibility on engraftment of bone marrow transplants in patients with leukemia or lymphoma. N Engl J Med 320:197–204
10. Martin PJ, et al. (1985) Effects of in vitro depletion of T cells in HLA-identical allogeneic marrow grafts. Blood 66:664–672
11. Petersen FB, et al. (1990) Autologous marrow transplantation for malignant lymphoma. A report of 101 cases from Seattle. J Clin Oncol 8:638–647
12. Riddell S, et al. (1988) High-dose cytarabine and total body irradiation with or without cyclophosphamide as a preparative regimen for marrow transplantation for acute leukemia. J Clin Oncol 6:576–582
13. Appelbaum FR, et al. (1988) Characterization of malignant lymphoma in dogs and use as a model for the development of treatment strategies. In: Baum SJ, Santos GW, Takaku F (eds) Recent advances and future directions in bone marrow transplantation (Experimental hematology today, 1987). Springer, Berlin Heidelberg New York, pp 31–35
14. Appelbaum FR, et al. (1989) Antibody-radionuclide conjugates as part of a myeloablative preparative regimen for marrow transplantation. Blood 73:2202–2208
15. Bianco JA, et al. (1989) Specific marrow localization of an ^{131}I-labeled anti-myeloid antibody in normal dogs: effects of a "cold" antibody pretreatment dose on marrow localization. Exp Hematol 17:929–934
16. Storb R, et al. (1988) Cyclosporine v methotrexate for graft-v-host disease prevention in patients given marrow grafts for leukemia: long-term follow-up of three controlled trials. Blood 71:293–298
17. Storb R, et al. (1986) Methotrexate and cyclosporine compared with cyclosporine alone for prophylaxis of acute graft versus host disease after marrow transplantation for leukemia. N Engl J Med 314:729–735
18. Butturini A, et al. (1988) T cell depletion in bone marrow transplantation for leukemia: current results and future directions. Bone Marrow Transplant 3:185–192
19. Meyers JD (1988) Prevention and treatment of cytomegalovirus infection after marrow transplantation. Bone Marrow Transplant 3:95–104

Allogeneic Bone Marrow Transplantation: State of the Art and Future Directions

J. M. GOLDMAN[1]

A relatively large numer of patients with chronic myeloid leukemia (CML) have now been treated in different centres by transplantation of bone marrow from HLA-identical sibling donors. The 4-year leukemia-free survival is 46% (40%–52%; 95% confidence limits). The major factors determining this probability are disease status at diagnosis, patient age, the occurrence of graft-versus-host disease after transplant and the use of T-cell depletion. The prognostic significance of residual or recurrent disease identified after transplant may on occasion be uncertain because there are various criteria for "relapse": (a) haematological relapse – the finding of leucocytosis and thrombocytosis; (b) cytogenetic relapse – the identification of Philadelphia chromosome-(Ph)-positivity in the marrow (in the absence of haematological abnormalities); and (c) molecular relapse – the identification only of mRNA with a BCR-ABL junction using the polymerase chain reaction. Haematological or cytogenetic relapse is rare in patients receiving transplants of T-replete marrow in chronic phase but common in the recipients of T-depleted donor marrow cells. The incidence of molecular relapse is not yet defined.

There are a number of other problems that apply particularly to CML. What can be done for patients who lack sibling donors? The use of matched unrelated donors gives preliminary results which may be comparable to those achieved with matched siblings. How can one determine the optimal timing of transplantation within the chronic phase? Improved methods for predicting the probability of survival with conventional treatment must be balanced against the calculated probability of transplant-related mortality and risk of relapse. It might be reasonable to offer to all patients eligible for transplant first the option of a therapeutic trial of alpha-interferon and to proceed to transplant only in those patients who obtain no cytogenetic benefit.

[1] Royal Postgraduate Medical School, London WI2 0NN, UK

Fleischer (Ed.) Leukemias
© Springer-Verlag Berlin Heidelberg 1993

Bone Marrow Transplantation for Leukemia in Europe

A. GRATWOHL,[1] for the Leukemia Working Party of the
European Group for Bone Marrow Transplantation

Introduction

Bone marrow transplantation (BMT) from an HLA-identical sibling donor
is today an accepted form of therapy. The methods are standardized and
defined and the major risks – transplant-related mortality (TRM) and relapse
of the primary disease – are well defined. BMT is the treatment of choice for
many patients with severe disorders of the bone marrow, e.g., leukemia. It
is the only curative form of therapy for patients with chronic myeloid
leukemia (CML), myelodysplastic syndromes, or chronic lymphocytic
leukemia and the most potent antileukemic therapy available for patients
with acute leukemia. Consensus exists that results are best if the transplant
is performed early in the disease, in first complete remission (1st CR) of
acute leukemia or in first chronic phase of CML (CML cp); however,
controversies exist about whether BMT should indeed be undertaken in all
patients with acute leukemia in 1st CR. A retrospective multicenter analysis
of transplant data cannot unequivocally answer such a question. It can,
however, by looking at the factors influencing outcome, be of help in
deciding the therapeutic strategy for prospective trials and in assessing the
risks for an individual patient.

The following analysis evaluates the various individual factors influencing outcome of leukemia-free survival (LFS), transplant related mortality
(TRM), and relapse incidence (RI) following allogeneic transplantation for
patients with leukemia.

Patients and Methods

The Leukemia Working Party of the European Group for Bone Marrow
Transplantation (EBMT) has collected patient data, with questionnaires,
from patients given transplants for leukemia in Europe since 1979. A new
data base management system was introduced in 1988. This analysis is still
restricted to the information on 2060 patients in the EBMT data base, given
transplants between 1979 and 1986, and updated as of December 1988 [1].

[1] Hematology Division, Department of Internal Medicine, Petersgraben 4,
CH-4031 Basel, Switzerland

Fleischer (Ed.) Leukemias
© Springer-Verlag Berlin Heidelberg 1993

This file includes: 616 patients with CML (mean age, 31 years; range, 1–53 years), 459 patients in CML cp (mean age, 30 years), and 157 patients not in CML cp (mean, 32 years); 745 patients with acute myeloid leukemia (AML) (mean age, 25 years; range, 1–50 years), 581 in 1st CR (mean, 25 years), and 164 not in 1st CR (mean, 26 years); 654 patients with acute lymphocytic leukemia (ALL) (mean, 18 years; range, 1–47 years), 267 in 1st CR (mean, 23 years), and 387 not 1st CR (mean, 15 years). Transplants were given to 45 patients for other leukemias, mainly myelodysplastic syndromes.

Information obtained for these transplants related to the following 13 fields:

1. Investigator information
2. Recipient information
   a) Name
   b) Sex
   c) Date of birth
3. Disease information
   a) Type and subtype
   b) Stage
   c) Date of diagnosis
   d) Date of last achieved hematological remission
   e) Cytogenetic abnormalities
   f) Extramedullary disease
4. Donor information
   a) Sex
   b) Date of birth
   c) Relationship
5. Transplant procedure
   a) Date
   b) Number of cells
6. Total body irradiation
   a) Dose
   b) Dose rate
   c) Lung dose
   d) Lung shielding
   e) Fractionation
   f) CNS irradiation
7. Graft-versus-host disease (GvHD)
   a) Prevention method
   b) Maximal grade
   c) Treatment
   d) Day of onset
8. Chronic GvHD
   a) Day of onset

      b) Severity

      c) Resolution

9. Interstitial pneumonitis

      a) Date of onset

      b) Etiology

      c) Severity

      d) Resolution

10. Relapse

      a) Date of onset

      b) Origin

11. Survival status and cause of death

12. Additional information

      a) Karnofsky performance

      b) Number of BMT

13. Follow-up, cataract, and secondary malignancies

These variables were analyzed by crosstabulation for differences within the cohorts and subgroups, for changes over time, and by diagnostic categories. Endpoints in multivariate analyses were LFS, RI, or TRM. Crosstables were analyzed by the Chi-square test. Differences in survival were examined with the Lee-Desu test. The Cox regression model was used for the multivariate analysis and to rank the influence of variables on the endpoints.

Results

Survival. On 1891 patients receiving transplants from an HLA-identical sibling donor for AML, ALL, or CML, complete information was obtained as of 1 January 1989. Of 829 patients who were alive (44%), 614 patients survived more than 3 years and 128 patients more than 6 years after the transplant; 1062 patients had died. The major factor influencing outcome was the stage of the disease at the time of the transplant. The survival rate was as follows: for CML cp, 67%, CML not cp, 33%; for AML 1st CR,

Table 1. Factors causing post-transplant death

	Acute GvHD (*n*)	Chronic GvHD		Intersitital pneumonitis (*n*)	Death		Alive	
		At any time (*n*)	Extensive (*n*)		TRM (*n*)	Relapse (*n*)	(*n*)	(%)
Absent	784	105	22	121	260	150	374	48
Mild	459	160	28	84	106	84	269	59
Moderate	351	140	37	96	150	53	148	42
Severe	292	94	59	111	243	11	38	13
Total	1891	499	146	412	531	298	829	44

50%, AML not 1st CR, 31%; for ALL 1st CR, 51%, for ALL not 1st CR, 33%.

The major post-transplant factor leading to death was GvHD. The presence and degree of acute GvHD influenced chronic GvHD, interstitial pneumonitis, and the relative cause of death. This is illustrated by the Table 1:

Historical Changes. There were considerable changes during the decade. CML became the most common indication and there was a clear trend to transplant in older patients. The methods of GvHD prevention changed as did the TBI techniques. Cyclosporine is the most frequent therapy for GvHD prevention now. About half of the teams use fractionated TBI and about half of the teams shield the lungs.

Investigator Information. Previous studies all have failed to show a center effect on transplant outcome. However, when centers are grouped by region the situation is different. The patient population varies considerably from region to region concerning disease, subtype, stage, GvHD prevention methods, and time intervals. In addition, a multivariate analysis shows that, independent of these differences in the population, LFS is not the same in all regions. This is not due to changes in TRM but due to a different RI. These findings suggest that pretransplant factors might be more important than previously thought.

Recipient Information. Age of the patient is the second most important factor influencing outcome. TRM increases decade by decade with a major breakpoint between the second and third decade of life. Very young children, from infancy to 3 years old, have also a relatively poor outcome. Sex of the recipient affects outcome in relation to the sex of the donor as well as independent of it. Male recipients in general have a worse prognosis than female recipients.

Disease. Stage of the disease is the most important single factor influencing LFS, TRM, and RI. Patients given transplants in first CR of their acute leukemia and in CML cp have a much better LFS, TRM, and RI than those receiving transplants at a later stage of their disease. There is no difference between the main three diagnostic categories AML, ALL, and CML. AML subtypes M4 and M5 have an increased RI. For ALL no such influence of subtype is yet significant.

There is an additional important factor concerning the disease. For patients with acute leukemia, results are influenced by the time intervals from diagnosis to first CR as well as by the time from first CR to the transplant. Patients entering late first CR (after more than 8 weeks) have a significantly higher, later TRM than those with rapid first CR. In contrast, patients receiving a transplant with a long delay between first CR and BMT have a reduced RI compared with patients who had a transplant soon after entering first CR (less than 3 months).

Total Body Irradiation. There have been changes over time in the number of patients receiving fractionated rather than single-dose total body irradiation (TBI) as well as in the number of patients given additional lung shielding. About 50% of the teams use either one of those approaches. This finding probably best illustrates that the irradiation techniques still need to be defined. The data have not yet allowed a clear assessment of the influence of individual TBI physical data upon outcome.

Graft-Versus-Host Disease. The most important cause of death and the factor contributing most to the development of interstitial pneumonitis (as illustrated in Table 1) is GvHD. The method of its prevention influences outcome. Cyclosporine reduces TRM compared to methotrexate. It increases RI in certain subgroups, but the advantage of a better LFS remains. T-cell depletion reduces TRM but increases the risk of relapse.

Relapse. The most important factor influencing RI is the stage of the disease at the time of transplant. Additional factors are subtype for AML, GvHD prevention methods, and the presence or absence of GvHD. Patients who relapse have a high risk of dying. Less than 20% respond to treatment with a prolonged sustained remission. All these patients return characteristically to donor-type normal hemopoiesis following reinduction therapy. A small subgroup might be cured.

Follow-up. The long follow-up of a large group of patients now allows assessment of late complications. Of a total of 648 patients surviving for at least 3 years, 48 died 3 or more years after BMT, 27 due to relapse, and 21 due to other causes. These numbers document that late complications occur and need to be addressed more closely in the future.

Discussion

These retrospective data can help to define the role of BMT in the treatment of leukemia. They help to elucidate mechanisms leading to failure, they are of importance when results of different studies have to be compared, and they are of value to assess the risks for individual patients. They cannot solve the dilemma of the physician in charge to decide whether an individual patient should be given a transplant or not. It is clear that certain factors are given: age, sex, and disease of a patient cannot be changed. Other factors such as GvHD prevention methods and donor age and sex can be changed under certain conditions. Donor factors will certainly become more important with the increased availability of unrelated matched donors. Despite these limitations, these data clearly show that BMT is a successful therapeutic modality leading to long-term cure rates in the order of 50% after 8 years for patients given transplants early, and 20%–30% for patients with refractory or relapsed leukemia.

Acknowledgements. The Working Party would like to thank the physicians of the following institutions for their cooperation in this report:

Austria: Dr. W. Hinterberger, Vienna; Belgium: Dr. A. Ferrant, Brussels, Dr. M.A. Boogaerts, Dr. G. Tricot, Louvain; Denmark: Dr. N. Jacobsen, Dr. P. Ernst, Copenhagen; Finland: Dr. T. Ruutu, Dr. M. Siimes, Helsinki, Dr. A. Toivanen, Turku; France: Dr. P. Hervé, Besançon, Dr. X. Troussard, Caen, Dr. J.P. Vernant, Creteil, Dr. M. Michallet, Grenoble, Dr. F. Bauters, Dr. J.P. Jouet, Lille, Dr. P. Bordigoni, Nancy, Dr. J.C. Harousseau, Nantes, Dr. D. Maraninchi, Marseille, Dr. E. Gluckman, Dr. N.C. Gorin, Dr. P. Rio, Paris, Dr. J. Reiffers, Pessac, Dr. F. Freycon, St. Etienne; Germany: Dr. W. Siegert, Berlin, Dr. U.W. Schaefer, Essen, Dr. G. Ehninger, Tübingen, Dr. W. Heit, Dr. B. Kubanek, Ulm, Dr. H.J. Kolb, Munich; Ireland: Dr. S.R. McCann, Dublin; Italy: Dr. S. Tura, Bologna, Dr. A. Marmont, Genova, Dr. F. Mandelli, Roma, Dr. G. Lucarelli, Pesaro, Dr. E. Polli, Dr. G. Lambertenghi, Dr. R. Mozzana, Milano; The Netherlands: Dr. F.E. Zwaan, Dr. J.M.J.J. Vossen, Leiden, Dr. T. de Witte, Nijmegen, Dr. B. Löwenberg, Rotterdam, Dr. L. Verdonck, Utrecht; Spain: Dr. A. Granena, Dr. S. Brunet-Mauri, Barcelona, Dr. A. Iriondo, Santander; Sweden: Dr. A. Fasth, Gothenburg, Dr. O. Ringden, Dr. G. Gahrton, Dr. B. Lundqvist, Huddinge; Switzerland: Dr. B. Speck, Basel, Dr. M. Jeannet, Dr. B. Chapuis, Geneva, Dr. J. Gmür, Zurich; United Kingdom: Dr. M. Franklin, Birmingham, Dr. A.C. Parker, Edinburgh, Dr. J.A. Barrett, Dr. J.M. Goldman, Dr. A.H. Goldstone, Dr. R. Levinsky, Dr. H.G. Prentice, Dr. D.G. Wardle, London, Dr. R. Powles, Sutton.

References

1. Leukemia Working Party of the European Group for Bone Marrow Transplantation (1988) Allogeneic bone marrow transplantation for leukemia in Europe. Lancet i:1379–1382
2. Leukemia Working Party (1989) Bone marrow transplantation for leukemia in Europe. Bone Marrow Transplant 4(suppl 2):1–12
3. Hermans J, Suciu S, Stijnen T, et al. (1989) Treatment of acute myelogenous leukemia. Eur J Clin Oncol 25:545–550

Bone Marrow Transplantation in Acute Leukemias and Chronic Myeloid Leukemia

U.W. Schaefer[1]

Bone marrow transplantation (BMT) has been used increasingly to treat patients with various hematological diseases. It is one method of overcoming dose-limiting myelosuppression, thereby allowing the administration of otherwise lethal doses of chemotherapy, total body irradition, or both. At the University of Essen a BMT program was instituted in December 1975. The current survey will review the results in acute myeloid leukemia (AML), acute lymphoblastic leukemia (ALL), and chronic myeloid leukemia (CML).

Patients and Methods

In this program, 102 patients with AML, 38 patients with ALL, and 63 patients with CML in chronic phase received an allogeneic bone marrow graft from HLA/MLC-identical relatives. Twenty-eight patients with AML in first complete remission (CR) were treated with cryopreserved autologous marrow. The median age of the patients undergoing allogeneic BMT was 31 years in AML, 25 years in ALL, and 33 years in CML. In the autologous setting the median age was 39 years. In AML and ALL the median time interval from diagnosis to transplantation in first CR was 7 months. In CML the median interval from diagnosis to transplantation in chronic phase was 14 months.

No attempts were made to remove, by ex vivo separation techniques, residual malignant cells in the autologous or T cells in the allogeneic setting. The majority of the patients undergoing allogeneic BMT were conditioned by total body irradiation (TBI) and high-dose cyclophosphamide (120 mg/kg administered over 2 consecutive days). Different TBI schedules were applied over the years [1]. Most patients received 4×2.5 Gy fractionated TBI with lung shielding (lung dose, 4×2.0 Gy) over 4 days (cobalt-60 source, dose rate 4 cGy/min). In the autologous setting all patients were pretreated with busulfan (4 mg/kg per day for 4 days) and cyclophosphamide (60 mg/kg per day for 2 days) [2].

---

[1] Department of Bone Marrow Transplantation, University Essen, Hufelandstraße 55, 4300 Essen, FRG

Fleischer (Ed.) Leukemias
© Springer-Verlag Berlin Heidelberg 1993

Strict gnotobiotic care was given to all patients using laminar air flow isolation or ultraclean barrier nursing rooms. Total gastrointestinal decontamination was attempted giving nonabsorbable antimycotics, antibiotics, and autoclaved food. Most patients received cytomegalovirus (CMV) hyperimmunoglobulins as well as CMV-negative blood products. For prophylaxis of acute graft-versus-host disease (GVH) patients were either treated with methotrexate (MTX) intermittently until day 102 or given a short course of MTX in combination with cyclosporine. Manifest GVH was treated with corticosteroids, ATG, or a monoclonal T-cell receptor antibody. Steroids, azathioprine, or cyclosporine were given as treatment for chronic GVH.

Results

In AML patients, 35 out of 63 (56%), 9 out of 16 (56%), or 2 out of 21 (10%) survived when the transplant was grafted in first CR, second CR, or in a later stage. The product-limit estimates of survival were 52% ± 7% by 6 years in first CR and 46% ± 14% by 4.6 years in second CR.

In ALL patients, 9 out of 16 (56%), 4 out of 13 (31%), and 2 out of 9 (22%) survived when transplanted in first CR, second CR, or in more advanced stages. The product-limit estimates of survival were 54% ± 13% by 4.4 years in first CR, 31% ± 13% by 6 years in second CR, and 22% ± 14% by 5 years in later stages of the disease.

The Kaplan-Meier estimates of relapse probability for AML patients in first CR and second CR, and ALL patients in first CR and second CR were 13% ± 11%, and 25% ± 15%, and 33% ± 19% and 72% ± 16%, respectively.

In CML we could demonstrate a significant influence of the GVH prophylaxis on patient survival. Ten out of 29 patients survived when MTX was used and 18 out of 26 when a short course of MTX in combination with cyclosporine was given. The product-limit estimates of survival were 34% ± 9%, or 68% ± 9% by 6 years and by 3.4 years, respectively; the relapse estimates in the two groups were 19% ± 12%, or 22% ± 16%.

The main cause of death after allogeneic BMT was interstitial pneumonia. A strong influence of the GVH prophylaxis was demonstrated. Among those patients who received MTX intermittently for 3 months 37% developed interstitial pneumonia. When the combination of a short course of MTX and cyclosporine was given, only 13% of the patients died from interstitial pneumonia.

The product-limit estimates for the incidence of acute GVH in acute leukemia and CML were 23% ± 6% and 56% ± 10% when MTX was used as prophylaxis. When the combination of MTX and cyclosporine was given the estimates were 15% ± 5% in acute leukemias and 33% ± 9% in CML.

Out of 28 patients with AML grafted during first CR with autologous marrow 21 survived. The Kaplan-Meier estimates for relapse-free survival and relapse probability were 57% ± 9% and 38% ± 10% by 3.6 years.

Discussion and Conclusions

In AML as well as in ALL more than half of the patients showed long-term survival if an allogeneic bone marrow transplantation was performed during first CR. In CML a strong influence of the GVH prophylaxis on the incidence of acute GVH and interstitial pneumonia and on survival could be demonstrated. After prolonged administration of MTX significantly more lethal interstitial pneumonias were observed than after a short course of MTX in combination with cyclosporine.

Autologous BMT in AML patients was followed by lower early morbidity and mortality and higher relapse rate than allogeneic BMT. Prospective trials are needed for better comparison of autologous BMT with allogeneic BMT and conventional chemotherapy.

References

1. Molls M, Bamberg M, Beelen DW, Mahmoud HK, Quast U, Schaefer UW (1987) Different TBI procedures in Essen: results and clinical considerations on the risk of leukemic relapse and interstitial pneumonitis. Strahlenther Onkol 163:237–240
2. Beelen DW, Quabeck K, Graeven U, Sayer HG, Mahmoud HK, Schaefer UW (1989) Acute toxicity and first clinical results of intensive postinduction therapy using a modified Busulfan and Cyclophosphamide regimen with autologous bone marrow rescue in first remission of acute myeloid leukemia. Blood 74:1507–1516

Bone Marrow Transplantation for Chronic Myeloid Leukemia in France. Results of the French Cooperative Group

A. Devergie,[1] J. Reiffers, J.P. Vernant, P. Hervé , D. Guyotat,
D. Maraninchi, M. Michallet, B. Rio, J.P. Jouet, P. Lehn,
and E. Gluckman

Transplants were performed in 281 patients (pts) with chronic myeloid leukemia (CML) in France between 1979 and 1986. The actuarial survival after 5 years is 55% for the patients receiving grafts in first chronic phase (CP), 43% for the patients given grafts in accelerated phase (AP) or second CP, and 35% for the patients receiving grafts in blastic crisis (BC). The main cause of death was interstitial pneumonitis and/or acute graft-versus-host disease (AGVHD). The incidence of AGVHD appears correlated with prophylactic treatment: 58% after methotrexate alone (MTX), 41% after cyclosporine (CSA), 26% after MTX + CSA, and only 14% after T-cell depletion. On the contrary, the relapse rate was much higher after T-cell depletion or syngeneic bone marrow transplantation (BMT) (70%) than after allogeneic non-T-cell-depleted BMT (18%). In this last group of patients, the relapse rate is correlated with the phase of CML at time of BMT: 10% for 102 patients in first CP and 30% for 77 patients in more advanced disease. Finally, the incidence of long-term disease-free survival is 55% for patients receiving grafts in first CP with a non-T-cell-depleted marrow. We conclude that the probability of cure after allogeneic BMT is very high, especially for patients in CP receiving non-T-cell-depleted marrow.

---

[1] GEGMO, UFGM, Hôpital Saint-Louis, 1 av. Claude Vellefaux, 75475 Paris Cedex, France

Fleischer (Ed.) Leukemias
© Springer-Verlag Berlin Heidelberg 1993

National and International Experiences with Autologous Bone Marrow Transplantation in Acute Leukemias

W. Helbig,[1] M. Kubel, R. Krahl, F.-A. Hoffmann, H. Schwenke, V. Thierbach, and M. Wötzel

At present autologous bone marrow transplantation (ABMT) is a post-remission treatment often used in acute leukemias. To estimate the current status of ABMT it is best to look into the results of the Leukemia Working Party of the European BMT Group (EBMTG), analyzed by Claude Gorin (Paris) [1] and first presented at the EBMTG meeting this year. These results include 1322 patients reported from 54 ABMT groups. Of acute myeloid leukemia (AML) patients within the total population studied, 14% were children and 15% were adults over 45 years. Purging of the autograft was done in one-third of the patients in first complete remission (CR 1) and more frequently in second CR (CR 2), especially in high-risk (HR) patients. The leukemia-free survival (LFS) was 36% in CR 1–standard-risk (SR) patients. There was a distinct trend of different survival in CR 1–SR patients according to the French-American-British Group (FAB) classification: about 50% LFS in M1 and M3, 40% in M2, but only 30% in M5, and 26% in M4. An influence of the pretransplant regimens on the LFS could also be found. The UCH regimen, consisting of cyclophosphamide, cytosine arabinoside, thioguanine, adriamycin and BCNU, seems to be better than others – the LFS was 61%.

In acute lymphoblastic leukemia (ALL) 43% of the total patient population were children, and two thirds of them were autografted for SR-ALL in CR 2. About 50% purged autografts were used in CR 1-SR-ALL, in contrast to about 80% in HR-ALL or CR 2. The LFS amounted to about 40% in CR 1 and in CR 2-SR, 31%; but in CR 2-HR the LFS was only 23%. In CR 2 the survival of children was twice as high as in adults: 42% in contrast to 20% at 52 and 34 months, respectively. There was also an influence of the conditioning regimen. Busulfan plus cyclophosphamide and fractionated total body irradiation (FTBI) seemed to be better than single-dose TBI or the UCH regimen.

As an interim result we can say that ABMT (for AML and ALL) is successful in 35%–40% of patients autografted in CR 1 and not much less for those autografted in CR 2, especially in the children. However, it has to

---

[1] Division of Hematology and Oncology, Department of Internal Medicine, University of Leipzig, O-7010 Leipzig, FRG

Fleischer (Ed.) Leukemias
© Springer-Verlag Berlin Heidelberg 1993

be considered that autografted patients are a selected population; thus, many questions are still open regarding the clinical efficacy of ABMT.

Critical issues of ABMT are:

1. Lack of a graft-versus-leukemia (GVL) effect
2. Difficulties in the detection of residual leukemic cells inside and outside the bone marrow (BM)
3. Importance of the in vitro purging (cytostatics; monoclonal antibodies
4. Importance of the in vivo purging (stronger consolidation)
5. Lack of randomized clinical studies (ABMT versus chemotherapy, CT)

The possibilities in the detection of minimal residual disease are limited. Usually we can detect in BM smears 2%–5% leukemic cells; single-marker analysis or gene rearrangements are only a little better. Double-marker labeling and the other methods are obviously more sensitive. Now it is hoped that molecular genetic methods including the polymerase chain reaction will solve the problem of minimal residual disease detection and allow us to estimate the quality of CR.

One of the most critical issues is the importance of in vitro purging. The very latest EBMT analysis from this year showed a higher disease-free probability (but not LFS) in patients with AML-CR 1–SR autografted with purged marrow, but this advantage was only caused by autografts which were purged by an adjusted dose of mafosfamide. In ALL survival only tended to be better in dose-adjusted purging. An ongoing prospective study of the EBMT working party on ABMT is studying the importance of marrow purging with mafosfamide for ABMT in AML and CR 2. The

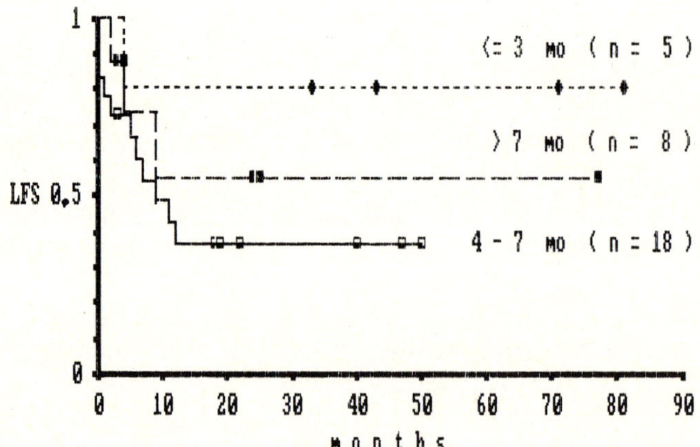

Fig. 1. LFS in patients who received autografts for ALL at different times between CR 1 and ABMT

second question is on the importance of consolidation before ABMT: Does strong consolidation act like an in vivo purging? This has been our working hypothesis, but other groups have not used it. Controversially, they use ABMT for consolidation of CR.

Gorin [1] found, in patients receiving autografts for ALL in CR 1, a different LFS regarding different periods between reaching CR and ABMT. The worst survival was observed if patients were given autografts soon after achieving CR, probably without or with weak consolidation. The best results were obtained if patients were given transplants after 7 months, but this group is probably a very select one, because early relapses are excluded. We did the same investigation and found similar results in groups given autografts between 4 and 6 months and later (Fig. 1), but the best LFS was in that group which received autografts within 3 months, meaning immediately after consolidation by three cycles of chemotherapy. This result is due to the fact that the small patient numbers are not statistically different as yet but probably provide some indication that strong consolidation is an in vivo purging.

The most important issue is the lack of randomized studies comparing ABMT and conventional postremission CT. There may be ongoing studies on ABMT versus CT in some West European countries. A multicenter trial was initiated in the GDR a few years ago. Because median follow-up is short and the number of patients in each arm small, though, the results are very preliminary.

In Table 1 (on the left side) the results of the pilot study until 1985 are compared with the prospective study (on the right side). The LFS of ABMT is unchanged in ALL, but in AML it is much worse. Considering all cases of our randomized study, there is a very bad LFS in ABMT for AML compared with the pilot study and the CT group.

Table 1. Leukemia-free survival after ABMT or CT for AML and ALL in first remission (GDR AL Study Group)

	Pilot study			Prospective study					
	(n)	$(\%)$	MFU (months)	All cases			Modified[a]		
				(n)	$(\%)$	MFU (months)	(n)	$(\%)$	MFU (months)
AML: ABMT	5	40	63	11	14	10	8	25	10
CT	–	–		19	28	12	13	38	15
ALL: ABMT	11	45	71	20	53	24	8	50	12
CT	–	–		13	24	8	6	67	11

ABMT, autologous bone marrow transplantation; CT, chemotherapy; AML, acute myeloid leukemia; ALL, acute lymphoblastic leukemia; MFU, mean follow-up
[a] Only patients with full dosage at induction therapy; all relapses within consolidation excluded.

In the prospective study of ABMT for ALL, the LFS is better than in the CT group and comparable with the pilot study. But these comparisons include two mistakes: (1) all patients with relapses between the CR and ABMT are excluded; (2) in another investigation we found that patients who did not receive the full dose of cytostatics during induction therapy had a significantly higher relapse rate and thus a survival like that of non-responders. Such patients did not fulfill the study protocol and, thus, they are to be considered as "off study." Therefore these patients and, for better comparison of ABMT with CT, all relapses within the consolidation therapy had to be excluded. With respect to these modified data one cannot find any advantage of ABMT as yet.

Conclusions

ABMT is probably a very good postremission therapy in AL, but so far there is no exact evidence that ABMT is superior. Some important open questions remain besides the value of ABMT itself: the determination of the quality of CR, the efficacy of in vitro und in vivo purging in ABMT, and the value of ABMT in comparison to allogeneic BMT using one-antigen-mismatched family donors or phenotypically HLA-identical unrelated donors.

References

1. Gorin NC, Aegerter P, Auvert B (1989) Autologous bone marrow transplantation (ABMT) for acute leukaemia in remission: an analysis on 1322 cases. Bone Marrow Transplant 4[Suppl 2]:3–5

CD48 Monoclonal Antibody K31 for Bone Marrow Transplantation: Functional Characteristics

P. Dreger,[1] B. Mueller, N. Schmitz, H. Löffler, and W. Müller-Ruchholtz

In clinical bone marrow (BM) transplantation, graft-versus-host reaction can be effectively prevented by depleting the graft of T cells. However, transplantation of T-depleted grafts is complicated by a high incidence of graft rejection due to residual immunological reactivity of the host and the immunogenicity of the graft [1]. Recent reports suggest that the immunogenicity of an organ graft is largely due to BM-derived "accessory cells" (AC) that are distributed in the organ, whereas the cells that are essential for the graft's function do not play nearly as important a role in immunogenicity [2]. In this context, we have been able to demonstrate that the CD48 monoclonal antibody (MoAb) K31 binds to almost all human lymphoid cells, and, in addition, to macrophage cells with high accessory capacity, such as monocytes, dendritic cells, and veiled accessory cells. On the other hand, no other hemopoietic or nonhemopietic cells, including progenitors, are labeled by K31 [3,4]. In the present paper, we report that K31 is cytotoxic with rabbit complement (C) but not with human C. Because it completely eliminates BM AC, K31 + C strongly reduces the allostimulatory capacity and thus the immunogenicity of BM mononuclear cells (BMNC). In contrast, the CDw52 MoAb CAMPATH-1 or T cell-specific MoAbs do not affect BM immunogenicity.

Materials and Methods

K31 (CD48) is a mouse IgM from our laboratory that recognizes a p180 antigen on all human lymphocytes and the vast majority of human lymphoid cell lines and lymphoid leukemias. Other hemopoietic or nonhemopoietic cells, including progenitors, do not express the antigen. CAMPATH-1 (CDw52) is a rat IgM MoAb that activates human C and binds to a glycoprotein on human lymphocytes and the majority of monocytes [5]. CT-2 is a CD2-specific mouse IgM MoAb [1]. 1AB3, from our laboratory, was used as anti-HLA-DR MoAb. Cytotoxicity with C was assessed in a standard

---

[1] Departments of Internal Medicine II and Immunology, University of Kiel, Chemnitzstrasszz, 2300 Kiel, FRG

Fleischer (Ed.) Leukemias
© Springer-Verlag Berlin Heidelberg 1993

chromium release assay: aliquots of 1×10^5 ^{51}Cr-labeled target cells were incubated with MoAb in 0.1 ml for 1 h at 4°C. The supernatants were removed, and the cells were resuspended in 0.1 ml C. After 1 h at 37°C, the supernatants were harvested and counted. Aliquots of ^{51}Cr-labeled cells were incubated with RPMI alone (for spontaneous release) or Triton × 100 (for maximum release). Assays were performed in triplicate. The [^{3}H]thymidine incorporation assays for the accessory capacity and the allostimulatory capacity have been described previously [3]. In brief, density-separated peripheral blood or BMNC were treated with MoAb + C or medium + C. To determine BM accessory capacity, 50 000 irradiated (25 Gy) antibody + C-treated BMNC were cocultured with an equal number of purified autologous T cells in the presence of phytohemagglutinin (PHA; Difco, Detroit, Michigan, USA). After a 96-h incubation period, 37 kBq [^{3}H]thymidine were added to each culture. Cells were incubated for another 16 h, harvested, and counted. To determine BM allostimulatory capacity,

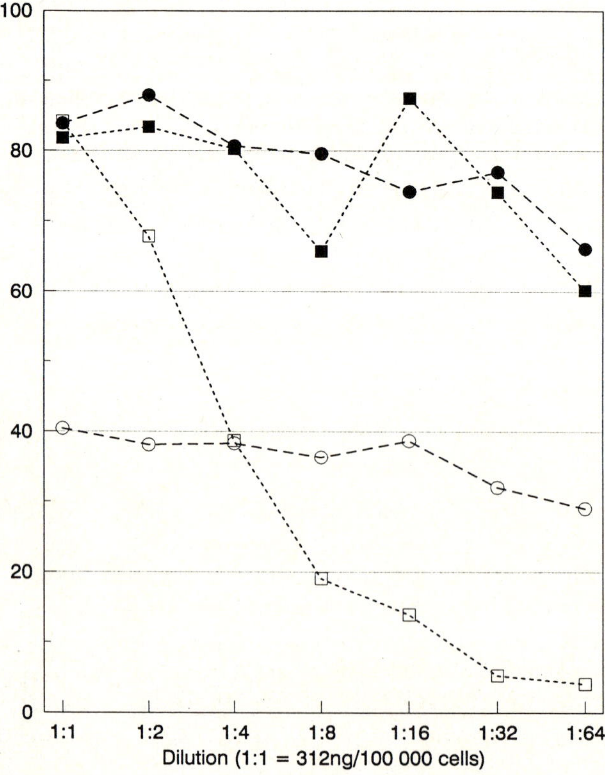

Fig. 1. ^{51}Cr release of K31 + rabbit C (--●--), K31 + human C (--○--), CAMPATH-1 + rabbit C (--■--), and CAMPATH-1 + human C (--□--) on peripheral blood mononuclear cells

10^5 fresh peripheral mononuclear cells (PMNC) from fully HLA-mismatched donors were stimulated with 5×10^4 irradiated MoAb + C-treated BMNC for 120 h, pulsed with [^{3}H]thymidine, cultured for another 16-h period, harvested, and counted. The number of HLA-DR-positive cells among BMNC was determined by the alkaline phosphatase anti-alkaline-phosphatase (APAAP) method [3].

Results

When applied with rabbit C, both K31 and CAMPATH-1 resulted in almost maximum release from PMNC, indicating virtually complete cell lysis. With human C, CAMPATH-1 again caused a complete kill, whereas K31 was not sufficiently effective (Fig. 1). With BMNC, K31 + rabbit C showed 19.2%–

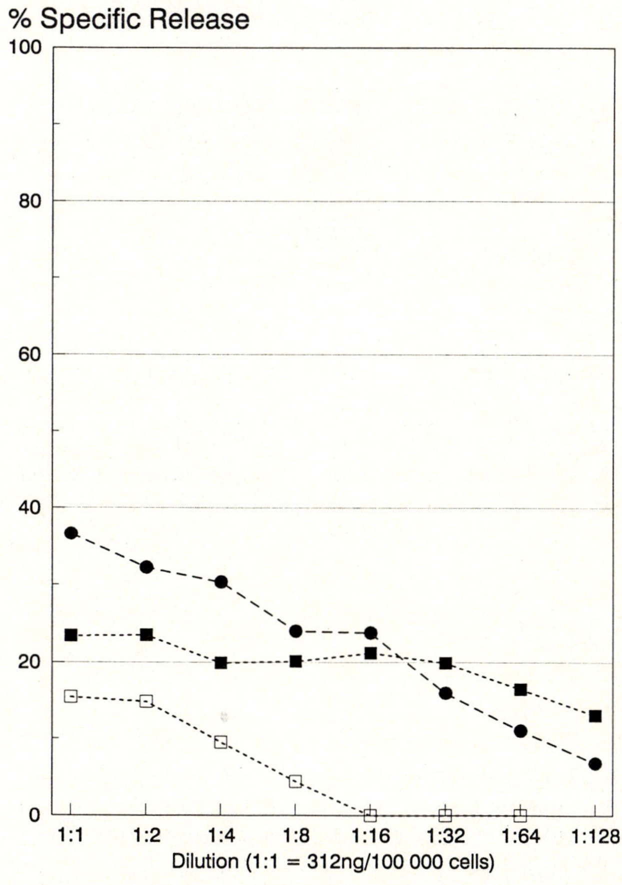

Fig. 2. ^{51}Cr release of K31 + rabbit C (--●--), CAMPATH-1 + rabbit C (--■--), and CAMPATH-1 + human C (--□--) on bone marrow mononuclear cells

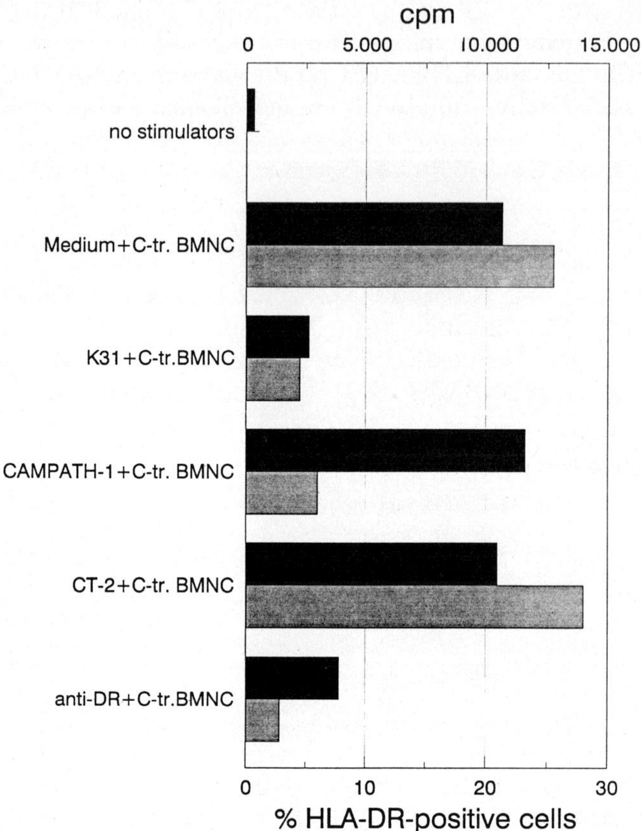

Fig. 3. Allostimulatory capacity of readjusted bone marrow mononuclear cells after treatment with various MoAb + rabbit C (*C-tr.*, C-treated). Note that the percentage of HLA-DR-positive cells (*grey shading*) does not correlate with the corresponding allostimulatory capacity (cpm in one-way MLC, shown by *black shading*)

57.1% specific release ($\bar{x} = 35.1\%$; $n = 5$). CAMPATH-1 + rabbit C killed a smaller cell volume ($7.3\%-27.4\%$; $\bar{x} = 23.5\%$; $n = 5$) but was more effective than CAMPATH-1 + human C ($9.9\%-22.9\%$; $\bar{x} = 13.2\%$; $n = 4$), as shown in Fig. 2.

Targeting and elimination of all functionally relevant BMAC by K31 + rabbit C was demonstrated by coculture of MoAb + C-pretreated BMNC and purified autologous T cells in the presence of PHA. Whereas K31 + C-pretreated BM cells were not able to support PHA-induced proliferation of autologous T cells ($0\%-11\%$ of the value obtained with BM treated with medium + C; $\bar{x} = 3\%$; $n = 6$), CAMPATH-1 + rabbit C resulted only in a moderate reduction of the BM's accessory capacity ($28\%-100\%$; $\bar{x} = 51$;

$n = 5$), indicating that residual cells with accessory function were still present. The elimination of AC by K31 + C correlated with a strong reduction of the BM's capacity to stimulate allogeneic PMNC in a mixed leukocyte culture- (MLC)-like fashion (0%–50% of the medium + C-treated control; $\bar{x} = 13\%$; $n = 58$). CAMPATH-1 + rabbit C (0%–100%; $\bar{x} = 71\%$; $n = 53$), CAMPATH-1 + human C (79%–100%; $\bar{x} = 99\%$; $n = 21$), and the CD2-specific MoAb CT-2 (75%–100%; $\bar{x} = 92\%$; $n = 10$) were much less effective in decreasing the BM's allostimulatory capacity (Fig. 3). The number of HLA-DR-positive cells among MoAb + C-treated BMNC did not correlate with the allostimulatory capacity, as measured in the MLC assay (Fig. 3).

Discussion

The complete lysis of PMNC that we observed with both K31 and CAMPATH-1 + rabbit C is consistent with the results of the labeling studies using flow cytometry that have been published [4,5]. With K31 + human C, only marginal cell lysis was achieved. Thus, we conclude that K31 does not sufficiently activate human C. Similar to PMNC, the proportion of BMNC that were killed by K31 or CAMPATH-1 was roughly within the range expected from the flow cytometry data [4,5]; however, although there was no signficant difference between K31 and CAMPATH-1 in the number of labeled BM cells in flow cytometry, K31+C lysed significantly more cells than CAMPATH-1 + rabbit or human C. The reason for this difference may be the resistance of certain cell subpopulations to CAMPATH-1-mediated C lysis [5]. As demonstrated in the T cell proliferation assays, the elimination of BMAC correlates with a strong reduction of the BM's allostimulatory capacity, indicating a decrease in its immunogenicity. This confirms and extends other in vivo and in vitro studies revealing that graft immunogenicity can be markedly decreased by elimination of AC [2]. Since K31 does not recognize hemopoietic progenitors or parenchymatous or stromal cells of liver, kidney, heart, pancreas, or small bowel [4], it appears to be a promising tool for reducing the immunogenicity of both BM and solid organ grafts [3]. The CDw52 MoAb CAMPATH-1 does not seem to be useful for these purposes.

References

1. Sondel PM, Hank JA, Trigg ME, Kohler PC, Finlay JL, Blank J, Meisner L, Borcherding W, Hong R, Steeves R, Billing R, Flynn B, Bozdech MJ (1986) Transplantation of HLA-haploidentical T-cell-depleted marrow for leukemia: autologous marrow recovery with specific immune sensitization to donor antigens. Exp Hematol 14:278

2. Lechler RI, Batchelor JR (1982) Restoration of immunogenicity to passenger cell-depleted kidney allografts by the addition of donor strain dendritic cells. J Exp Med 155:31
3. Dreger P, Müller-Ruchholtz W (1990) Evidence that reduction of immunogenicity of T-depleted bone marrow depends on additional depletion of accessory cells. Implications for prevention of graft rejection. Transplantation 49:622
4. Dreger P, Viehmann K, Löffler H, Müller-Ruchholtz W (1990) A CD48 monoclonal antibody for reduction of graft immunogenicity. Transplant Proc 22:1930
5. Hale G, Bright S, Chumbley G, Hoang T, Metcalf D, Munro AJ, Waldmann H (1983) Removal of T cells from bone marrow for transplantation: a monoclonal anti-lymphocyte antibody that fixes human complement. Blood 62:873

Comparison of the Growth of Xenografted Human Bone Marrow with the Growth of Xenografted Acute Myeloid Leukemia Cells and Marrow Repopulating Capacity Following Transplantation into Allogeneic Recipients

R.D. Clutterbuck,[1] R.L. Powles, and J.L. Millar

Introduction

Blast cells from the peripheral blood of patients with acute myeloid leukemia (AML) have been shown to be capable of forming discrete subcutaneous tumours when inoculated into immune-deprived mice [2]. The proliferative potential of these tumours is limited and in the great majority of cases, regression ensues. One possible cause for tumour regression is the maturation of blast cells, producing a cell population with an abolished capacity for proliferation [7,1]. This process is to a certain extent analogous to the cell kinetics of normal haemopoiesis. It was considered that normal human bone marrow cells might therefore also undergo a phase of proliferation when implanted into immune-deprived mice.

The growth of normal human bone marrow as subcutaneous xenografts was therefore investigated and compared with the growth of xenografted AML cells. A comparison was also made between the growth of bone marrows as xenografts from a series of normal donors and the repopulating abilities of these same bone marrow cells in preconditioned leukaemia patients.

Materials and Methods

Bone Marrow. Bone marrow was taken into heparin from anaesthetised healthy donors by multiple puncture of the iliac crest. Mononuclear cells were separated from erythrocytes and granulocytes by centrifugation over lymphoprep (Nycomed; density 1.077) at $400\,g$ for $30\,\text{min}$. Interface cells were collected and the cell concentration was adjusted to 2×10^8 cells/ml Hams F12 medium.

---

[1] Institute of Cancer Research and Royal Marsden Hospital, Section of Medicine, Belmont, Sutton, Surrey SM2 5NG, UK

Fleischer (Ed.) Leukemias
© Springer-Verlag Berlin Heidelberg 1993

Table 1. The growth of normal human bone marrow xenografts compared with haemopoietic recovery in patients following allogeneic bone marrow transplantation (from *Leukemia* 3(9):637–642, 1989)

Patient	Sex	Age	Disease	Sex match	Conditioning	Xenograft growth		Patient recovery	
						Maximum volume (mm^3)	AUC (mm^3 days ×10^3)	Neutrophils[a] (days)	Platelets[b] (days)
1	M	33	CGL	Yes	CY/TBI	116	1.78	20	>70[c]
2	M	42	CGL	Yes	CY/TBI	114	4.16	33	70
3	M	24	AML	No	CY/TBI	103	2.26	16	18
4	F	42	CGL	Yes	ME/BU	97	1.79	11	12
5	M	24	ALL	No	ME/TBI	96	2.38	16	26
6	M	32	ALL	Yes	CY/TBI	84	1.85	17	20
7	M	40	AML	Yes	BU/CY	84	0.95	15	35
8	M	14	ALL	Yes	ME/TBI	71	1.27	14	35
9	M	33	AML	Yes	ME/TBI	51	0.81	15	26
10	M	11	AML	Yes	CY/TBI	50	1.12	38	>40[c]
11	M	32	CGL	Yes	CY/TBI	40	1.25	23	>86[c]
12	F	29	CGL	Yes	CY/TBI	34	0.74	19	16

ALL, acute lymphocytic leukemia; CGL, chronic granulocytic leukemia; CY, cyclophosphamide; ME, melphalan; BU, busulfan
[a] Time taken for peripheral blood neutrophil count to reach 0.5 × 10^9/l.
[b] Time taken for peripheral blood platelet count to reach 50 × 10^9/l.
[c] Patient died before platelets reached 50 × 10^9/l.

Xenografts. Male CBA mice were immune-suppressed by thymectomy at 3 weeks of age followed 5–8 weeks later by 9 Gy total body irradiation (TBI), the lethal effects of which were prevented by pretreatment with 200 mg/kg cytosine arabinoside given 48 h previously [5]. Immediately following TBI, 3–5 mice were given subcutaneous implants with 2×10^7 mononuclear bone marrow cells or AML cells in a volume of 0.1 ml Hams F12. AML cells were thawed from stock cell populations frozen in liquid nitrogen and separated over lymphoprep. Xenograft growth was monitored daily by measuring, using calipers.

Patients. Leukemia patients receiving bone marrow transplants were HLA-matched siblings of the bone marrow donors. Ten were sex-matched and all were Caucasian. Details of age, sex and leukemia are given in Table 1. From 12 patients, 7 were conditioned pre-transplant by cyclophosphamide ($1.8 \, g/m^2$) and TBI, 3 by melphalan ($110 \, mg/m^2$) and TBI, one by melphalan and busulfan ($16 \times 1 \, mg/kg$), and one by cyclophosphamide and busulfan (Table 1). TBI was given as single fraction from a cobalt-60 source. The average mid-line dose was between 10 and 11.7 Gy; lung shielding was not used.

Results

In all donor marrows tested implantation into immune-deprived mice gave rise to subcutaneous nodules. The mean maximum nodule size ranged between 116 and 34 mm^3 (Table 1). The pattern of growth was similar to that observed for human AML xenografts; that is, a growth phase followed by regression. The growth observed from the implantation of AML cells was significantly greater than that produced by the implantation of normal mononuclear bone marrow cells (Table 2).

The growth of human bone marrow xenografts, as assessed by mean maximum nodule volume or area under the growth curve (AUC), appeared not to be correlated with the rate of haemopoietic recovery in patients who had been transplanted with the bulk of the same marrow. Criteria for neutrophil and platelet repopulation are given in Table 1. Correlation

Table 2. Comparative growth of human AML cells and normal human mononuclear bone marrow cells in immune-deprived mice

	Mean maximum vol. (mm^3) $\pm$ SD	n
AML cells	170 $\pm$ 89	18 patients
Normal BM cells	78 $\pm$ 29	12 donors

BM, bone marrow
$p < 0.002$ (Student's t test).

coefficients (r) between mean maximum xenograft volume and rates of patient neutrophil recovery or platelet recovery were 0.02 and 0.06 respectively; r values for AUC correlated with neutrophil or platelet recoveries were 0.30 and 0.27 respectively. These values were not significant (Student's t test).

Three experiments were performed to investigate the effect of intra-peritoneal administration of recombinant human granulocyte-macrophage–colony-stimulating factor (rhGM-CSF; Sandoz, Basel) on bone marrow xenografts. rhGM-CSF (100 µg/kg) was administered for 6 days post-implantation. Results from these preliminary experiments indicate that nodules appeared more rapidly in rhGM-CSF-treated mice than in saline-treated mice, but that the maximum volume attained was not increased and nodule regression was not delayed.

Discussion

Several recent reports have described the survival and/or proliferation of normal human haemopoietic cells following infusion into immune-deprived mice [3,4,6]. We have shown that normal human mononuclear bone marrow cells will grow for a limited period in thymectomised and irradiated mice as subcutaneous nodules which ultimately regress. In this respect xenografted normal bone marrow and xenografted human AML cells behave in a similar manner. However, the nodule size produced by the implantation of normal bone marrow cells is less than that observed following the implant of AML cells (although there is considerable variation within each of these two groups). This may indicate a greater overall in vivo proliferative potential on the part of AML cell populations.

Although variation in extent of xenograft growth was observed between different donors this did not prove to be indicative of the success of the graft in reconstituting the marrow of patients conditioned by high-dose chemoradiotherapy. At the outset of these investigations it was considered that the growth of xenografted human bone marrow might provide an indicator of the repopulating potential of allogeneic transplanted bone marrow. The lack of significant correlation between xenograft growth and repopulation may be because the marrow cell types responsible for xenograft growth possess limited "stemness" and are not those cells necessary for marrow reconstitution in patients [8]. HLA matching of donor and recipient does not ensure complete histocompatibility. It is likely that donor marrow proliferative capacity is a relatively more important factor in the context of autografted bone marrow where host-versus-graft immunological reactions are absent. A closer relationship may therefore exist between the growth of bone marrow as a xenograft and its autologous repopulating ability.

References

1. Clutterbuck RD, Hills CA, Hoey P, Alexander P, Powles RL, Millar JL (1985) Studies on the development of human acute myeloid leukemia xenografts in immune-deprived mice: comparison with cells in short-term culture. Leuk Res 9:1511–1518
2. Franks CR, Bishop D, Balkwill FR, Oliver RTD, Spector WG (1977) Growth of acute myeloid leukaemia as discrete sudcutaneous tumours in immune-deprived mice. Br J Cancer 35:697–700
3. Kamel-Reid S, Dick JE (1988) Engraftment of immune-deprived mice with human haematopoietic stem cells. Science 242:1706–1709
4. McCune JM, Namikawa R, Kaneshima H, Schulz LD, Lieberman M, Weissman IL (1988) The SCID-hu mouse: murine model for the analysis of human haematolymphoid differentiation and function. Science 241:1632–1639
5. Millar JL, Blackett NM, Hudspith BN (1978) Enhanced post-irradiation recovery of the haemopoietic system in animals pretreated with a variety of cytotoxic agents. Cell Tiss Kinet 11:543–553
6. Mosier DE, Gulizia RJ, Baird SM, Wilson DB (1988) Transfer of a functional human immune system to mice with severe combined immuno-deficiency. Nature 335:256–259
7. Palu G, Selby P, Powles R, Alexander P (1979) Spontaneous regression of acute myeloid leukemia xenografts and phenotypic evidence for maturation. Br J Cancer 40:731–735
8. Spangrude GJ (1989) Enrichment of murine haemopoietic cells: diverging roads. Immunol Today 10:344–350

Chemotherapy of Acute Leukemias

Cellular Pharmacokinetics of Daunomycin in Human Leukemic Blasts In Vitro and In Vivo*

M.E. Scheulen,[1] B. Kramer, M. Skorzec, and W.K. Reich

Introduction

The description of a decrease in the intracellular accumulation of a number of cytostatics, such as anthracyclines, vinca alkaloids, epipodophyllotoxins, and actinomycin D, in drug-resistant malignant cells, which was first demonstrated for colchicine in Chinese hamster ovary cells [4], has substantially contributed to the understanding of "multidrug resistance" [6]. This process is caused by an energy-dependent outward pump in connection with the expression of the 170 000-Da plasma membrane glycoprotein P170 [2].

Accordingly, the responsiveness of malignant cells to these cytotoxic drugs may more critically depend on their cellular tumor pharmacokinetics and metabolism than on their plasma pharmacokinetics, which in general only poorly correlates with their pharmacodynamics [7].

We have determined the cellular pharmacokinetics and metabolism of the anthracycline daunomycin (DNM) in leukemic blasts from peripheral blood of 30 patients with acute myelogenous leukemia treated according to the TAD protocol with 6-thioguanine, cytosine arabinoside, and DNM [1] in vivo and in isolated leukemic blasts in vitro. The aim of the study was to evaluate the clinical relevance of a decreased intracellular accumulation of DNM in vivo for multidrug resistance and to possibly predict the response of individual patients from in vitro parameters.

Material and Methods

Leukemic blasts were isolated from peripheral blood by Ficoll gradient centrifugation and lysis of red blood cells up to 4 h after intravenous bolus injection of 60 mg/m^2 DNM, washed and analyzed for DNM and metabolites by high-performance liquid chromatography (HPLC) with fluorescence detection after extraction [10]. DNM content was calculated by internal

* Supported by Deutsche Forschungsgemeinschaft, Bonn-Bad Godesberg, Sonderforschungsbereich 102.
[1] Department of Internal Medicine (Cancer Research), West German Tumor Center, University of Essen Medical School, W-4300 Essen, FRG

Fleischer (Ed.) Leukemias
© Springer-Verlag Berlin Heidelberg 1993

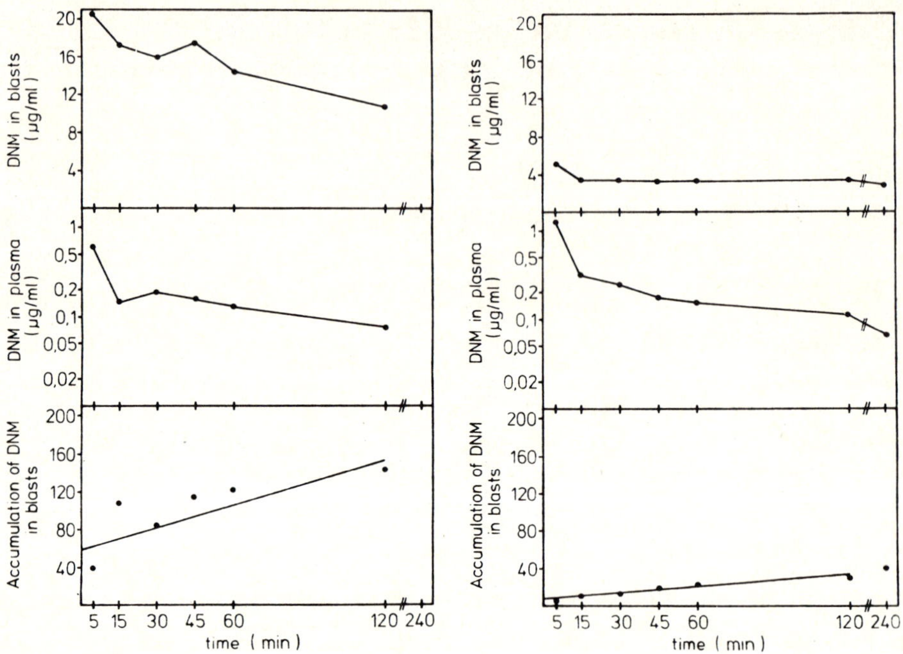

Fig. 1. Cellular and plasma pharmacokinetics and intracellular accumulation of daunomycin (*DNM*) in leukemic blasts in two patients (L.S., *left*; M.H. (a), *right*) in vivo

standardization with adriamycin (doxorubicin) and expressed in micrograms per milliliter after determination of cellular volume by morphometry. Plasma DNM kinetics was simultaneously measured. Accumulation of DNM in leukemic blasts was defined by the quotient of the intracellular and DNM plasma concentration for each time point of the kinetics (Fig. 1). For in vitro experiments, leukemic blasts were isolated in the same way before treatment and incubated with 0.02–6.0 µg/ml DNM up to 1 h before washing and HPLC analysis, including efflux studies by reincubation of leukemic blasts in DMN-free medium.

Outcome of TAD treatment was quantified by the relative reduction of leukemic blasts in bone marrow calculated from the percentages of blasts immediately before and on day 21 after treatment.

Results

According to the in vitro experiments, there was no significant correlation between the cellular uptake of DNM by isolated leukemic blasts and the response to TAD treatment (data not shown).

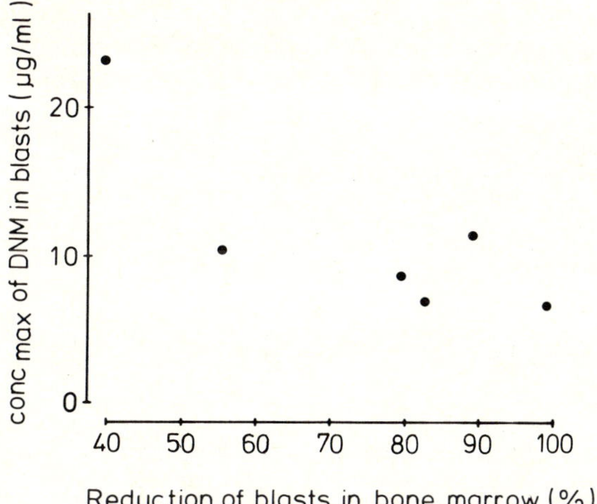

Fig. 2. Correlation between the maximal intracellular daunomycin (*DNM*) concentrations in vivo and the outcome of induction TAD therapy

An example of the differences in the cellular pharmacokinetics of DNM in vivo during TAD induction therapy among the diverse acute myelogenous leukemias is given in Fig. 1. In spite of the nearly identical plasma kinetics of DNM in both patients, intracellular concentrations vary strongly, resulting in a significant change in the intracellular accumulation of the drug. In the same way, there are great *inter*individual differences in the maximal intracellular DNM concentrations, between 4.0 and 23.1 µg/ml, and in the areas under the concentration time curves (AUC) for DNM during the first 2 h after administration, between 6.8 and 30.7 µg/h for the first TAD induction therapy in vivo. A significant correlation either between the maximal intracellular DNM concentrations or between the AUC in vivo and the outcome of TAD induction therapy did not exist in a series of six patients (Fig. 2). Also, there was no significant relationship between the in vitro and in vivo parameters for the cellular pharmacokinetics of DNM (Fig. 3).

DNM metabolites such as daunomycinol (DNMol) or aglycones were not detected in leukemic blasts in significant amounts.

Discussion

Our investigations of the cellular pharmacokinetics and metabolism of DNM in leukemic blasts in the peripheral blood of patients with acute myelogenous leukemia treated according to the TAD protocol show great *inter*individual differences. We found no significant correlation between: the in vitro pharmacokinetic parameters and the response to initial TAD therapy; the in

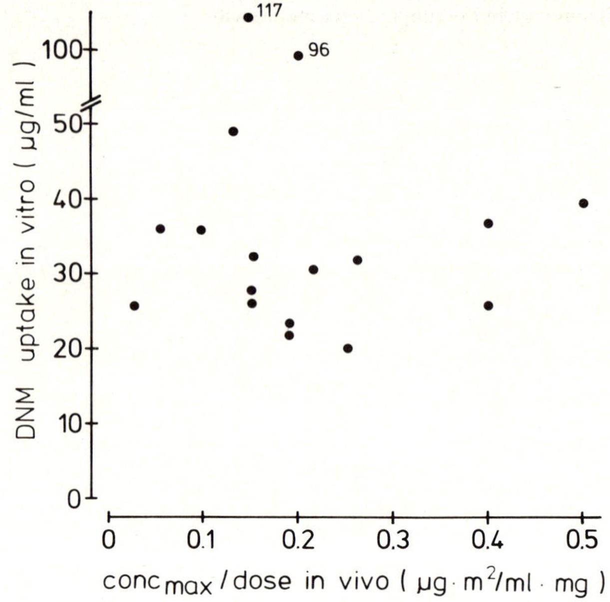

Fig. 3. Correlation between the daunomycin (*DNM*) uptake by leukemic blasts in vitro and the maximal intracellular DNM concentrations per dose in vivo

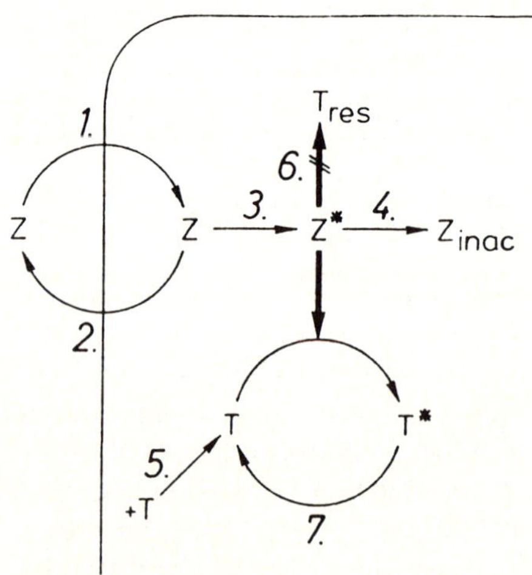

Fig. 4. Potential mechanisms of drug (*Z*) resistance:

    1. Reduction of intracellular uptake
    2. Increase in extracellular efflux (e.g., multidrug resistance)
    3. Reduction of intracellular activation (Z^*, activated drug)
    4. Increase in intracellular inactivation (Z_{inac}, inactivated drug)
    5. Increase in cellular target (*T*)
    6. Development of resistant cellular target (T_{res})
    7. Increase in repair of damaged cellular target (T^*)
    8. Shortening of drug-sensitive phase of cell cycle (not shown)
    9. Reduction of number of proliferating cells (not shown)

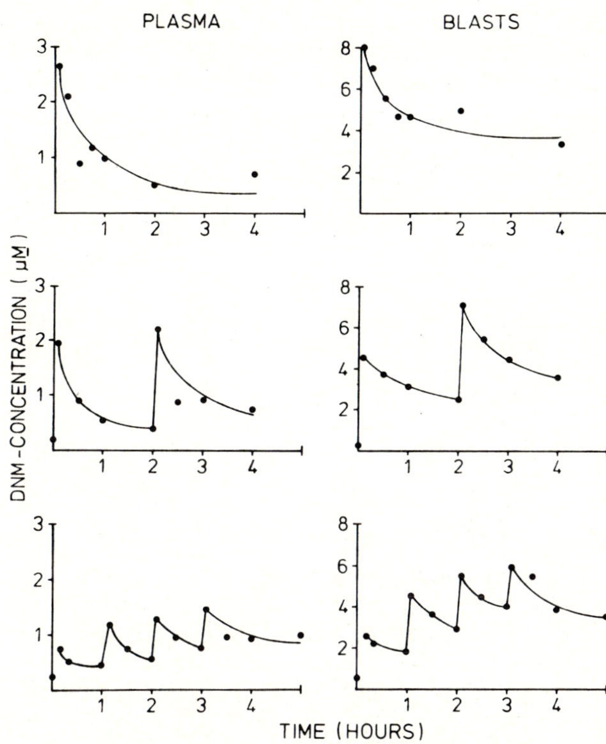

Fig. 5. Influence of the fractionation of daunomycin (*DNM*) on the cellular and plasma pharmacokinetics of DNM in the same patient (*top*, 60 mg/m^2 on day 1; *middle*, 2 × 30 mg/m^2 at 0 and 2 h on day 2; *bottom*, 4 × 15 mg/m^2 at 0, 1, 2 and 3 h on day 3)

vivo pharmacokinetic parameters and the response to initial TAD therapy; and the in vitro and in vivo pharmacokinetic parameters.

The lack of conformity of the intracellular uptake of DNM with the outcome of treatment is in agreement with the results of Kokenberg et al. [3]. However, it has to be considered as a potential restriction of the significance of our findings that the impact of the cellular pharmacokinetics of cytosine arabinoside and 6-thioguanine combined with DNM on the response to this combination chemotherapy has not been determined simultaneously. Thus, only resistance to the TAD regimen is identical with DNM resistance, while response to the TAD regimen may not necessarily correspond to DNM efficacy.

Nevertheless, the feasibility of the analysis of the cellular pharmacokinetics and metabolism of DNM in leukemic blasts in vitro and in vivo as a "predicitive test" for the response to treatment is questionable. In the same way, though the expression of the plasma membrane glycoprotein P170 has been demonstrated in two acute nonlymphoblastic leukemias [5], the multidrug resistant phenotype may be rare in the clinics. Thus, reduced susceptibility of acute myelogenous leukemias may be more critically influenced by other factors (Fig. 4) [9].

However, the *intra*individual comparison of the cellular pharmacokinetics and metabolism of DNM in leukemic blasts in the peripheral blood of patients with acute myelogenous leukemia may be a helpful tool for the assessment of: (a) different treatment schedules, e.g., dose fractionation (Fig. 5) or continuous infusion [11]; (b) concomitant cardio- or myelo-protective measures; or (c) concomitant chemosensibilization [8] to ameliorate the chemotherapy with anthracyclines and reduce toxic side effects.

References

1. Büchner T, Urbanitz D, Hiddemann W, Rühl H, Ludwig WD, Fischer J, Aul HC, Vaupel HA, Kuse R, Zeile G, Nowrousian MR, König HJ, Walter M, Wendt FC, Sodomann H, Hossfeld DK, von Paleske A, Löffler H, Gassmann W, Hellriegel KP, Fülle HH, Lunscken C, Emmerich B, Pralle H, Pees HW, Pfreundschuh M, Bartels H, Koeppen KM, Schwerdtfeger R, Donhuijsen-Ant R, Mainzer K, Bonfert B, Köppler H, Zurborn KH, Ranft K, Thiel E, Heinecke A (1985) Intensified induction and consolidation with or without maintenance chemotherapy for acute myeloid leukemia (AML): two multicenter studies of the German AML Cooperative Group. J Clin Oncol 3:1583–1589
2. Kartner N, Riordan JR, Ling V (1983) Cell surface P-glycoprotein associated with multidrug resistance in mammalian cell lines. Science 221:1285–1288
3. Kokenberg E, van der Steuyt K, Löwenberg B, Sonneveld P (1987) Pharmacokinetics of daunorubicin as a determinant of response in acute myeloid leukemia. In: Büchner T, Schellong G, Hiddemann W, Urbanitz D, Ritter J (eds) Acute leukemias. Prognostic factors and treatment strategies. Springer, Berlin Heidelberg New York, pp 283–287 (Haematology and Blood Transfusion, vol 30)
4. Ling V, Thompson LH (1974) Reduced permeability in CHO cells as a mechanism of resistance to colchicine. J Cell Physiol 83:103–116
5. Ma DDF, Scurr RD, Davey RA, Mackertich SM, Harman DH, Dowden G, Isbister JP, Bell DR (1987) Detection of a multidrug resistant phenotype in acute non-lymphoblastic leukemia. Lancet 1:135–137
6. Pastan I, Gottesman M (1987) Multiple-drug resistance in human cancer. N Engl J Med 316:1388–1393
7. Powis G (1985) Anticancer drug pharmacodynamics. Cancer Chemother Pharmacol 14:177–183
8. Scheulen ME, Osieka R (1987) Increased activity of adriamycin against a human testicular cancer xenograft by cyclosporine A. Proc Am Assoc Cancer Res 28:409
9. Scheulen ME, Hoensch H, Kappus H, Seeber S, Schmidt CG (1987) Positive correlation between decreased cellular uptake, NADPH-glutathione reductase activity and adriamycin resistance in Ehrlich ascites tumor lines. Arch Toxicol 60:154–157
10. Scheulen ME, Lennartz K, Heidrich T, Host G, Kramer B (1987) Determination of the cellular uptake of daunorubicin in human leukemia in vivo. Method of examination and first results. In: Büchner T, Schellong G, Hiddemann W, Urbanitz D, Ritter J (eds) Acute Leukemias. Prognostic factors and treatment strategies. Springer, Berlin Heidelberg New York, pp 298–301 (Haematology and blood transfusion, vol 30)
11. Speth PAJ, Linssen PCM, Boezeman JBM, Wessels HMC, Haanen C (1987) Leukemic cell and plasma daunomycin concentrations after bolus injection and 72 h infusion. Cancer Chemother Pharmacol 20:311–315

Detection of the Multidrug Resistance Phenotype in Leukemic Cells with an In Vitro Chemosensitivity Assay*

T. Lion,[1] F. Prischl, F. Tichelmann, S. Kürkciyan, and J. Schwarzmeier

Detection of the pattern of resistance of tumor cells to chemotherapeutic agents is an important task in the treatment of patients with malignant diseases. In our laboratory, we established and optimized an in vitro chemosensitivity assay based on the incorporation of radioactively labeled nucleotides in the presence of various drugs. Using this assay, we analyzed the pattern of resistance in 62 patients with leukemia.

In a retrospective study, we were able to demonstrate the good predictive value of our test system. Furthermore, we addressed the question of whether this test detects the multidrug resistance phenotype (MDR) conferred by overexpression of a membrane protein (P-glycoprotein) which is encoded by the *mdr-1* gene. As a model, we utilized two epithelial tumor cell lines KB3-1 and KB-C1. The former is a drug-sensitive parental cell line from which the latter, a highly resistant cell line displaying the MDR phenotype, has been selected by culturing in increasing concentrations of colchicine. We demonstrated that our test system reliably detects MDR.

To assess the usefulness of this test in distinguishing between MDR and other types of drug resistance we are investigating the possibility of suppressing MDR in vitro by monoclonal antibodies or calcium antagonists. These results may have an impact on the therapeutic approach and contribute to an improvement of the efficacy of treatment.

* Supported by Fonds zur Förderung der wissenschaftliche Forschung, project no. P 6814, Anton Dreher Gedächtnis-Stiftung für medizinische Forschung and Hochschuljubiläumsstiftung der Stadt Wien.
[1] 1st Department of Medicine, University of Vienna, Lazarettg. 14, A-1090 Vienna, Austria

Chemotherapy for Adult Acute Myeloid Leukemia: Study Results from the Acute Myeloid Leukemia Cooperative Group and Overview*

T. Büchner,[1] W. Hiddemann, H. Löffler, D. Urbanitz, P. Koch,
G. Maschmeyer, F. Wendt, R. Kuse, A. Mohr, W.D. Ludwig, E. Thiel,
H. Seibt, W. Gassmann, C. Aul, H. Fuhr, R. Mertelsmann,
C.H. Anders, M.R. Nowrousian, K. Straif, K.A. Vaupel, D. Hossfeld,
A. von Paleske, A. Ho, H.H. Fülle, K.-P. Hellriegel, H.J. König,
B. Emmerich, E. Lengfelder, W. Siegert, H. Bartels, J. Schwammborn,
R. Bonhuijsen-Ant, F. Overkamp, M. Planker, G. Middelhoff,
K. Mainzer, K.H. Zurborn, H. Köppler, L. Nowicki, W. Augener,
J. Karow, M. Schroeder, H. Eimermacher, A. Heinecke,
and M.C. Sauerland

Introduction

In 1978 the Acute Myeloid Leukemia Cooperative Group (AMLCG) started its work. We take this opportunity to summarize the major results of the 10 years' work of this study group and combine it with an overview of results from other multicenter study results as published during the past decade. What are the lessons learned from clinical study data during the 1980s resulting from more than 5000 patients treated for AML?

Intensity of Induction Treatment and Response

Table 1 gives an overview of complete remission (CR) incidences achieved in ten multicenter studies. After increasing the remission rate to more than 50% in the early decade, substantial progress occurred. The average remission rate of 61% for the total of the studies appears realistic up to the present and is only exceeded in studies including children, using upper age limits, defining CR by bone marrow criteria only, or excluding very early death. Thus, it is important to show that in the AMLCG 62% CR could be achieved in as many as 1338 adult patients of all ages using both (bone marrow and peripheral blood) CR criteria.

* Supported by grants 01 ZP 012/3 and 01 ZP 8701/9 from Ministry for Research and Technology of the FRG.
[1] AML Cooperative Group, Department of Internal Medicine, Hematology/Oncology, University, Albert-Schweitzer-Strasse 33, D-4400 Münster, FRG

Fleischer (Ed.) Leukemias
© Springer-Verlag Berlin Heidelberg 1993

Table 1. Complete remissions (CR) in 10 multicenter studies: CALGB 81 [1], CALGB 82 [2], SAKK 84 [3], SECSG 84 [4], ECOG 84 [5], EORTC 86 [6], BMRC 86 [7], CALGB 87 [8], ECOG 88 [9], and AMLCG 89 [10]

Study	Patients (*n*)	CR (%)	Age range (years)
CALGB 81	211	46–55	0–
CALGB 82	653	49–59	0–
SAKK 84	162	72	7–65[a]
SECSG 84	508	66	15–[b]
ECOG 84	285	65	16–69
EORTC 86	295	64	10–65
BMRC 86	1045	66	10–65[a]
CALGB 87	668	53–57	14–
ECOG 88	191	66	15–65
AMLCG 89	1338	62	16–
	5356	61	

[a] Bone marrow-CR, [b] Early deaths in 1st week excluded.

What is the role of the intensity of induction chemotherapy for response? Our group has been using TAD9 [10] as the uniform induction chemotherapy regimen since 1978. Dose modifications of this standard regimen have been investigated in two groups of patients. In the 1985 study in patients of 60 years and over patients randomly received TAD9 at full- or half-dose for daunorubicin. Table 2 shows data of response to the two alternatives. We conclude that even in elderly patients an induction chemotherapy dose reduction appears to decrease the CR rate and to increase the early death rate. This effect is explained by a more frequent requirement of two induction courses in the reduced-dose group (54%) than in the full-dose group (31%).

What about an intensification of induction treatment and its effect on response and tolerability? We investigated this effect in our 1985 study in patients up to the age of 60 years. In this group patients received a uniform two-course preremission regimen with the second course being started on day 21 of therapy nonadapted to response to the first course and administered even in aplasia without blasts (double induction). For double induction patients received either two courses of TAD9 or TAD9 followed by a combination of high-dose Ara-C and mitoxantrone (HAM). HAM had proven highly effective in relapsed or resistant AML in a phase II study of our group [14]. Table 3 compares complete remission and early death incidences in the 1985 study using double induction to those in the 1981 study using conventional, mostly one-course induction. It is shown that double induction appears not to increase but even to decrease the risk of induction therapy and to improve response of AML. The unexpectedly good practicability of double induction may be explained (1) by the fact that a second induction course is well tolerated because most patients are not yet contaminated by infections, and (2) a standard double induction circumvents

Table 2. 1985 study in patients of 60 years and older. Comparison of response to induction by TAD9 randomly at full (6) or reduced (3) dose of daunorubicin

	TAD9 (60 mg/m^2)	TAD9 (30 mg/m^2)
Patients 60+ years (n)	70	77
Complete remission (%)	51	36
Early death (%)	21	29

Table 3. Comparison of response to induction treatment in patients up to 60 years in two consecutive studies representing conventional induction by mostly one-course (1981) and double induction (1985)

	1981	1985
Patients 16–60 years (n)	506	272
Complete remission (%)	65	73
Early death (%)	16	10

the common problem of diagnosis of adequate blast reduction after the first course, often leading to substantial delays in the treatment schedule.

Summarizing the two 1985 studies in elderly and younger patients: Induction dose reduction may worsen both the response and tolerability of induction treatment; on the other hand, further intensification, as by double induction, may further improve both response and tolerability of induction treatment.

Postremission Chemotherapy and Remission Duration

From most of the comparative multicenter studies published during the 1980s (Fig. 1) the role of postremission treatment alternatives remained unclear. In our 1978 study patients received TAD9 for induction and after achieving CR received induction-type consolidation and/or monthly myelo-suppressive maintenance chemotherapy or no further treatment. In this nonrandomized study the probability of ongoing CR after 9 years is 18% in patients receiving any postremission therapy, whereas relapses occurred within 2 years in all patients not receiving further treatment. The important role of at least some postremission chemotherapy becomes evident. In our 1981 study we addressed the important question about the role of a long-term monthly myelosuppressive chemotherapy [11,12]. Patients achiev-ing CR after one or two courses of TAD9 were randomized to receive one course of induction-type consolidation with or without subsequent maintenance for 3 years. Figure 2 shows the results for remission duration

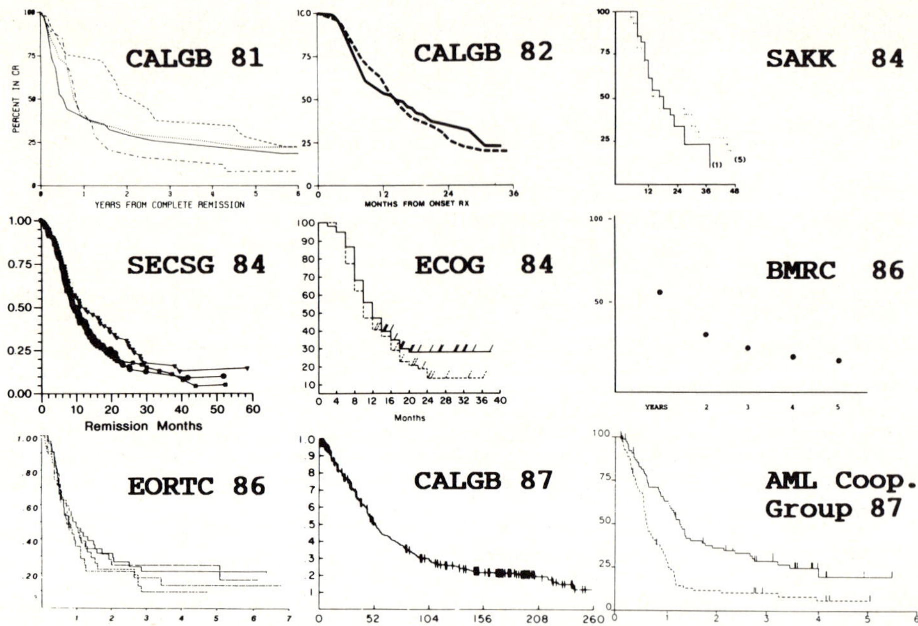

Fig. 1. Overview of AML remission duration in nine multicenter studies. For references see Table 1

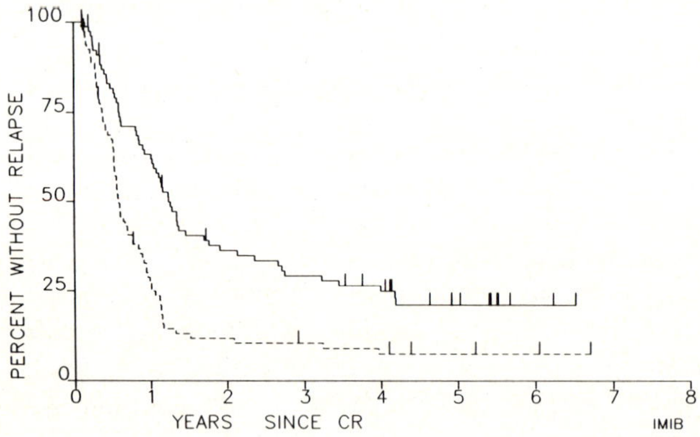

Fig. 2. AML Cooperative Group study 1981 (update 1989): remission duration in patients receiving postremission chemotherapy by consolidation randomly with (*continuous line*; *n* = 79; censored, 21) or without (*broken line*; *n* = 82; censored, 10) monthly maintenance

which in the maintenance arm appears twice that in the nonmaintenance arm. With a 21% probability of ongoing CR after 6 years the result of monthly maintenance compares favorably to those of almost all other multi-center studies and is exceeded in only one arm of the CALGB study [1]

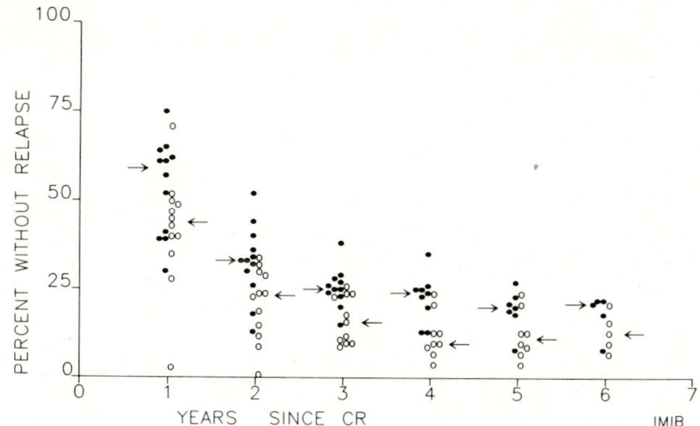

Fig. 3. Interstudy comparison of remission duration in patient groups receiving monthly or bimonthly myelosuppressive maintenance chemotherapy (*solid circles*) or no comparable myelosuppressive maintenance (*open circles*). *Arrows* indicate medians of probabilities. (The values compared are published in references 1–9 and in present article)

using monthly maintenance almost identically to our study. As in remission duration ($p = 0.0001$), also in survival ($p = 0.02$), maintenance is clearly superior to no maintenance in our 1981 study. In addition to the randomized intrastudy comparison we did an interstudy comparison of patient groups with and without maintenance treatment comparable to that used in our study. This analysis of 20 patient groups in 10 multicenter studies is shown in Fig. 3. There is a marked trend in favor of maintenance. After 3 years the medians of probabilities of ongoing CR for groups with maintenance are twice that of groups without maintenance. Again, there is a trend in favor of postremission treatment for 2 years or longer with median values after 3 years and later in the longer-treatment groups twice that of those in the shorter-treatment groups. Summarizing our 1981 study and the interstudy comparison we conclude that long-term chemotherapy in remission shows an important impact on remission duration. The gain in ongoing remissions after 5 years may amount to 100%.

Postremission Chemotherapy and Induction of Drug Resistance. In our 1981 study the incidence of second CR after relapse is 36% in the maintenance vs 38% in the no maintenance arm. Fig. 4 shows survival of all treated patients after relapse for the two randomized groups. After the first relapse median survival is 6 months and 3 years survival 12% in both groups. Thus, progressive drug resistance may be an effect of the natural course of the disease rather than induced by long-term postremission chemotherapy.

Intensity of Induction Treatment and Remission Duration. Fig. 15 shows remission duration for patients over the age of 60 years receiving randomly full-dose or reduced-dose TAD9 induction followed by uniform reduced-

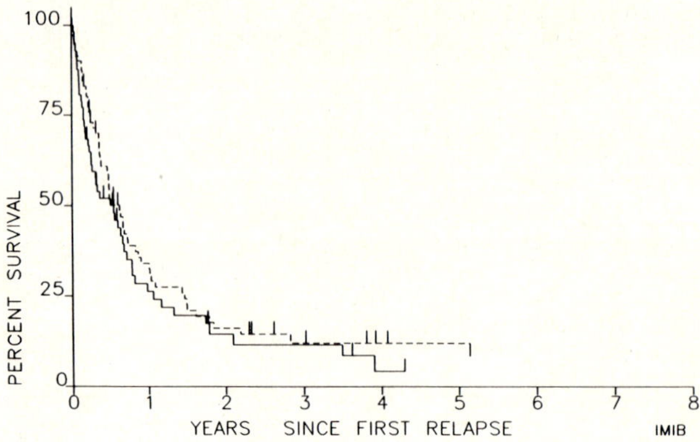

Fig. 4. 1981 AML study (update 1989): comparison of survival after first relapse for patients having been treated randomly by consolidation with (*solid line*; $n = 79$; censored, 28) or without (*broken line*; $n = 82$; censored, 22) monthly maintenance during first remission

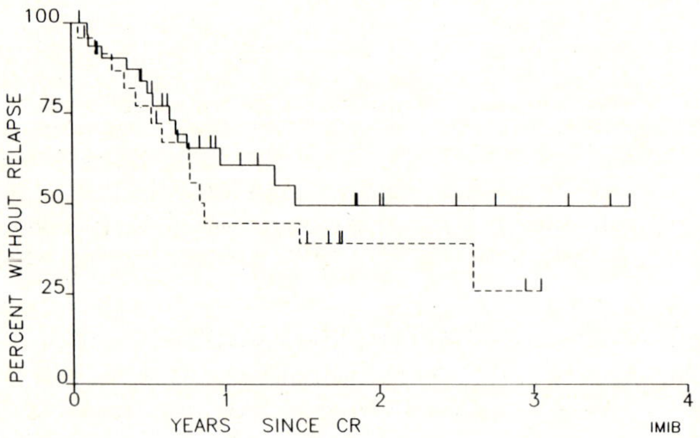

Fig. 5. 1985 AML study in patients of 60 years and over. Comparison of remission duration in patients (responders only) randomly receiving TAD9 induction at full (*solid line*; $n = 32$; censored, 19) or reduced (*broken line*; $n = 24$; censored, 11) dose for daunorubicin

dose TAD9 consolidation and standard monthly myelosuppressive maintenance for 3 years. There is a trend to longer remissions in favor of full-dose TAD9. Fig. 6 shows remission duration in the 1985 study in patients up to 60 years of age compared with the same age group in the 1981 study as a historical control. At this update there is no significant advantage in favor of double induction to conventional induction followed by the identical consolidation and monthly maintenance [13]. Thus, another 1–2 years are required to show whether differences in induction intensity affect remission duration and whether double induction in addition to a gain in response results in a gain in long-term remissions.

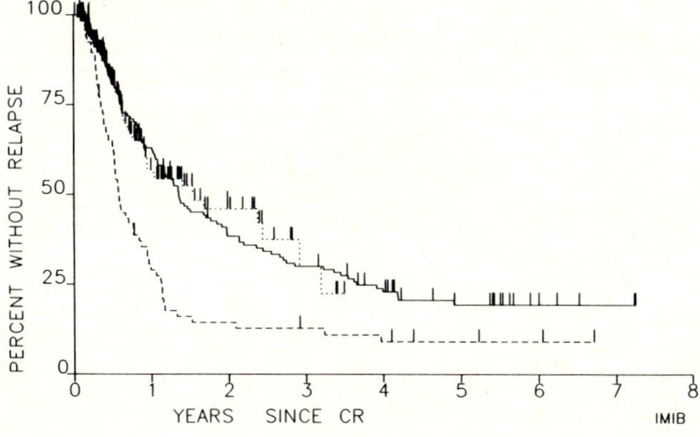

Fig. 6. 1985 AML study in patients of up to 60 years. Comparison of remission duration in the 1981 study applying conventional induction by mostly one-course and monthly maintenance (*solid line*, maintenance; $n = 129$; censored, 32; *broken line*, no maintenance; $n = 68$; censored, 10) and 1985 study applying double induction and monthly maintenance (*dotted line*; $n = 182$; censored, 119)

The Role of Hematopoietic Growth Factors in Chemotherapy for AML

Human recombinant granulocyte–colony-stimulating factor (G-CSF) and granulocyte-macrophage–colony-stimulating factor (GM-CSF) have recently become available by gene-technology methods. First clinical studies showed an effective stimulation of neutrophil recovery in both bone marrow failures and therapy-induced myelosuppression. In acute leukemias, however, there is not much experience so far. As from in vitro leukemic colony assays there is a stimulation of blasts from most of the patients with AML. Thus, the first step taken to explore GM-CSF in AML had to be restricted to patients in aplasia and at high risk of early death, such as patients after early or multiple relapses or patients 65 years of age and over. In this high-risk group continuous infusion of GM-CSF started on day 4 after the end of chemotherapy if bone marrow was aplastic without blasts. Dosage reduction and discontinuation of GM-CSF were adapted to neutrophil recovery. A typical time course of white blood cells is shown in Fig. 7, with an early recovery of neutrophils. Figure 8 shows Kaplan-Meier plots of neutrophil recovery time in the GM-CSF group compared with a control group without GM-CSF. The median recovery time appears reduced by 1 week under GM-CSF. 23 high-risk patients entered this study and 12 patients achieved a CR. Median age of responders is 61 (17–84) years. We observed 3 cases of AML with leukemic regrowth under GM-CSF. Under discontinuation the regrowth was reversible in one patient, appeared uninfluenced by the discontinuation, and spontaneous rather than GM-CSF-induced. Remission

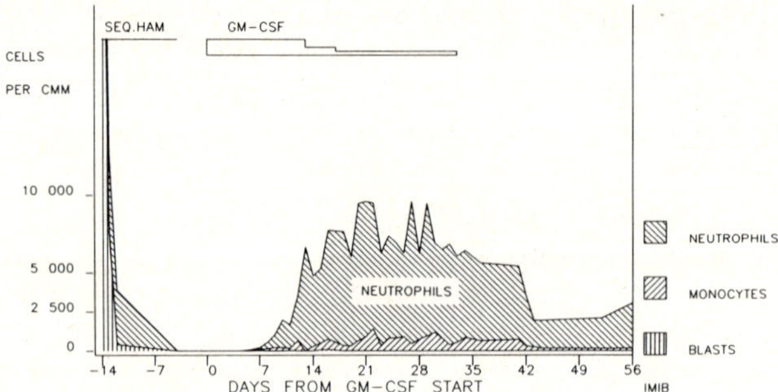

Fig. 7. Typical time course of white blood cell counts in a patient with second relapse of AML treated with sequential HAM followed by GM-CSF

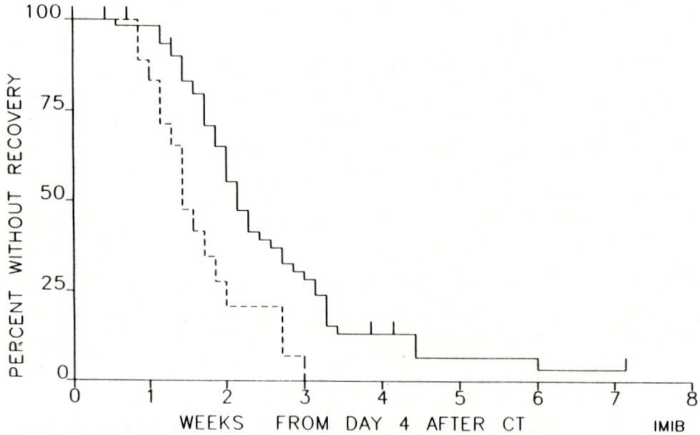

Fig. 8. Kaplan-Meier plots of neutrophil recovery time in high-risk patients receiving chemotherapy followed by GM-CSF (*broken line*; n = 19; censored, 3) compared with a control group without GM-CSF (*solid line*; n = 63; censored, 15)

duration of the responders does not appear reduced by GM-CSF. The data of this first study on GM-CSF in AML [15] require a longer observation time and a confirmation by a prospectively controlled study.

Future Directions

As inferred from our 1981 study results together with the interstudy analyses of representative multicenter trials, cure from AML appears to be a multiple-step long-term process rather than the result of a short-term highly intensive treatment in the majority of long-term survivals. Thus, in addition to a long-term, monthly myelosuppressive maintenance chemotherapy, courses of intensive postremission consolidation may further improve the results. The new approach of double induction as the earliest possible intensification may add to this concept. New, effective non-cross-resistant drug combinations can be expected from second-line treatment studies, and should have their place in primary treatment. An intensive multiple step concept, however, is clearly limited by toxicity and an increasing incidence of remission death as observed from postremission intensification protocols [8]. It has to be noted, too, that complete remission rates in adult AML are still unsatisfactory and are mainly explained by a high early death rate. Thus, a substantial fraction of patients don't have a chance to benefit from the curative potential of intensified multiple-step chemotherapy. As myelosuppression and especially extended phases of critical neutropenia represent the most limiting toxicity of antileukemic chemotherapy, reducing the neutropenic phases would reduce early lethality and would allow an increase in the antileukemic activity of chemotherapy. The new hematopoietic growth factors such as GM-CSF may open a way to such an improvement. As we showed in a first pilot study, GM-CSF appears to effectively accelerate neutrophil recovery after chemotherapy. On the other hand, the risk of stimulating the disease may be lower than it is expected to be from in vitro data.

Conclusions

The data from 10 years' work of the AML Cooperative Group together with interstudy analyses of ten representative multicenter trials support a multiple-step long-term chemotherapy concept for adult AML. In our 1981 randomized study monthly myelosuppressive maintenance produced twice as many long-term remissions as no maintenance. This finding is confirmed by a marked trend in favour of maintenance and, similarly, of a longer post-remission chemotherapy in the ten trials. The long-term results may further be improved by introducing postremission intensification courses and the new approach of double induction. Myelotoxicity and especially critical neutropenia as the most limiting toxicity of an intensified multiple-step antileukemic therapy may today be controlled by the new hematopoietic growth factors. Thus, human recombinant GM-CSF proved effective in reducing neutrophil recovery time in high-risk patients with AML in a first study of our group.

References

1. Rai KR, Holland JF, Glidewell OJ, et al. (1981) Treatment of acute myelocytic leukemia: a study by cancer and leukemia group B. Blood 58:1203
2. Yates J, Glidewell O, Wiernik P, et al. (1982) Cytosine arabinoside with daunorubicin or adriamycin for therapy of acute myelocytic leukemia: a CALGB Study. Blood 60:454

3. Sauter C, Fopp M, Imbach P, et al. (1984) Acute myelogenous leukemia: maintenance chemotherapy after early consolidation treatment does not prolong survival. Lancet I:379

4. Vogler WR, Winton EF, Gordon DS, et al. (1984) A randomized comparison of postremission therapy in acute myelogenous leukemia: a southeastern cancer study group trial. Blood 63:1039

5. Cassileth PA, Begg CB, Bennett JM, et al. (1984) A randomized study of the efficacy of consolidation therapy in adult acute nonlymphocytic leukemia. Blood 63:843

6. Hayat M, Jehn U, Willemze R, et al. (1986) A randomized comparison of maintenance treatment with androgens, immunotherapy, and chemotherapy in adult acute myelogenous leukemia. A leukemia-lymphoma group trial of the EORTC. Cancer 58:617

7. Rees JKH, Swirsky D, Gray RG, Hayhoe FGJ (1986) Principal results of the medical research council's 8th acute myeloid leukemia trial. Lancet II:1236

8. Preisler H, Davis RB, Kirshner J, et al. (1987) Comparison of three remission induction regimens and two postinduction strategies for the treatment of acute nonlymphocytic leukemia: a cancer and leukemia group B study. Blood 69:1441

9. Cassileth PA, Harrington DP, Hines JD, et al. (1988) Maintenance chemotherapy prolongs remission duration in adult acute nonlymphocytic leukemia. J Clin Oncol 6:538

10. Büchner T, Urbanitz D, Hiddemann W, et al. (1985) Intensified induction and consolidation with or without maintenance chemotherapy for acute myeloid leukemia (AML): two multicenter studies of the German AML cooperative group. J Clin Oncol 3:1583

11. Büchner T, Hiddemann W, Koch P, et al. (1988) The role of myelosuppressive maintenance, immunotherapy, induction dose reduction in higher age, and double induction in adult acute myeloid leukemia (AML). Four studies of the AML cooperative group. In: Kimura K, et al. (eds) Cancer Chemotherapy: Challenges for the furture. Excerpta Medica, Tokyo, p 119

12. Büchner T, Urbanitz D, Rühl H, et al. (1985) Role of chemotherapy for AML in remission. Lancet I:1224

13. Büchner T, Hiddemann W, Wendt F, et al. (1987) Early intensification by double induction (DI) in adult AML: a multicenter study of the AML cooperative group. Blood 70[Suppl 1]:752

14. Hiddemann W, Kreutzmann H, Straif K, et al. (1987) High-dose cytosine arabinoside and mitoxantrone (HAM): a highly effective regimen in refractory acute myeloid leukemia. Blood 69:744

15. Büchner T, Hiddemann W, Koenigsmann M, et al. (1988) Human recombinant granulocyte-macrophage colony-stimulating factor (GM-CSF) for acute leukemias in aplasia and at high risk of early death. Blood 72[Suppl 1]:354

Mitoxantrone and Cytosine Arabinoside as First-Line Therapy in Elderly Patients with Acute Myeloid Leukemia

I.W. Delamore,[1] P. Johnson, J.L. Yin, J.M. Davies, N. Flannagan, M. Lewis, and D. Gorst

Since May 1986, we have treated 98 patients with acute myeloid leukemia (AML) on a protocol consisting of induction with mitoxantrone ($10\,\text{mg/m}^2$) for 4 days and cytosine arabinoside (Ara-C) ($100\,\text{mg/m}^2$ bd) for 5 days and consolidation with 1 or 2 courses of mitoxantrone for 2 days and Ara-C for 5 days at the same dosages. Maintenance therapy with cyclophosphamide and 6-thioguanine administered orally was optional. The age range was 60–79 years, with a median of 68 years. There were 54 males and 44 females. Results from tests on 90 patients were evaluated for response; 58 patients (64%) achieved a complete remission (CR) (Fig. 1). Of 72 patients with de novo AML, 52 (72%) achieved CR; also, 15 patients had a documented pre-existing myelodysplastic syndrome, of whom 6 (40%) achieved CR. The median time to CR was 29 days (range, 12–88 days). In the CR group, 34 of 58 (59%) patients have relapsed and the median disease-free survival is 14

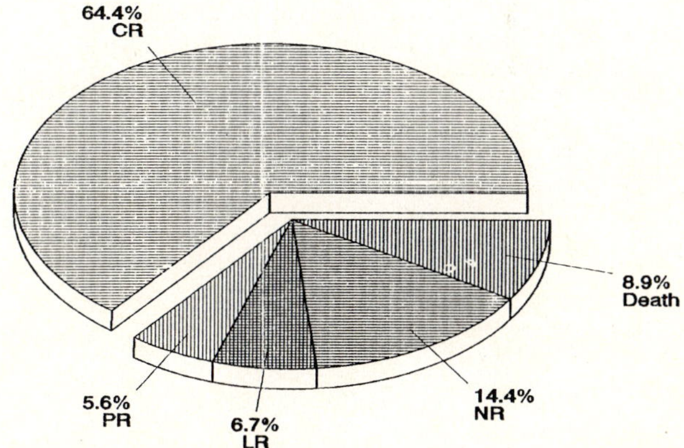

Fig. 1. Overall response of AML patients to a treatment regimen with mitoxantrone and Ara-C ($n = 90$). *CR*, complete remission; *PR*, partial response; *LR*, limited remission; *NR*, no response

---

[1] Manchester Royal Infirmary, Department of Haematology, University of Manchester, Manchester, UK

Fleischer (Ed.) Leukemias
© Springer-Verlag Berlin Heidelberg 1993

months, with an overall median survival of 20 months. The median survival in all 98 patients recruited is 12 months, with an actuarial survival of 28% at 3 years. Non-haematological toxicity was mild to moderate in severity and the treatment was generally well tolerated. Responders enjoyed a good quality of life. We conclude that a combination of mitoxantrone and Ara-C is an effective and well-tolerated regimen in elderly patients with AML.

Intermediate-Dose Cytosine Arabinoside and Amsacrine for Remission Induction and High-Dose Cytosine Arabinoside and Amsacrine for Intensive Consolidation in Relapsed and Refractory Adult Acute Myelogenous Leukemia[*]

U. Jehn[1] and V. Heinemann

Introduction

High-dose cytosine arabinoside (Ara-C) regimens (HD-Ara-C) designed as intermittent infusions of $3 \, g/m^2$ over $1-3 \, h$ at 12-h intervals have shown good efficacy either as single-drug treatment or in combination with anthracyclines, amsacrine (m-AMSA), or L-asparaginase [1–5]. However, remission induction has been achieved at the expense of a considerable treatment-associated death rate. In our present approach we examine intermediate-dose Ara-C (ID-Ara-C) for treatment of refractory and relapsed acute myelogeuous leukemia (AML). The dose reduction to $1 \, g/m^2$ performed in ID-Ara-C was anticipated to decrease treatment-related toxicity, while treatment efficacy should not be impaired [6–8].

Patient Characteristics and Methods

Patients of all age-groups and French-American-British (FAB) subtypes with relapsed or primary refractory AML were included in this phase II study. The majority of relapsed patients experienced their relapse during or after completion of intensive maintenance treatment according to the European Organisation for Research on Treatment of Cancer- (EORTC)-AML 6 study [9,10]: they had been randomized to either repeated courses of the induction type (daunorubicin, DNR, $45 \, mg/m^2$ i.v. on day 1 plus Ara-C $100 \, mg/m^2$ s.c. on days 1–5) or to non-cross-resistant drugs alternating m-AMSA ($150 \, mg/m^2$ i.v. on day 1) plus Ara-C ($3 \, g/m^2$ i.v. q 12 h on days 1 and 2) with m-AMSA plus 5-azacytidine (5-AZA $150 \, mg/m^2$ i.v. on days 1–3). A total of six intensive maintenance courses were given every 6 weeks. Retractory patients were defined as being resistant to two courses of

[*] Presented at the Leukemia Symposium of the International Society of Hematology in Dresden, May 1989, and previously published in *Haematology and blood transfusion*, vol. 33, pp. 333–338 (Springer, Berlin Heidelberg New York)
[1] Department of Internal Medicine, Hematology/Oncology, Klinikum Grosshadern, Ludwig-Maximilians-Universität, W-8000 München 70, FRG

Fleischer (Ed.) Leukemias
© Springer-Verlag Berlin Heidelberg 1993

an anthracycline-containing induction regimen totaling 6 doses of DNR (6 × 45 mg/m^2) combined with 14 doses of Ara-C (14 × 200 mg/m^2). Patients with a history of myelodysplastic syndrome (MDS) or a second malignancy were included.

The remission induction regimen consisted of ID-Ara-C. 1 g/m^2 i.v. every 12 h by a 2-h infusion for 6 days and m-AMSA, 120 mg/m^2 i.v. on days 5, 6, and 7. One or two cycles for induction were given. When complete remission (CR) was reached, one consolidation course was administered consisting of HD-Ara-C, 3 g/m^2 i.v. every 12 h by a 2-h infusion for 4 days, and m-AMSA, 120 mg/m^2 i.v. on day 5. The treatment-free interval between 2 induction cycles was 3 weeks. The interval between the end of induction and the beginning of consolidation was 4 weeks. No further therapy was given thereafter.

Results

A total of 34 patients entered the study: 6 were refractory and failed previous standard remission induction treatment, 28 were treated for relapse (26 in first and 2 in second relapse). One relapsed and one refractory patient had a previous history of MDS, another patient suffered, in addition to refractory AML, from a cervical cancer stage II–III. The median age was 44 years. The patient characteristics are shown in Table 1.

Table 1. Patient characteristics

Total number	34
Age (years), median (range)	44 (18–66)
FAB M1	1
M2	13
M3	4
M4	10
M5	5
Refractory	6
Relapsed	28
First	26
Second	2
Duration of preceding remission (months, median)	8
Time from last chemotherapy to relapse (months, median)	3.1
Type of preceding maintenance	
Intensive (EORTC-AML 6):	
DNR, Ara-C (induction type)	13
HD-Ara-C, mAMSA/5-AZA, mAMSA	8
Conventional (EORTC-AML 5)	1
No maintenance	6

Table 2. Response to treatment

Total number	34
Refractory	6
Complete remission (one cycle)	1
Failure (refractory)	2
Hypoplastic death	3
Relapsed	28
Complete remission	22/28 (79%)
After one cycle	21
After two cycles	1
Failure (refractory)	3
Hypoplastic death	3
Hypoplastic death in CR (after consolidation)	3

One out of six refractory patients achieved CR after one cycle of ID-Ara-C and m-AMSA. Two patients remained refractory to two reinduction cycles and three died in hypoplasia, one with concomitant cervical cancer and one with a history of MDS. Twenty-two out of 28 relapsed patients (79%) reached CR, 17 after 1 cycle of ID-Ara-C. Three patients were refractory to two courses of this regimen; three died during hypoplasia without evidence of leukemic regrowth. Three patients died in CR after intensive consolidation with HD-Ara-C (Table 2). Three patients were recipients of transplants in second remission, two of them received an allograft and are in continued CR 14 and 21.5 months after bone marrow transplantation (BMT), and one patient received an autograft but died shortly thereafter.

Table 3 shows that responding patients had a longer duration of preceding remission (9.5 vs. 4.5 months) and a longer interval from last chemotherapy to relapse (3.5 vs. 2 months) than nonresponders. The type of preceding maintenance (induction-type vs. HD-Ara-C-containing regimen) had, most remarkably, no impact on achieving another CR or not. It is noteworthy that two patients in first relapse, who reached a second remission of 10 months and 24 months duration respectively with this program, achieved a third remission with the identical regimen and are still in CR at more than 6 and 7 months, respectively. The median disease-free survival (DFS) of relapsed and refractory patients was 3.3 months, the median survival of responders, 4.6 months (Fig. 1), and the overall survival, 4.7 months (Table 4). Patients receiving BMT were excluded from this analysis at the time of BMT.

The major toxicity seen in these patients was a noncardiogenic pulmonary edema due to ID- or HD-Ara-C as substantiated in detail elsewhere [11,12]. So far 7 out of 34 patients (20%) experienced this type of lung toxicity either in combination with or without infection (3 patients have not yet received consolidation therapy using HD-Ara-C). Three patients

Table 3. Remission incidence according to pretreatment characteristics

Total relapsed	28
Complete remission	22
Duration of preceding remission (months, median)	9.5
Time from last chemotherapy to relapse (months, median)	3.5
Type of preceding maintenance	
Intensive (EORTC-AML 6):	
DNR/Ara-C (induction type)	11
HD-Ara-C, m-AMSA/5-AZA, m-AMSA	6
Conventional	1
No maintenance	4
Failure	6
Duration of preceding remission (months, median)	4.5
Time from last chemotherapy to relapse (months, median)	2
Type of preceding maintenance	
Intensive	
DNR/Ara-C (induction type)	2
HD-Ara-C, m-AMSA/5-AZA	2
No maintenance	2

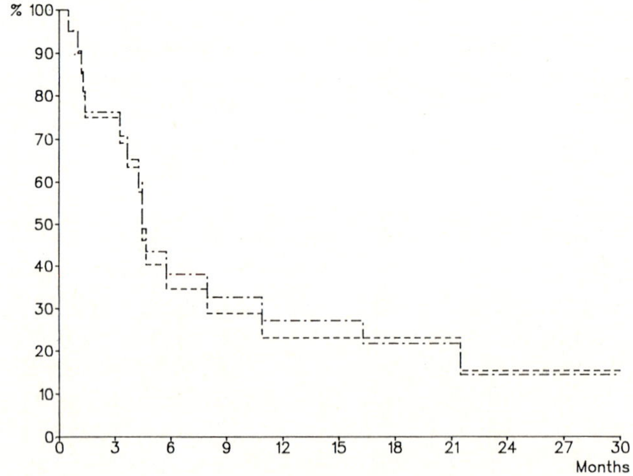

Fig. 1. DFS in 20 relapsed AML patients (----) and 21 relapsed plus refractory AML patients (-·-·-·-·-)

recovered, and four died. From our data, the incidence of pulmonary edema was significantly related to the type of preceding intensive maintenance: 2 our of 13 cases (15%) arising from the induction type, and 3 out of 8 cases (38%; $P \leq 0.05$) pretreated with the HD-Ara-C-containing maintenance. One patient with this type of toxicity underwent a previous "low-dose"

Table 4. Response to treatment

Disease-free survival (months, median)	
Relapsed ($n = 20$)	3.3
Relapsed + refractory ($n = 21$)	3.3
Survival CR	
Relapsed	4.5
Relapsed + refractory	4.5
Survival all	
Relapsed ($n = 25$)	4.7
Relapsed + refractory ($n = 31$)	4.5

Patients receiving BMT ($n = 3$) were excluded at the time of BMT.

Table 5. Lung toxicity

	Number of patients	
	(n)	(%)
Total	7/34	
Recovery	3	
Death	4	
Type of preceding maintenance		
Intensive (EORTC AML 6)		
DNR, Ara-C (induction type)	2/13	15
HD-Ara-C, m-AMSA/5-AZA, m-AMSA	3/8	38
Conventional (after consolidation)	1/1	
No maintenance (after second cycle of induction)	1/6	16

$P = 0.05$ for DNR, Ara-C (induction type) and HD-Ara-C, m-AMSA/5-AZA, m-AMSA.

Three patients had not yet received therapy using HD-Ara-C, so are not included in this evaluation.

conventional maintenance program, 3 years in duration, and developed a lethal noncardiogenic pulmonary edema after the HD-Ara-C consolidation course. Another relapsed patient died of this complication without having any previous exposure to ID-Ara-C or HD-Ara-C after two cycles of induction with ID-Ara-C (Table 5).

Discussion

Leukemic relapse occurs in the vast majority of responding AML patients within the first 1–2 years after achievement of CR [13,14]. Reinduction with HD-Ara-C as single drug or in combination with anthracyclines, m-AMSA, or L-asparaginase achieves CR rates between 60% and 70% [1,3–5]. However, HD-Ara-C-containing regimens are associated with severe toxicity, contributing to a substantial treatment-induced mortality. In fact, Ara-C-induced toxicity correlates directly with the cumulative amount of drug administered [15,16].

Sufficient pharmacological data have been accumulated to advocate that reduction of Ara-C to intermediate-dose regimens ($1\,g/m^2$ per 2 h) will not impair maximal accumulation of the active Ara cytidine triphosphate (CTP) in leukemia cells [6,8,17] and thereby the treatment outcome. Following this approach we investigated a regimen consisting of ID Ara-C and m-AMSA for its efficacy in relapsed and primary refractory leukemia ($n = 29$; Table 2). Complete remission was achieved in nearly 80% (18/23) of patients with relapsed AML. This observation is in accordance with recent reports showing CR rates of 71%–83% induced by ID-Ara-C [18–20] which are equivalent to those reached with HD-Ara-C-containing regimens.

A treatment-related mortality of 11% in our study compares favorably with mortality rates between 27% and 33% observed in HD-Ara-C regimens [4,5,21]. Interestingly, despite a marked reduction of treatment-related mortality using ID-Ara-C, the remission incidence is at least equivalent to or superior to HD-Ara-C in relapsed AML. Duration of preceding remission or time from last chemotherapy to relapse appear to be prognostic factors for remission induction. In patients achieving CR, the duration of preceding remission was 9.5 months vs. 4.5 months in failing patients (Table 3). Comparably, the time from last chemotherapy to relapse amounted to 3.5 months in responding patients vs. 2 months in failing patients. The type of maintenance therapy preceding relapse had no influence on the outcome of the reinduction therapy (Table 3). Thus treatment failures were equally distributed between patients who had undergone either no maintenance or induction-type maintenance (DNR and Ara-C) or HD-Ara-C-containing maintenance. The significance of this observation will have to be evaluated with greater numbers of patients.

Despite a good CR rate using ID-Ara-C and m-AMSA, and despite intensive consolidation with HD-Ara-C, DFS was short and the overall survival time 4.7 months. It should be stressed, however, that three patients receiving BMT were exluded at the time of transplantation. In view of considerable toxicity seen after the consolidation treatment (3/18 toxic deaths), the value of an intensive consolidation regimen for prolongation of DFS and survival appears questionable in patients with relapsed leukemia.

In primary refractory patients only one out of six achieved CR after treatment with ID-Ara-C and m-AMSA (Table 2). It should be noted that the incidence of hypoplastic death in this group was considerable at 50% (3/6). Previous studies using HD-Ara-C in refractory AML, either as single-drug regimen or in combination, induced CR rates of 14%–56% [1,3,18,21]. Although the number of patients in this analysis is too small to allow final conclusions, it appears that ID-Ara-C and m-AMSA is insufficient as treatment of refractory AML. Life-threatening toxicity occurred as non-cardiogenic pulmonary edema [12,22,23] in 20% (7/34) of the patients (Table 4). The incidence of pulmonary edema was significantly related to the type of preceding maintenance treatment.

In conclusion, guided by pharmacokinetic studies, we have reduced the Ara-C dosage in relapsed and refractory AML patients and thereby reduced the treatment-related death rate markedly without loss of treatment efficacy in respect to CR rate.

References

1. Herzig RH, Wolff SN, Lazarus HM, Phillips GL, Karanes C, Herzig GP (1983) High-dose cytosine arabinoside therapy for refractory leukemia. Blood 62:361–369
2. Kantarjian HM, Estey EH, Plunkett W, Keating MJ, Walters RS, Iacoboni S, McCredie KB, Freireich EJ (1986) Phase I–II clinical pharmacologic studies of high-dose cytosine arabinoside in refractory leukemia. Am J Med 81:387–394
3. Herzig RH, Lazarus HM, Wolff SN, Phillips GL, Herzig GP (1985) High-dose cytosine arabinoside therapy with and without anthracycline antibiotics for remission induction of acute non-lymphoblastic leukemia. J Clin Oncol 3:992–997
4. Hines JD, Oken MM, Mazza JJ, Keller AM, Streeter RR, Glick JH (1984) High-dose cytosine arabinoside and m-AMSA is effective therapy in relapsed acute non-lymphocytic leukemia. J Clin Oncol 2:545–549
5. Capizzi RL, Davis R, Powell B, Cuttner J, Ellison RR, Cooper MR, Dillman R, Major WB, Dupre E, McIntyre OR (1988) Synergy between high-dose cytarabine and asparaginase in the treatment of adults with refractory and relapsed acute myelogeneous leukemai – a cancer and leukemia group B study. J Clin Oncol 6:499–508
6. Plunkett W, Iacoboni S, Keating MJ (1986) Cellular pharmacology and optimal therapeutic concentrations of 1-β-D-arabinofuranosylcytosine 5′-triphosphate in leukemic blasts during treatment of refractory leukemia with high-dose 1-β-D-arabinosylcytosine. Scand J Haematol 36[Suppl 44]:51–59
7. Rustum YM, Preisler HD (1979) Correlation between leukemic cell retention of 1-β-D-arabinofuranosyl-cytosine 5′-triphosphate and response to therapy. Cancer Res 39:42–49
8. Plunkett W, Liliemark JO, Adams TM, Nowak B, Estey E, Kantarjian H, Keating JM (1987) Saturation of 1-β-D-arabinofuranosylcytosine 5′-triphosphate accumulation in leukemia cells during high-dose 1-β-D-arabinofuranosylcytosine therapy. Cancer Res 47:3005–3011
9. Jehn U, Zittoun R (for the EORTC Leukemia Lymphoma Study Group) (1985) AML-6 Studie zum Wert einer zyklisch alternierenden Chemotherapie während der Remission bei akuter myeloischer leukämie. Onkologie 8:94
10. Zittoun R, Jehn U, Fiere D, Haanen C, Löwenberg B, Willemze R, Abels J, Bury J, Suciu S, Solbu G. Stryckmans P (1989) Alternating versus repeated postremission treatment in adult acute leukemia: a randomized study of the EORTC Leukemia Cooperative Group. Blood 73:896
11. Jehn U, Ruckdeschel G, Sauer H, Clemm C, Wilmanns W (1981) Vergleichende Studie zum Wert der selektiven Darmdekontamination (SDD) bei der Behandlung akuter Leukämien. Klin Wochenschr 59:1093
12. Jehn U, Göldel N, Rienmüller R, Wilmanns W (1988) Noncardiogenic pulmonary edema complicating intermediate and high-dose ara-C treatment for relapsed leukemia. Med Oncol Tumor Pharmacother 5:41
13. Freireich EJ (1984) Acute leukemia: a prototype of disseminated cancer. Cancer 53:2026–2033
14. Keating M, Estey E, Kantarjian HM, Walters R, Smith T, McCredie KB, Freireich EJ (1987) Comparison of results of salvage therapy in adult acute myelogeneous leukemia. Acta Haematol 78[Suppl 1]:120–126

15. Lazarus HM, Herzig RH, Herzig GP, Phillips GP. Roessman U, Fishman DJ (1981) Central nervous system toxicity of high-dose systemic cytosine arabinoside. Cancer 48:2577–2582
16. Willemze R, Fibbe WE, Zwaan FE (1983) Experience with intermediate and high-dose cytosine arabinoside in relapsed and refractory acute leukemia. Neth J Med 26:215–219
17. Heinemann V, Estey E, McMullen G, Plunkett W (1988) Patient specific dose rate for continuous infusion high-dose cytarabine (ara-C) in relapsed acute leukemia. Proc Am Assoc Cancer Res Am Soc Clin Oncol 24:258
18. Willemze R. Peters WG, van Hennik MB, Fibbe WE, Kootte AMM, van Berkel M, Lie R. Rodenburg CJ, Veltkamp JJ (1985) Intermediate and high-dose ara-C and m-AMSA (or daunorubicin) as remission and consolidation treatment for patients with relapsed acute leukemia and lymphoblastic non-Hodgkin lymphoma. Scand J Haematol 34:83–87
19. Van Prooyen HC, Dekker AW, Punt K (1984) The use of intermediate-dose cytosine arabinoside in the treatment of acute nonlymphoblastic leukemia in relapse. Br J Haematol 57:291–299
20. Amadori S, Papa G, Miniero R, Petti MC, Meloni G, Mandelli F (1988) A phase II study of intermediate-dose ara-C (IDAC) with sequential mitoxantrone in acute myelogeneous leukemia. In: 22nd Congr Int Soc hematol, p 455
21. Walters RS, Kantarjian HM, Keating MJ, Plunkett W, Estey EH, Andersson B, Beran M, McCredie KB, Freireich EJ (1988) Mitoxantrone and high-dose cytosine arabinoside in refractory acute myelogeneous leukemia. Cancer 62:677–682
22. Haupt HM, Hutchins GM, Moore GW (1981) Ara-C lung: noncardiogenic pulmonary edema complicating arabinoside therapy of leukemia. Am J Med 70:256–261
23. Andersson BS. Cogan BM, Keating MJ, Estey EH, McCredie KB, Freireich EJ (1985) Subacute pulmonary failure complicating therapy with high-dose ara-C in acute leukemia. Cancer 56:2181–2184

Aclacinomycin A Therapy in Acute Nonlymphoblastic Leukemia*

L. Konopka,[1] S. Pawelski, P. Obląkowski, P. Kohutnicki, D. Apel, B. Mariańska, and S. Maj

Anthracycline antibiotics used in combination with other agents can produce complete remission (CR) in about 70%–80% previously untreated and possibly selected group of patients with acute nonlymphoblastic leukemia (ANLL) [2,3].

In larger studies, response rates were lower (in the mid-40%–mid-60% range) particularly in group studies with largely unselected patients [2,8]. These studies also demonstrated that a small proportion of patients may remain in long-term CR for 5 or more years.

Although relapses do occur in these patients, the majority occur within a year of discontinuation of chemotherapy. The risk of relapse never returns to zero, but the probability of relapse per unit time in patients 4–5 years in CR and off therapy for 2–3 years continues to be extremely low [8]. The potential for long-term survival and cure is, therefore, clearly demonstrated, particularly in patients under the age of 50. In older patients long-term administration of these compounds and especially of Adriamycin (ADR) is also limited by their cardiotoxicity, which is directly related to the cumulative dose [1,4].

On the basis of a study performed by Praga et al. [10] the incidence of both "definite" (congestive heart failure, CHF) and "possible" (other cardiac complications, such as myocardial infarction, cardiogenic shock, cardiac arrest, increased heart size, and symptomatic cardiac arrhythmia) ADR cardiomyopathy (ADR-CMP), analyzed after logit transformation in 1273 patients showed a highly significant curvilinear regression for definite ADR-CMP, while possible ADR-CMP was not found to be dose related and is represented by a line corresponding to the overall incidence (3%) in this group (Fig. 1).

Among the different anthracyclines, Aclacinomycin A (ACM) has by far the lowest cardiotoxicity in humans. Preclinical evaluation of ACM has shown also several important positive differences in comparison to doxorubicin. Cellular uptake of ACM occurs more rapidly than doxorubicin

---

* Some of the results included in this paper are from work carried out under IGCI study group (Vienna, Austria), Chairman, Prof. Dr. D. Lutz [6].
[1] Institute of Haematology, 00-957 Warsaw, Chocimska 5, Poland

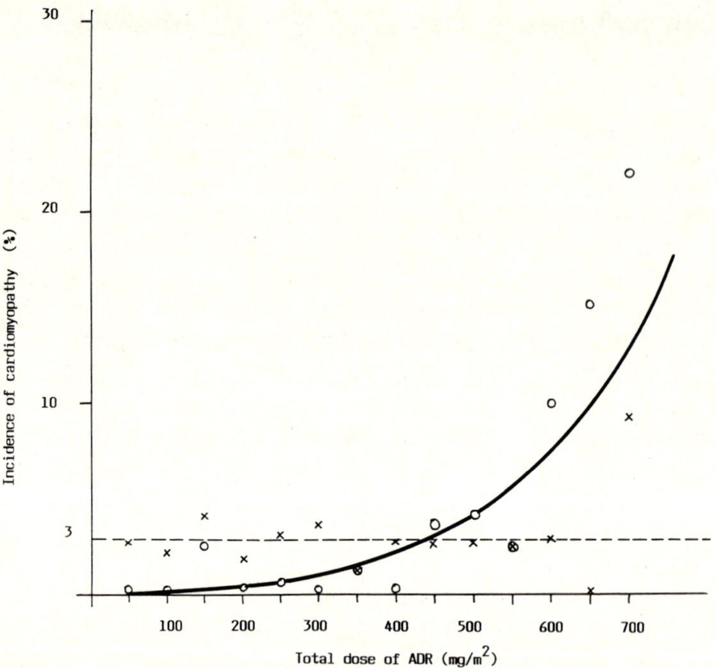

Fig. 1. Effect of total dose on incidence of CMP (definite ADR-CMP, *open circles*; possible ADR-CMP, *crosses*) in 1273 patients receiving ADR (from [10])

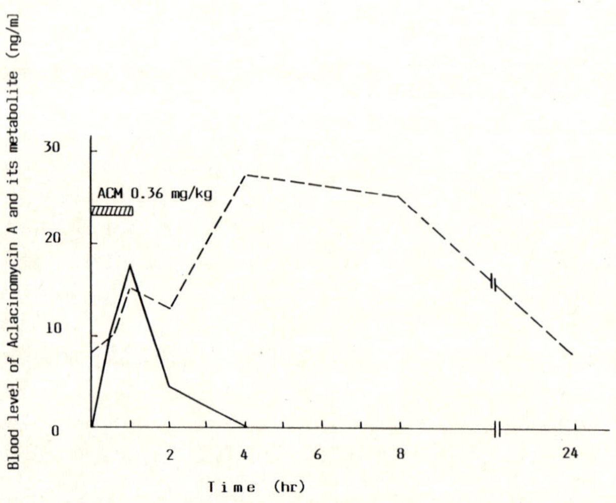

Fig. 2. Serial analysis of the concentration of ACM (*solid line*) and its active metabolites (MA 144 M$_1$ and MA 144 N$_1$, *broken line*, produced by the reduction of the keto group of L-cinerulose of ACM to L-aminocetose and L-rhodinose respectively) in the blood (from [11])

and its final concentration is higher. ACM is also a more potent inhibitor of RNA synthesis and is less mutagenic [13]. Initial clinical trials confirmed that ACM can be effective for achieving remission in adults with refractory leukemia even in patients heavily pretreated with doxorubicin [6,9,11].

ACM is rapidly metabolized in vivo, as shown in Fig. 2 [11]. After intravenous infusion of ACM in a dose of 0.36 mg/kg body weight, the blood level of ACM was 17.8 µg/ml at the end of infusion; it decreased thereafter and was down to zero 4 h later. The level of its active metabolites MA 144 M_1 and MA 144 N_1, which are formed by the reduction of the keto group of L-cinerulose of ACM to L-amicetose and L-rhodinose, respectively, rose for the first 4 h (27.7 ng/ml), reached a plateau, then decreased. They were detectable for 24 h. These clinico- and pharmacokinetics indicate that ACM is a promising agent for the treatment of acute leukemia.

In this report we present our experience in intensive treatment with ACM in 26 patients with ANLL.

Material and Methods

Nine untreated patients with ANLL and 17 persons with refractory and/or relapsing ANLL were entered in this study (Table 1).

Sixteen patients were female and ten were male. The median age was 42.6 years, with a distribution of 18–65.

Table 1. Characteristics of ANLL patients

Characteristic	ANLL patients	
	Untreated ($n = 9$)	Refractory and/or relapsing ($n = 17$)
Age in years (range)		
Women	6 (18–34)	10 (25–65)
Men	3 (20–41)	7 (18–58)
Cytochemical type of ANLL (FAB classification)		
M0	–	1
M1	2	2
M2	7	13
M6	–	1
Karnofsky performance status		
50 or more	2	14
30–40	7	3
Median number of previous induction attempts (range)	–	2–6
Median cumulative total dose of prior ADR (range; mg)	–	300–900

Patients were classified according to the French-American-British Group (FAB) classification, as follows: M0 – 1 case, M1 – 4 cases, M2 – 20 cases, and M6 – 1 case.

The patients with refractory and/or relapsing ANLL, in response to conventional therapy (17 patients), failed to improve after standard chemotherapy, including ADR, cytosine arabinoside (Ara-C), and/or 6-thioguanine (Tg), for remission induction (12 cases), or relapsed during maintenance treatment with Ara-C and Tg, Ara-C and Oncovin and Prednisone, or Ara-C and ADR (5 cases).

All patients had adequate hepatic and renal function. More than one-half of the patients had an initial Karnofsky performance status of at least 50.

Involvement of central nervous system (CNS) due to ANLL was observed in four patients then treated with methotrexate, administered intrathecally. Three patients without cytological changes in cerebrospinal fluid were submitted to prophylactic intrathecal treatment.

Untreated patients received a single or double course of induction therapy consisting of $18\,mg/m^2$ per day ACM administered for 7 days by 30-min i.v. infusion together with $100\,mg/m^2$ per day Ara-C, for 7 days by continuous 20-h i.v. infusion (Table 2).

In 17 relapsing or refractory ANLL patients, ACM was given daily by 1-h i.v. infusion with dose $25\,mg/m^2$ administered together with 20-h i.v. infusion of Ara-C $(100\,mg/m^2)$ and with Tg $(100\,mg/m^2)$ per os for 5 consecutive days.

These courses were repeated on day 21 or after bone marrow recovery in the case of post-therapeutic bone marrow aplasia or hypoplasia. The program was discontinued usually if 3 cycles did not induce complete remission (CR) or partial (PR) remission.

Induction of CR was followed by further chemotherapy (Ara-C and Tg, Ara-C and Oncovin plus Prednisone, and Ara-C and ACM) as main-

Table 2. Therapy programs

Drug	1st group (Untreated patients)	2nd group (Refractory or relapsing patients)
Aclacinomycin	$18\,mg/m^2$ for 7 days (in 30-min i.v. drip infusion)	$25\,mg/m^2$ for 5 days (in 1-h i.v. infusion)
Arabinoside-cytosine	$100\,mg/m^2$ for 7 days (in 20-h i.v. infusion)	$100\,mg/m^2$ for 5 days (in 20-h i.v. infusion)
6-Thioguanine	–	$100\,mg/m^2$ p.o. for 5 days
Courses	1 or 2 courses	Repeated on day 21 or after bone marrow recovery of post-therapeutic bone marrow aplasia or hypoplasia (no more than 3 courses)

tenance therapy. Evaluation during therapy included the monitoring of hematologic values, hepatic and renal function, and electrocardiogram (ECG).

CR was defined by criteria proposed by the Cancer and Acute Leukemia Group [4] as a state of less than 5% blasts in the bone marrow nucleated cells and normal hematopoietic components as well as no signs attributable to leukemia. PR meant over 50% reduction of blast cells in the bone marrow and recovery of normal hematopoietic components.

Results

Of the 26 patients entered in this study, 7 were considered not to have received an adequate trial (Table 3), 3 because of death in less than 4 weeks or just after ending of the first course, 1 because he refused therapy after a single course of ACM plus Ara-C and Tg therapy. In another 3 patients therapy was discontinued after the first course because of severe arrythmia due to the treatment (2 cases) and, in 1 case, abscess of the breast. The rest of the patients (19 persons) received two or three courses of these programs. The total dose of ACM ranged from 185 to 600 mg.

Twelve of 26 patients achieved CR or PR. CR was achieved by 5 out of 9 (55%) untreated ANLL patients and 4 out of 17 (23.5%) refractory or relapsing ANLL patients. In the last group of patients PR was achieved in three cases (18%) additionally (Table 4). The days required for achieving CR ranged from 42 to 78 days (median, 33 days). Durations of CR ranged from 6 to 24 months (median, 12.5+ months).

Out of nine patients with CR, seven are still alive, five with CR lasting from 6 to 17 months; two others, after 6 and 7 months of CR, relapsed during the combination of chemotherapy. One patient of these two then died because of a tumor of the brain (autopsy was not performed).

Table 3. Number of chemotherapy courses with ACM plus ARA-C and Tg or ACM and ARA-C

	Number of patients
Number of cycles	
2 or 3	19
1	7
Causes of discontinuation of therapy	
Early death	2
Death after the first course (bleeding, infection)	1
Severe arrhythmia due to treatment	2
Abscess of the breast	1
Further treatment refused	1

Table 4. Clinical response to the programs with ACM

	Group I: untreated patients		Group II: refractory or relapsed patients	
	(*n*)	(%)	(*n*)	(%)
Total	9		17	
Complete remission	5	55	4	23.5
Partial remission	–		3	18

Complete remission rate in both groups of patients, 34.6%.

Three refractory patients with PR obtained after ACM plus Ara-C and Tg program relapsed after 2–4 months of PR and then died in spite of reinduction therapy with a combination of different cytostatics.

With respect to side effects of ACM, gastrointestinal symptoms such as anorexia, nausea, and vomiting were most frequently seen in 50%–70% of the patients and could be successfully suppressed by antiemetics. Stomatitis and diarrhea occurred in four and three patients, respectively. Reversible ECG abnormalities (cardiac ventricular arrhythmia) were observed in two cases, but only in one case was discontinuation of therapy necessary.

At the dose level of cytostatics in ACM plus Ara-C or plus Tg programs all patients developed, after treatment, marked granulocytopenia (i.e., wbc count of $500/mm^3$) and thrombocytopenia (median nadir of $12\,000/mm^3$ on the fifth day after the end of the treatment). Marrow aplasia or reversible hypoplasia was observed in all treated patients and lasted from 15 days to 3 months. Beside two early deaths during the therapy and one other 1 month after the end of the treatment, recovery from hypo- or aplasia of the bone marrow was achieved in the rest of the patients.

Discussion

The results of this study indicate that ACM in combination with Ara-C or/and with Tg produced CR in 55% of untreated and in 23.5% of previously treated refractory ANLL patients. The CR rates are comparable to rates reported by other authors [5,7,9,14]. Yamada et al. [15] reported CR rates of 35% in 20 previously untreated and 18% in 33 previously treated patients with ANLL. The schedule of ACM used as a single drug in their trial consisted of daily administration of $15\,mg/m^2$ until toxicity developed. Most CRs were attained by patients who received a total dose of more than $200\,mg/m^2$ of ACM. However, our results indicate that short treatment cycles (5 or 7 days only) with moderate daily dose ($18–25\,mg/m^2$) and the total amount of ACM per course not exceeding $200\,mg$ led to CR or PR and also in this way avoided severe drug-induced toxicity.

In a paper presented recently, Hansen et al. [5] obtained even more encouraging results. In a series of 86 patients with untreated ANLL, CR after ACM and Ara-C was achieved in 71% of patients. ACM in their program was given in a dosage of $75\,mg/m^2$ per day for 3 days together with 7 days of Ara-C in a dosage of $100\,mg/m^2$ per day. Of patients on Ara-C and ACM in this trial, 75% obtained CR after one course of this program.

It appears that a cumulative dose of $250-500\,mg/m^2$ ACM is necessary for patients to achieve CR. This closely agrees with the results found by other investigators [12,14]. Moreover, 7 out of 17 patients, who were previously resistant to intensive induction regimens comprised of ADR or daunorubicin (DNR), Ara-C and/or Tg, attained a CR or PR with ACM instead of ADR. These results support previous clinical studies which suggest that there is no cross-resistance between ADR and ACM.

The incidence and severity of the toxic effects of the administered drug were related to the dose given during each course of therapy. Myeloid hypoplasia or aplasia were severe in all patients and recovery of myelo-poiesis required 15–60 days given that all were supported by transfusion with granulocyte and thrombocyte concentrates. The incidence of other side effects during the treatment with ACM plus Ara-C and Tg program (mucositis, diarrhea, vomiting, and infection) was significantly high but similar to that observed during combination chemotherapy with doxorubicin. Cardiac toxicity was limited to extrasystolic arrhythmias in two patients, which in one person was mild and transient. CHF attributable to cytostatics used in the program has not been observed. However, a full assessement of the risk of chronic anthracycline cardiotoxicity is not possible now until accurate cardiac monitoring has been carried out in a much larger group of patients treated with a higher cumulative dose of ACM.

In conclusion, the combination of ACM plus Ara-C and/or Tg is effective in untreated as well as in some patients with relapsing or refractory ANLL and can be a salvage treatment in heavily pretreated patients. Therefore, further evaluation of ACM in this combined chemotherapy is indicated.

Conclusions

Combination of ACM with Ara-C and/or with Tg is effective in untreated (CR, 55%) as well as in some (CR, 23.5%) patients with relapsing or refractory ANLL.

References

1. Bonghton BJ, Franklin IM, Apperley J, et al. (1984) Non-cardiotoxic anthracycline regimens in the treatment of acute myeloblastic leukaemia. Br J Haemat 54: 378

2. Clarkson B, Gee T, Arlin Z, et al. (1984) Current status of treatment· of acute leukemia in adults: an overview. In: Büchner Th, Urbanitz D, van de Loo J (eds) Therapie der Akuten Leukämien. Springer Berlin, Heidelberg New York, p 1
3. Freireich EJ, Keating MJ, Gehan EA, et al. (1978) Therapy of acute myelogenous leukemia. Cancer 42:874
4. Goldberg J, Grunwald H, Vogler WR, et al. (1965) Treatment of patients with acute nonlymphocytic leukemia in relapse: a leukemia intergroup study. Am J Hematol 19:167
5. Hansen OP, Ellegaard J, Bastrup-Madsen P, et al. (1988) Aclarubicin plus cytosine arabinoside versus daunorubicin plus cytosine arabinoside in chemotherapy of de-novo acute myelocytic leukemia. A Danish national trial (abstract). XXII Congress of the International Society of Hematology, 28 Aug–2 Sept 1988, Milan, Italy, TU-6-3, p 47
6. Holowiecki J, Konopka L, Maj S, et al. (1984) Aclacinomycin, Cytosinoarabinoside, 6-Thioguanine therapy for relapsing or treatment resistant acute non-lymphocytic leukemia. Results of a multicenter phase II – trial (IGCI) (abstract). New trends in antimicrobial and anticancer chemotherapy. Prague, 15–19 April, p 65
7. Kimura K, Nagur E, Kawashima K, et al. (1988) A controlled randomized clinical trial of adult acute leukemia using Behenyol Ara-C (BH-AC) + DNR + GMP + PSL versus BH-AC + Aclacinomycin (ACR) + GMP + PSL for AML and ADR + VCR + PSL versus L-Asparaginase + ADR + VCR + PSL for ALL (abstract). XXII Congress of the International Society of Hematology, 28 Aug–2 Sept 1988, Milan, Italy, OP-TU-15-4, p 208
8. McCredie KB, Gehan EA, Freireich EJ, et al. (1983) Management of adult acute leukemia. A Southwest Oncology Group study. Cancer 52:958
9. Mitrou PS (1983) Aclacinomycin A (ACM) in the treatment of relapsing acute leukaemia. 13th International Congress of Chemotheoapy. Vienna symposium aclacinomycin A, 28 Aug–2 Sept 1983 (84, Part 211, pp 45–48)
10. Praga C, Beretta G, Vigo PL, et al. (1979) Adriamycin cardiotoxicity: a survey of 1273 patients. Cancer Treat Rep 63:827
11. Suzuki H, Kawashima K, Yamada K, et al. (1980) Phase I and preliminary phase II studies on Aclacinomycin A in patients with acute leukemia. Jpn J Clin Oncol 10:111
12. Takahashi I, Hara M, Adachi T, et al. (1980) Treatment of refractory acute leukemia with Aclacinomycin-A. Acta Med Okayama 34:349
13. Tapiero H, Fourcade A, Farhi JJ, et al.: Structure activity relationship of Aclacinomycin-A and its metabolites on sensitive and Adriamycin resistant friend leukemic cells. 13th International Congress of Chemotheoapy. Vienna symposium Aclacinomycin A. 28 Aug–2 Sept 1983 (84, Part 21, pp 9–14)
14. Warrel RP Jr, Arlin ZA, Kempin SJ, Young CW (1982) Phase I–II evaluation of a new anthracycline antibiotic, Aclacinomycin A in adults with refractory leukaemia. Cancer Treat Rep 66:1619–1623
15. Yamada K, Nakamura T, Tsuruo T, et al. (1983) Phase II–III study of Aclacinomycin A in acute leukemia in adults. In: Proceeding of the 13th International Congress of Chemotheoapy. Vienna symposium Aclacinomycin A. 28 Aug–2 Sept 1983 (84, Part 211, pp 49–53)

Therapy of Blastic Transformation of Chronic Myeloid Leukemia

S. Pawelski,[1] L. Konopka, K. Szczepanik, and H. Zdziechowska

Since 1865 the basic treatment of chronic myeloid leukemia (CML) has been chemotherapy: arsenic, urethan, busulphan and other alkylating agents, hydroxyurea and only recently, radiotherapy of the spleen or use of radioactive $[^{32}P]$ phosphate. The most frequent and optimal was treatment with busulphan, causing remission of CML, but only in rare cases could partial elimination of clonal Ph^1+ cells be observed. However statistical data indicate that these kinds of monotherapy do not prolong the median survival of patients with CML, which has remained 3–4 years [2,14,21,22]. Beginning in the second year of illness the death rate averages 20%–30% per year [7], caused by disease acceleration and blastic (myeloblastic or less frequently lymphoblastic) transformation (BT). Acceleration of CML is marked by: increase of leucocyte number, excess of blasts (or blasts and promyelocytes) in peripheral blood and bone marrow (5%–10%), thrombocytopenia, progressive splenomegaly, extramedullary leukemic involvement (CNS, lymph nodes, testicles, lungs, bones, etc.), fever, bone pains, cytogenetic abnormalities apart from Ph^1 chromosome, and increase of granulocyte alkaline phosphatase activity. BT demonstrates the same symptoms as above and an increase of peripheral and bone marrow blasts over 30%. (Lymphoblastic forms are characterized by increase of PAS reaction and terminal deoxynucleotidyltransferase (TdT) activity of the cells.) Myeloblastic transformation is more refractory to treatment and leads to death after several months (in 2–3 or 3–5 months). Therefore in recent years many efforts have been undertaken to delay BT such as intensive chemotherapy, splenectomy, interferon treatment, and bone marrow transplantation.

Unfortunately intensive cytostatic treatment consisting of araC and thioguanine and/or doxorubicin; cyclophosphamide, 6-mercaptopurine and hydroxyurea (HU); or intermittent use of different cytostatics in an attempt to eliminate Ph^1+ myeloid population did not influence the duration of the chronic phase of CML nor survival of the patients [7,8]. Similar negative results were observed after splenectomy removing the main site of BT, or spleen irradiation, splenectomy and chemotherapy [13], though after such

[1] Institute of Haematology, P-00-957 Warsaw, Chocinska 5, Poland

Fleischer (Ed.) Leukemias
© Springer-Verlag Berlin Heidelberg 1993

treatment 12 of 37 patients of Cunningham et al. revealed reduction of Ph[1]+ cells and lived longer than the remaining patients [3].

Natural or recombinant interferons (IFN), IFN-α, IFN-β and IFN-γ, act like hormones and show antiproliferative activity by inhibition of the growth factor and expression regulation of certain oncogenes. They also have immunostimulant and antiviral properties. Clinical use of IFN-α was estimated at first as very effective in hairy-cell leukaemia and in recent years also in CML and essential thrombocythaemia. Antileukemic effect of recombinant IFN-γ was confirmed by in vitro studies in which IFN-γ added to Ph[1]+ stem cell culture caused their growth inhibition and increase of Ph[1]− metaphases, which is important for reconstitution of normal hemopoiesis [19]. The present reports [2,5,6,10,17,18,19] on the treatment of about 200 patients in the chronic phase of CML by IFN-α state that in 70%–80% of them there is a positive haematological response and in 60%– 70% complete remission (CR). Outside of full haematological normalization of leucocytes and their precursors in the bone marrow, concentrations of serum lactic dehydrogenase and vitamin B_{12} also returned to normal values, as did spleen size. And what is most important, in about 50% of patients with CR the percentage of Ph[1]+ cells decreased below 35% with the tendency toward complete eradication of these pathological cells during long-term maintenance therapy [12,16]. According to Talpaz et al. [18], who have the most experience in this field, 94% of complete responders maintained on IFN-α and only 45% of patients not treated with this drug attained the 3-year survival expected. The immediate future will show if this kind of natural treatment with relatively mild toxicity is curative at least for some group of these patients. There are also trials going on to test whether combinations of different IFNs and/or cytostatics could be more helpful in prolonging the chronic phase of those CML patients refractory to treatment with single IFN.

But most promising are the results obtained in patients with CML after syngeneic, twin bone marrow transplantations (BMT) begun by Fefer et al. [4] and followed by allogenic BMT, performed now in more than 2000 cases. Very incouraging and effective are the results of the Seattle Group [18] and European Group of BMT (Table 1) [9]. Better prognostic factors are found in patients under 30 years of age, in the early phase of the disease (before acceleration), and without the severe form of graft-versus-host disease [9]. Of 198 transplant patients in the chronic phase of CML, 71 are alive without Ph[1]+ cells 1–9 years after BMT [20]. The results suggest that most patients benefit from BMT and some of them may be cured. It is a notable landmark in the history of this disease. But in spite of this fascinating progress only relatively few patients with CML could be treated by BMT (no suitable donor, over 40 years of age etc.) or by interferon (great costs, limited availability). Most of the patients are treated long term with busulphan or hydroxyurea and undergo acceleration and then BT. The lymphoblastic forms of BT, accounting for about 20% of patients, respond a little better

Table 1. Results of BMT in 454 patients in the chronic phase (CP) and 152 patients in the acceleration phase (AP) of CML (European Group of BMT)

	Up to 1 year (%)		After 2–5 years (%)	
	CP	AP	CP	Ap
Leukemia-free survival	60	40	50	30
Transplant-related mortality	30	40	35–45	48–60
Relapse incidence	12	30	22	50

Table 2. HAR program for BT of CML

Day 1	Days 2–5	Day 5
Hydroxyurea 5.5 g/m^2 in continuous intravenous infusion: 40% of the dose during 1 h in 500 ml of 0.9% NaCl solution and the rest during 12 h in 1500 ml of 0.9% NaCl		
AraC 60 mg/m^2 during next 12 h in continuous infusion	AraC 60 mg/m^2 twice daily in 12-h infusions	Rubidomycin 50 mg/m^2 intravenously

than myeloblastic forms to cytotoxic drugs effective in acute lymphoblastic leukemia. But duration of CR is only a little longer. In myeloblastic transformation such schemes as COAP, ROP, and HMP did not increase the frequency of CR. Also the very intensive TRAMPCO(L) program consisting of seven cytostatics used by Spiers et al. [15] and in our department [16] did not improve remission rate and its duration and caused many serious adverse toxic effects. Therefore every new trial is worthy of consideration. Recently, Koller and Miller [11] published very good results after treatment with intravenous mithramycin (plicamycin) and oral hydroxyurea: six out of nine patients with BT achieved CR and returned to a chronic phase lasting longer (5–19 months) than after other programs. These results were not confirmed by other authors.

Basing our work on Belt et al.'s [1] treatment of cancer patients with continuous infusion of HU, which is specific for the S phase of the cell cycle, we introduced in 29 patients with BT of CML an original program of hydroxyurea and ara-C (HAR; Table 2). The patients' ages ranged from 27 to 59. All had a well-defined preceding period of chronic phase CML (ranging from 12 months to 5 years), for which they had received busulfan (20 patients) or hydroxyurea (4) or both (5). No other prior HAR chemotherapy regimens had been used to treat the blast phase of the disease (Table 3). The blastic phase was defined as involving the presence of at least 20% blasts and promyelocytes in the bone marrow and peripheral blood. The myeloid nature of blast cells was confirmed by morphology and cyto-

Table 3. Patients' characteristics before treatment with HAR program

Length of chronic phase of CML-BT (months)	M:F	Age of patients (years)	WBC ($\times 10^3$)	Blasts (peripheral blood) (%)	LDH at BT (U/l)
≤12	2:3	35–57	35–78	20–60	109–715
13–36	5:3	27–48	49–167	20–80	310–1365
37–60	8:4	31–59	77–117	35–70	307–1172
>60 (5 years)	3:1	42–50	37–167	40–78	170–1058

M, male; F, female; LDH, lactate dehydrogenase.

chemistry (peroxidase, Sudan black). Terminal deoxynucleotidyltransferase (TdT) activity was measured only in three cases and it was negative. The mean number of HAR cycles ranged in 18 patients from 2 to 3, in 3 patients 4 or 5 cycles were given, and only in 8 patients was just 1 course of the HAR program introduced. In five patients treatment had to be discontinued after the first cycle of chemotherapy because of serious haematological complications (granulocytopenia or thrombocytopenia followed by haemorrhage into CNS or from gastrointestinal tract). Positive response after treatment was evaluated as a return to the second chronic phase. Reduction in the percentage of blasts but no return to the chronic phase was defined as a partial response.

Results

Out of all 29 patients treated, 5 patients (17.2%) responded during 3–4 weeks of HAR program (Table 4). The patients became asymptomatic with decrease of spleen size. The second chronic phase was then maintained with

Table 4. Response of patients to HAR treatment

Number of HAR cycles	Results		
	Return to chronic phase	PR	NR
1	1	1	6
2–3	4	4	10
4–5	–	2	1
Total	5	7	17
(% of patients)	(17.2)	(24.0)	(58.6)

PR, partial response: short term stabilization of disease and no return to chronic phase; NR, no response to treatment with progression of BT.

oral hydroxyurea, busulfan or 6-mercaptopurine. In one (P.A.; see Table 5) of these five responders in 5th month of duration of the second chronic phase, splenectomy and 1 month later successful allogeneic bone marrow transplantation were performed. Unfortunately, 4 months later this patient relapsed with extensive lymph node and skin infiltrations and with an increase of blasts to 58% in the bone marrow. The patient died within 4 weeks after relapse. The survival of the other four responders ranged between 5 and 12 months. Only one patients is still alive with the continous chronic phase of CML lasting 12 months (Table 5). Six of seven patients with partial response were maintained for 2–4 months with 6-mercaptopurine or hydroxyurea but the disease progressed as it did in the last patient from this group, who was treated afterwards with recombinant human IFN-α (Intron).

The toxic effects observed during HAR treatment are listed in Table 6 in order of frequency. Leukopenia and thrombocytopenia were recognized in all the patients, 16 of whom were subject to septic and haemorrhagic complications. Gastrointestinal side effects such as nausea, vomiting and anorexia were very frequently seen but they never caused stopping the

Table 5. Second chronic phase after HAR program

Initials (age/sex)	Duration (months)			Survival from the beginning of the disease (months)
	Chronic phase I	BT	Chronic phase II	
K.J. (42/M)	12	3	9[a]	39
S.D. (54/M)	48	2	5	56
P.A. (39/M)	18 years	4	10	19.5 years
K.E. (41/F)	61	3	6	70
G.Z. (38/M)	42	2	12	57

[a] In this patient in the fifth month after HAR treatment, allogeneic bone marrow transplantation was performed.

Table 6. Adverse reactions to HAR program

Complication	Patients	
	n	(%)
Leukopenia[a]	29	(100)
Thrombocytopenia[b]	29	(100)
Mucositis	16	(55.2)
Severe infections	16	(55.2)
Hepatotoxicity (up to three times the	8	(27.5)
upper normal level of enzymes)	2	(6.8)
Kidney failure		

[a] $<1.0/\mu l$ and granulocytopenia $<500/\mu l$.
[b] $<50\,000/\mu l$.

treatment. Serious mucositis (present in 55.2% of patients) occurred only in patients who received three or more cycles of HAR program. Transient elevation of serum glutamine-oxaloacetic transaminase (108–240 U/l) and glutaminic pyruvic transaminase (120–180 U/l) was noted in eight patients. All these toxic signs were controlled by symptomatic treatment and did not require cessation of HAR program.

Discussion

There is no effective therapy for patients in blast transformation of CML. Different kinds of intensive chemotherapy employed for acute myeloblastic leukemia (AML) as well as aggressive polychemotherapy (TRAMPCOL regimen) or alternate-day plicamycin and daily hydroxyurea did not change the fate of the patients. Only the minority of patients with TdT and PAS positive lymphoblasts respond transiently to regimens containing vincristine and prednisone, but remissions are short and usually incomplete. The combination of hydroxyurea, cytosine arabinoside and daunorubicin proposed by us seemed to exert synergistic effects probably by blast differentiation and cytotoxic influence. Unfortunately, in our series of patients treated with HAR regimen, only in five cases was return to the second chronic phase of CML and in another seven persons short-lasting stabilization of CML-BT observed. Toxicity of this treatment is rather serious. Our results obtained in the treatment of BT are similar to the observations of other authors [7,8,11,15,16].

The resistance to different intensive cytostatic treatments is possibly caused by low sensitivity of blasts to cytostatics and by the lack of hemopoietic progenitor cells in the bone marrow of these patients. Real progress would be obtained by prolongation of the chronic phase of CML by performing allogeneic bone marrow transplantation in selected cases or employing interferon treatment in others.

Conclusions

1. Presently, there is no effective treatment of CML-BT.
2. The theoretically promising HAR program also failed, causing serious adverse effects.
3. The only present treatment of CML is to delay BT (or cure CML?) by allogenic bone marrow transplantation or by long-term use of interferons.
4. Final evaluation of these modern methods requires several years of observation of the treated patients.

References

1. Belt RJ, Hass CD, Kennedy J, Taylor S (1980) Studies on hydroxyurea administered by continuous infusion. Cancer 46:455
2. Bergsagel DE, Haas RH, Messner HA (1986) Interferon alpha-2b in the treatment of chronic granulocytic leukemia. Semin Oncol 13:29
3. Cunningham I, Gee T, Dowling M, et al. (1979) Results of treatment of PH[1]+ chronic myelogenous leukemia with an intensive treatment regimen (L-5 Protocol). Blood 53:375
4. Fefer A, Cheerer MA, Greenberg PD, et al. (1982) Treatment of chronic granulocytic leukemia with chemotherapy and transplantation of marrow from identical twins. N Engl J Med 306:63
5. Friche E, Hansen MM, Wieslander S (1988) Refractoriness to alpha-interferon (Intron A) in previously chemotherapy treated patients with chronic myelocytic leukemia. Eur J Haematol 40:305
6. Gastl G, Aulitzky Q, Tilg H, et al. (1987) Dose related effectiveness of alpha interferon in chronic myelogenous leukemia. Blut 54:251
7. Goldman JM (1978) Modern approaches to the management of chronic granulocytic leukemia. Semin Hematol 15:420
8. Goldman JM, Lu Dao-Pei (1982) New approaches in chronic granulocytic leukemia–origin, prognosis and treatment. Semin Hematol 19:241
9. Gratwohl A, Hermans J, Barrett AJ, et al. (European Group for Bone Marrow Transplantation) (1988) Allogeneic bone marrow transplantation for leukemia in Europe. Lancet I:1379
10. Hehlmann R, Anger B, Messerer D, et al. (1988) Randomized study on the treatment of chronic myeloid leukemia (CML) in chronic phase with busulfan versus hydroxyurea versus interferon alpha. Blut 56:87
11. Koller CA, Miller DM (1986) Preliminary observations on the therapy of the myeloid blast phase of chronic granulocytic leukemia with plicamycin and hydroxyurea. N Engl J Med 215:1433
12. Kloke O, Becher R, Niederle N (1987) Response to the combined administration of interferons alpha and gamma after failure of single interferon therapy in chronic myelogenous leukemia. Blut 55:453
13. Medical research council's working party for Therapeutic Trials in Leukemia (1983) Randomized trial of splenectomy in Ph positive chronic granulocytic leukemia, including an analysis of prognostic features. Br J Haematol 54:415
14. Pawelski S, Leszko B, Sobczyńska-Czechowska Z, Wolosewicz-Zdziechowska H (1961) Wyniki leczenia 210 przypadków różnych postaci bialaczek. Pol Tyg Lek 16:1279
15. Spiers ADS, Coslello C, Catousky D, et al. (1974) Chronic granulocytic leukemia: multiple drug chemo-therapy for acute transformation. Br Med J 3:77
16. Sylwestrowicz T, Pawelski S, Maj S, Żywicka-Lopaciuk H, Zdziechowska H, Sobczyńska Z. Apel D (1980) Wyniki leczenia zaostrzenia przewleklej bialaczki szpikowej wedlug programu TRAMPCO. Pol Tyg Lek 35:1062
17. Talpaz M, McCredie KB, Kantarjian HP, et al. (1986) Chronic myelogenous leukemia: haematological remissions with alpha interferon. Brit J Haematol 64:87
18. Talpaz M, Kantarjian HP, McCredie KB, et al. (1987) Clinical investigation of human alpha interferon in chronic myelogenous leukemia. Blood 69:1280
19. Talpaz M (1988) Interferons in CML. Book of abstracts of the XXII congress of the intern soc of haematology, Milan
20. Thomas ED, Clift RA, Fefer A, et al. (1986) Marrow transplantation for the treatment of chronic myelogenous leukemia. Ann Int Med 104:155
21. Williams WJ, Beutler E, Erslev AJ, et al. (1977) Haematology. Mc Graw-Hill, New York
22. Wintrobe MM, Lee GR, Boggs DR, Bithell TC, Athens JW, Foerster J (eds.) (1984) Clinical Haematology. Lea Febiger, Philadelphia

Chronic Myeloproliferative Diseases and Chronic Lymphatic Leukemia

Hanover Classification of Chronic Myeloproliferative Diseases by Histopathology of the Bone Marrow

A. Georgii,[1] K.F. Vykoupil, T. Buhr, M. Dominis, U. Döhler, and S. Delventhal

Introduction

Whereas acute leukemias may be reliably classified according to hematological criteria, supported by the application of immunophenotyping, a systematic classification of chronic myeloproliferative disorders (CMPD) can be based only on histopathology from biopsies of the bone marrow. In the current classification of the WHO and textbooks [24], chronic myelocytic leukemia (CML), polycythemia (PV), and primary thrombocythemia (PTH) are the main groups of the CMPDs, besides agnogenic myeloid metaplasia. The aim of this article is to explain a system for classifying the CMPDs according to histopathology of bone marrow biopsies showing correlations between histopathological features and the hematologic appearance of the various groups. The introduction of two further groups seems necessary to provide more profound understanding of the conspicuous hematological finding of increased platelet counts [20,23]. The first is CML with an increase of megakaryocytes (CML.MI), the other is chronic megakaryocytic-granulocytic myelosis (CMGM) [10]; these are meant to substitute for the terms "agnogenic myeloid metaplasia" [24] and "idiopathic myelofibrosis" [4], respectively. Moreover, in addition to this introduction of two new main groups, the natural course of development within the progress of the different entities should be regarded, characterized by fiber increase or increasing blastic excess phenomena which are not always clearly expressed by overt hematological or clinical criteria [3,15,29].

Material and Methods

From 20 000 bone marrow biopsies sampled in the years from 1985 to 1988, 1500 diagnoses of CMPD have been reclassified and evaluated. The classification was pragmatically established during this period. A panel of four of the authors have reclassified 500 of the 1500. All biopsies had been

[1] Pathologisches Institut, Medizinische Hochschule Hannover, Konstanty-Gutschow-Straße 8, 3000 Hannover 61, FRG

Fleischer (Ed.) Leukemias
© Springer-Verlag Berlin Heidelberg 1993

embedded without decalcification in a mixture of methyl-methacrylate after fixation in Schaffer's solution. Sections of 2–3 µm thickness were cut on Reichert's Ultracut, and five stains were applied routinely: Giemsa–gallamin blue, Goldner's trichrome, Gomori's silver methylpyronine, and Prussian blue. Immun-histochemistry was used only to characterize megakaryocytes and myeloid cells on smear preparations, not on sections [18]. Hematological findings and clinical courses were extracted from the patient registers of the Hematology Department of Hanover Medical School as well as from affiliated hospitals and registered within the Statistical Package for Social Sciences (SPSS) system for statistical analysis.

Entities Classified

Chronic Myeloid Leukemia (CML)

CML has to be divided into two groups, which are distinguished by the number of megakaryocytes found within the bone marrow (Table 1). The common type (CML.CT) can be distinguished from the type with

Table 1. Hanover Classification of chronic myeloproliferative disorders by histopathology of bone marrow biopsies

	Acronyms		N	%
Primary Stages				
Chronic Myelocytic Leukemia	CML (CGL)		661	38.7
1.1. Common Type	CML.CT	365		
1.2. Megakaryocytic Increase	CML.MI	176		
1.3. Megakaryocytic Predominance	CML.MP	38		
1.4. Overlapping Type	CML.OT	82		
Polycythemia rubra vera	PV		359	21.0
Megakaryocytic Myelosis (MM) consistent with Primary Thrombocythemia (PTH)	MM or PTH		306	17.9
Chronic Megakaryocytic Granulocytic Myelosis			383	22.4
Total			1,709	100
Advanced Stages				
Early myelosclerosis with recognizable basic disorder	.EMS		128	
Myelosclerosis – Myelofibrosis with or without recognizable primary stage	.MF/MS		90	
Advanced MF with bone sclerosis – with or without recognizable primary stage	.AMF		90	
3.1. Hypercellular				
3.2. Atrophic				
Excess of blasts within primary or advanced stages	.EB		1	
Other Disorders				
CMPD not classifiable without further data	.CMPD.UC		163	

megakaryocytic increase (CML.MI) and possibly even with megakaryocytic predominance (CML.MP). CML.MI as well as CML.MP shows a significant increase of platelets in peripheral blood and a tendency to progress by transformation into myelosclerosis by early fiber increase (CML.MI.EMS) [3,4]. However, only slight differences were found concerning life expectancy, and they have been statistically insignificant until now [2]. Both types are positive for Philadelphia (Ph[1]) chromosome. Pseudo-Gaucher cells or sea-blue histiocytes occur equally frequently in both groups. In CML patients, pseudo-Gaucher cells were found in 40% of biopsies before and in 72.6% of biopsies after busulfan or hydroxyurea treatment [7]. Patients with these histocytes could be shown to have significantly better survival [7,25].

Primary Thrombocythemia (PTH)

This clinical entity is characterized histologically by a pure megakaryocytic proliferation, by enlarged cells with only slight pleomorphy, and by cluster-like localization in the middle of the marrow spaces. PTH could therefore be termed "pure-line megakaryocytic myelosis." The disease ist practically always Ph[1] negative. In very few cases, early or fully developed myelo-scleroses may be observed, whereas advanced types of myelofibrosis with bone increase probably do not occur.

Polycythemia Vera (PV)

The characteristic feature is a proliferation of all three lineages of hemopoiesis, among which the megakaryocytes are especially enlarged, but of only little pleomorphy, and the hyperplasia of erythropoiesis is rather conspicuous. The sinus system is hyperplastic; it is enlarged and dilated. Myelosclerosis ist seldom observed and occurs very late, and acute leukemias (blast crises) are rare.

Chronic Megakaryocytic-Granulocytic Myelosis (CMGM)

Proliferation of both megakaryocytes and granulocytes, without consider-able total increase of hematopoieses, is characteristic [10]. Pleomorphy of the enlarged megakaryocytes, being most pronounced among the CMPDs, is a hallmark of this disease. Of the CMGMs, 30% are found to be without increase of fibers on primary diagnosis and may remain so for years in the subsequent course of the disease. Nevertheless, the tendency to fiber in-crease is the strongest among the various groups of CMPDs. Hematological findings are merely of slight leukocytosis with an increase of early stages of maturity of the lineage, and sometimes of thrombocythemic platelet counts, whereas no significant increase of the median diameter of platelets is observed. Life expectancy is significantly better than in CML patients, but worse than in PTH or PV. Similar to PTH and PV, CMGM is cytogenetically always Ph^1 negative.

Myelosclerosis (MS) and Myelofibrosis (MF)

A distinction should be made between pure reticulin fiber sclerosis (EMS) and collagenous fibrosis (MS/MF), a distinction that can be reliably based on simple staining and polarization-optical criteria. According to these criteria, fiber increase in the bone marrow can be subdivided into four groups (Table 2), which are defined according to density and breadth of the fibers, replacement of hematopoietic tissue, and sclerosis of the bone. In many cases, especially in CML or CMGM patients, the basic disease can still be reliably indentified even in fully developed myelofibrosis, and always in early myelofibrosis (EMS). Therefore, the diagnosis may take recourse to designations connecting the type of basic disorder with the degree of myelosclerosis. The term "advanced myelosclerosis" (AMF) designates cases in which broad bundles of collagenous fibers occupy large parts of the bone marrow spaces so that hematopoiesis appears to have been replaced or be atrophic. Additionally, in a certain number of cases, endophytic bone sclerosis will ensue in later stages of disease.

The natural progress of CML into its accelerated and, finally, blastic phases may sometimes be difficult to recognize from clinical and hematological symptoms. The morphological increase of blasts should therefore be carefully observed, which is certainly a task that histopathology from bone marrow biopsies is dedicated to. The acceleration from chronic phase to blast crisis in CML is taken account of by adding the suffix "excess of blasts" (CML.EB), or "blast crisis" (CML.BC) to the acronym of the basic disease. The same acronyms may designate the progress of the disease in CMGM, PV, and even PTH, if it is actually found to occur in these diseases.

Table 2. Grading or staging of myelosclerosis and myelofibrosis within the Hanover classification of CMPD

Grading:	I	II	III
Acronym:	EMS	MS/MF	AMF
Fiber quality	Reticulin	Reticulin plus collagen	Collagen
Fiber distribution	Focal, patchy	Diffuse; network with patches of collagen	Diffuse
Sinus walls	No	Sclerosed and dilated	Fibrosed and extended
Bone sclerosis	No	Rare	By definition
Hematopoiesis	Unchanged	Mostly unchanged	Mostly reduced

Discussion

CMPD may be explained as a neoplastic transformation of hemopoietic stem cells, which is based upon two phenomena: First, the loss of an isoenzyme of G-6-PD in heterozygote female patients is observed in hemopoietic cells only, whereas fibroblasts still carry both isoenzymes [9]. This phenomenon was also shown in CML [8], PV [1] and myeloid metaplasia [12]. Secondly, in CML patients, the Ph^1 translocation [18,22] is also restricted to hemopoietic cells, whereas fibroblasts are unchanged [17].

In contrast to expanding knowledge in cellular and molecular biology, the understanding of the morphological basis of these disorders has been rather modest as yet, although characteristic morphological changes, e.g., of megakaryopoiesis [27], can easily be demonstrated. In addition, such morphological changes are related to characteristic cytogenetic findings [29]. There are several reports dedicated to the individual disease entities, especially to CML and PTH [25,26], but only two laboratories are approaching a systematic classification of this complex of various entities [5,11,12,13,14].

The proposed term, CMGM, seems to be more helpful than "primary" or "idiopathic myelofibrosis," even when the latter are described as the hyperplastic stage, since there is no increase of any kind of fibers in 50% of the patients with these myeloproliferative disorders. Neither does the term "agnogenic myeloid metaplasia" really cover the nature of the disorder designated, since there is no myeloid metaplasia, e.g., extramedullary hematopoiesis, of liver, spleen, and other organs, provided early stages are analyzed.

Acknowledgements. The authors express their thanks to Professor Dr. Hubert Poliwoda, Department of Hematology and Oncology, Medizinische Hochschule Hannover, and Professor Dr. K. Mainzer, Chief, Department of Hematology and Oncology, Allgemeines Krankenhaus Hamburg-Altona, for their stimulating support and cooperation over many years. The authors are moreover obliged to Harald Choritz, Chief, Section of Documentation, in our Department, for his continuous care for our project. The support of our English assistant, Mrs. Renate Schmidt, is highly appreciated.

References

1. Adamson JW, Fialkow PJ, Murphy S, Prchal JF, Steinmann L (1976) Polycythemia vera: stem-cell probable clonal origin of the disease. N Engl J Med 295:913–916
2. Buhr T, Delventhal S, Freund M, Vykoupil KF, Georgii A (1987) Chronische myeloische Leukämien mit hohem Gehalt an Megakaryocyten – eine eigene Gruppe innerhalb der myeloproliferativen Erkrankungen. Verh Dtsch Ges Pathol 71:480

3. Buhr T, Choritz H, Georgii A (1992) The impact of megakaryocyte proliferation for the evolution of myelofibrosis. Histological follow-up study in 186 patients with chronic myeloid leukemia. Virchows Archiv A 420:473–478
4. Buhr T, Georgii A, Choritz H (1992) Myelofibrosis in chronic myeloproliferative disorders: incidence among subtypes according to the Hannover classification. Path Res Pract 1347 (in press)
5. Burkhardt R, Bartl R, Jäger K, Frisch B, Kettner G, Mahl G, Sund M (1984) Chronic myeloproliferative disorders (CMPD). Pathol Res Pract 179:131–186
6. Buyssens N, Bourgeois NH (1977) Chronic myelocytic leukemia versus idiopathic myelofibrosis. A diagnostic problem in bone marrow biopsies. Cancer 40:1548–1561
7. Delventhal S, Buhr T, Georgii A (1987) Gaucher-like cells are characteristic only for CML and not for other CMPDs. Blut 55:392
8. Fialkow PJ, Jacobson RJ, Papayannopoulou T (1977) Chronic myelocytic leukemia: clonal origin in a stem cell common to the granulocyte, erythrocyte, platelet and monocyte/macrophage. Am J Med 63:125–130
9. Fialkow PJ, Denman AM, Singer J, Jacobson RJ, Lowenthal MN (1978) Human myeloproliferative disorders: clonal origin in pluripotent stem cells. Cold Spring Harbor Conf Cell Proliferation 5:131
10. Georgii A, Vykoupil KF, Thiele J (1980) Chronic megakaryocytic granulocytic myelosis – CMGM. A subtype of chronic myeloid leukemia. Virchows Arch (Pathol Anat) 389:253–268
11. Georgii A, Vykoupil KF, Thiele J (1984) Classification of chronic myeloproliferative disease by bone marrow biopsies. Hematological and cytogenetic findings and clinical course. In: Frisch B, Bartl R (eds) Bone marrow biopsies updated, new prospects for clinical diagnostics. Karger, Basel, pp 41–56 (Bibliotheca haematologica, vol 50)
12. Georgii A, Vykoupil KF, Thiele J (1984) Histopathology of bone marrow and clinical findings in chronic myeloproliferative disorders. In: Lennert K, Hübner K (eds) Pathology of the bone marrow. Fischer, Stuttgart, pp 147–169
13. Georgii A, Vykoupil KF, Buhr T, et al. (1990) Chronic myeloproliferative disorders in bone marrow biopsies. Path Res Pract 186:3–27
14. Georgii A, Thiele J, Hehlmann R, Buhr T (1992) Histopathology of chronic myelogenous leukemia: Results from diagnostic bone marrow biopsies patients from the German CML-Trial. -in preparation-
15. Goldman JM and Lu DP (1982) New approaches in chronic granulocytic leukaemia: origin, prognosis and treatment. Semin Hematol 19:241–256
16. Jacobson RJ, Salo A, Fialkow PJ (1987) Agnogenic myeloid metaplasia: a clonal proliferation of hematopoietic stem cells with secondary myelofibrosis. Blood 51: 189–193
17. Kaloutsi V, Fritsch RS, Buhr T, Restrepo-Specht I, Widjaja W, Georgii A (1991) Megakaryocytes in chronic myeloproliferative disorders. I. Numerical density correlated between different entities. Virchows Archiv A 418:493–497
18. Kemnitz J, Helmke M, Freund M, Buhr T, Dominis M, Choritz H (1987) Heterogeneity of the phenotype of leukemic cells. Tumor Diagn Ther 8:237–245
19. Maniatis AK, Amsel S, Mitus WJ, Coleman N (1969) Chromosome pattern of bone marrow fibroblasts in patients with chronic granulocytic leukaemia. Nature 22:1278
20. Murphy S, Davis JL, Walsh PN, Gardner FH (1978) Template bleeding time and clinical hemorrhage in myeloproliferative disease. Arch Intern Med 138:1251–1253
21. Nafe R, Georgii A, Kaloutsi V, Fritsch RS, Choritz H (1991) Planimetric analysis of megakaryocytes and the four main groups of chronic myeloproliferative disorders. Virchows Archiv B (in press)
22. Rowley JD (1984) Biological implication of constistent chromosome rearrangement in leukemia and lymphoma. Cancer Res 44:3159–3168
23. Schafer A (1984) Bleeding and thrombosis in the myeloproliferative disorders. Blood 64:1–12
24. Silverstein MN (1983) Agnogenic myeloid metaplasia. In: Wiliams WJ, Beutler E, Erslev AJ, Lichtman MA (eds) Hematology, 3rd edn. McGraw-Hill, New York, pp 214–218

25. Thiele J, Fohlmeister I, Vonneguth B, Zankovich R, Fischer R (1986) The prognostic implication of clinical and histological features in Ph^{1+} chronic myelocytic leukaemia (CML). Anticancer Res 8:1401–1410
26. Thiele J, Moedder B, Kremer B, Zankovich R, Fischer R (1987) Chronic myeloproliferative disease with an elevated platelet count (in excess of $1\,000\,000/\mu m$): a clinicopathological study on 46 patients with special emphasis on primary (essential) thrombocythemia. Hematol Pathol 1(4):227–237
27. Thiele J, Fischer R (1991) Megakaryocytopoiesis in haematological disorders: diagnostic features of bone marrow biopsies. Virchows Archiv A (Pathol Anat) 418:87–97
28. Tura S, Baccaroni M, Corbelli G, The Italian Cooperative Study Group on Chronic Myeloid Leukaemia (1981) Staging of chronic myeloid leukaemia. Br J Haematol 47:105–119
29. Werner M, Kaloutsi V, Buhr T, Delventhal S, Vykoupil KF, Georgii A (1991) Cytogenetics of chronic myelogenous leukemia (CML) correlated to the histopathology of bone marrow biopsies. Anal Haematol (in press)

Chronic Myeloproliferative Syndromes: Initial Findings, Evolution, and Prognosis in 489 Patients

H. HEIMPEL,[1] U. HAUG, R. SEIDLER, and B. ANGER

Introduction

Chronic myeloproliferative syndromes (c-MPS) comprise a group of clonal diseases of hematopoietic stem cells. Conventionally, they are subclassified into polycythemia vera (PV), chronic myeloid leukemia (CML), essential thrombocythemia (ET), and idiopathic myelofibrosisis (IMF). This contribution reports data collected over a 20-year period in one institution and then retrospectively analyzed. Both diagnostic procedures and treatment modalities had been prospectively defined as standard routines.

Patients and Methods

Files from all patients coded as having CML, PV, IMF, ET or c-MPS were analyzed. These included all patients who were seen for the first time between 1967 and 1986 and in whom sufficient follow-up data were available. The patiens were classified according to their ultimate diagnosis, derived from all data obtained during follow-up and using definitions as shown in Table 1.

Guidelines for diagnostic and therapeutic procedures had been established in 1968. They remained valid throughout the period of recruitment of data as indicated above, except for allogeneic bone marrow transplantation for CML, which was introduced in 1980, and for replacement of busulphan by hydroxyurea in half of the patients with CML and in the other subtypes if cytostatic therapy was indicated.

Spleen size was estimated clinically and expressed in centimeters below the left costal margin. Laboratory investigations always included a complete blood count with differential, centrifuge hematocrit for patients with erythrocytosis, alkaline leukocyte phosphatase (ALP), lactate dehydrogenase (LDH), and bone marrow aspiration and/or iliac crest biopsy. Patients were seen in our institution at least once a year but more frequently for the

---

[1] Abteilung Innere Medizin III, Medizinische Klink und Poliklinik der Universität Ulm, Robert-Koch-Strasse 8, W-900 Ulm, FRG

Fleischer (Ed.) Leukemias
© Springer-Verlag Berlin Heidelberg 1993

Table 1. Phenotypic parameters used for classification of chronic myeloproliferative syndrome subtypes

Parameter	CML	PV	IMF	ET
Red cells (T/l)	<5.5	>6.5	<5.5	<5.5
WBC (G/l)	>30	<50	<50	<50
Platelets (G/l)	n or ↑	n or ↑	n or ↑	>600
Myelofibrosis	(+)	−	+++	+
Splenomegaly	++	+	+++	+
ALP score	↓	↑	↑	↑ or n
Ph-chromosome	+	−	−	−

CML, chronic myeloid leukemia; PV, polycythemia vera; IMF, idiopathic myelofibrosis; ET, essential thrombocythemia; n, normal; ↑, increased; ↓, decreased.

majority of patients, in particular those with CML. Bone marrow was usually obtained at 1-year intervals. Cytogenetic examinations were carried out according to standard techniques, with growth factors used for stimulation of mitogenic activity if peripheral cells were analyzed intead of bone marrow cells. (Most results were obtained by B. Heinze, Abteilung für klinsische Physiologie und Arbeitsmedizin der Universität Ulm.)

Busulphan was administered for primary cytoreductive therapy of CML up to 1983. The drug was withdrawn when leukocytes fell below 15 G/l, but was used for maintenance if the doubling time of peripheral leukocytes was less than 70 days. Since 1983 all patients were randomized for studies comparing busulfan versus hydroxyurea [12]. Patients less then 40 years old were transplanted if an HLA identical sibling donor was available [4,15].

Phlebotomy was the primary therapy for patients with PV. In general hematocrit values were kept below 45%, but maximal hematocrit values were adjusted in each patient according to his or her complaints and risk of vascular injury. Secondary treatment consisted of small doses of busulfan (usually less than 2 mg daily) or, since 1983, hydroxyurea (0.5–2.0 g). Cytostatic treatment was initiated if platelets increased to more than 1500 G/l, in patients with large spleens causing symptomes, and in a few patients who either did not tolerate or did not agree to repeated phlebotomy [2].

No primary treatment was given to asymptomatic patients with ET. Aspirin was given if platelets were continuously more than 1000 G/l or if there were symptoms of impaired microcirculation. Busulfan and, since 1983, hydroxyurea in the same doses as those used for treating PV were given to a few patients with extremely high platelet counts and/or repeated vascular accidents.

Patients with IMF received supportive therapy if necessary, including red cell substitution and androgens in a minority of patients up to 1980. A few patients were treated with low doses of busulfan or underwent splenectomy or splenic irradiation [6].

Results

Basic data are given in Table 2. Observation time was longer for ET and PV patients than for those with IMF and CML, due to the longer survival times in the former groups. The interval between initial symptoms of the particular diseases, as verified by history, and the diagnosis was found to be longer in PV patients than in patients with the other subtypes.

The most pertinent laboratory values of all patients at the time of diagnosis are shown in Figs. 1–4. At this time 43/489 (8.8%) of all patients could not definitely be assigned to one of the subtypes and were provisionally classified as having c-MPS. The WBC was significantly ($p < 0.01$) higher in CML patients than in those with any of the other subtypes, but in a few patients with the other subtypes WBCs higher than 50 G/l were found (Fig. 1). As expected, red cell counts were significantly higher in patients with PV, but again there were some patients with comparable numbers of red cells initially who were ultimately diagnosed as having one of the other subtypes (Fig. 2). An even more distinct overlap was seen for platelet counts (Fig. 3). ALP scores were below 20 in all but one patients, but subnormal scores were also found in a minority of other c-MPS patients (Fig. 4). Initial splenomegaly was observed in all subtypes, but very large spleens were definitely more common in IMF and CML patients.

Survival probabilities of all groups are shown in Fig. 5. There was no significant difference between PV and IT patients, but when data from these two groups were combined, differences were significant with the PV/ET group showing the longest and CML the shortest survival times.

Thromboembolic events were observed more often in PV, IMF, and ET patients than in CML patients, even in those with initially high platelet counts. There were 18 patients who suffered from thromboses of the portal and caval system, including the Budd–Chiari syndrome. These data have been described in detail previously [7]. Blastic transformation was most often seen in CML patients. Among the other groups, differences were not significant. In the first bone marrow biopsy suggesting the diagnosis of

Table 2. Distribution of subtypes and basic data of patients with chronic myeloproliferative syndrome subtypes

Ultimate diagnosis	CML	PV	IMF	ET
Number of patients	223	141	103	22
Male/female ratio	1.4	0.8	0.9	0.6
Observation time (years)	2.9	5.0	3.0	6.9
Diagnostic delay (years)	0.2	1.3	0.6	0.7
Median survival (years)	3.5	9.4	4.3	11.2

CML, chronic myeloid leukemia; PV, polycythemia vera; IMF, idiopathic myelofibrosis; ET, essential thrombocythemia.

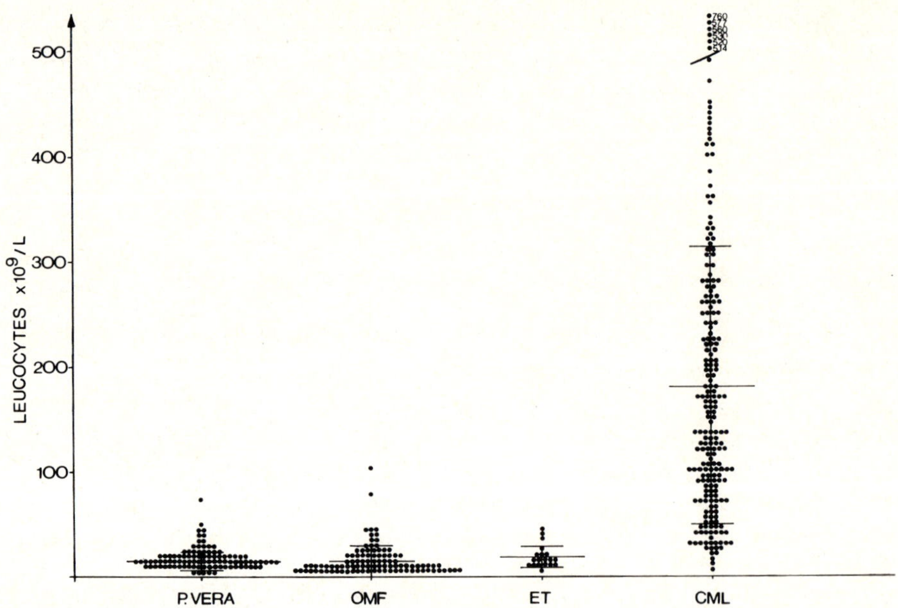

Fig. 1. WBC in the four subtypes of chronic myeloproliferative syndrome (c-MPS) at the time of diagnosis. *P.vera*, polycythemia vera; *OMF*, ostemyelofibrosis; *ET*, essential thrombocythemia; *CML*, chronic myeloid leukemia

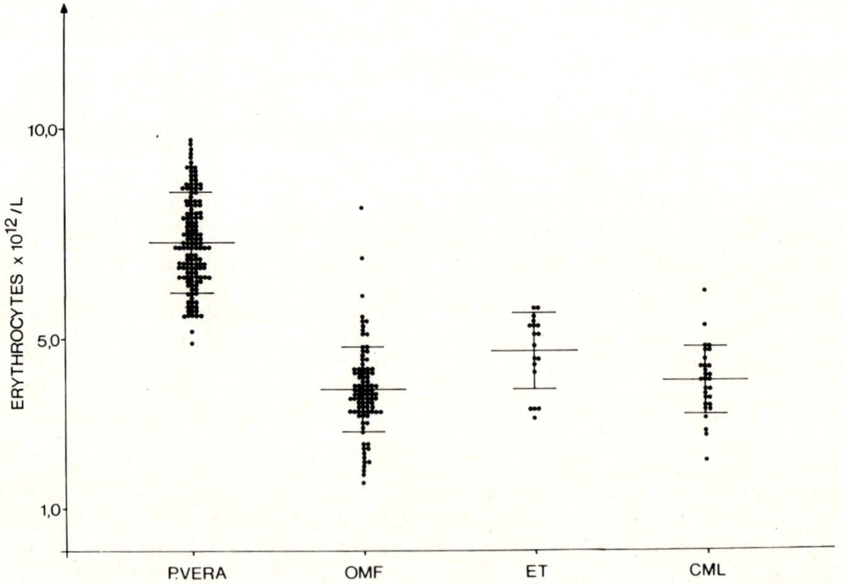

Fig. 2. Red cell count in the four subtypes of chronic myeloproliferative syndrome (c-MPS) at the time of diagnosis. *P.vera*, polycythemia vera; *OMF*, osteomyelofibrosis; *ET*, essential thrombocythemia; *CML*, chronic myeloid leukemia

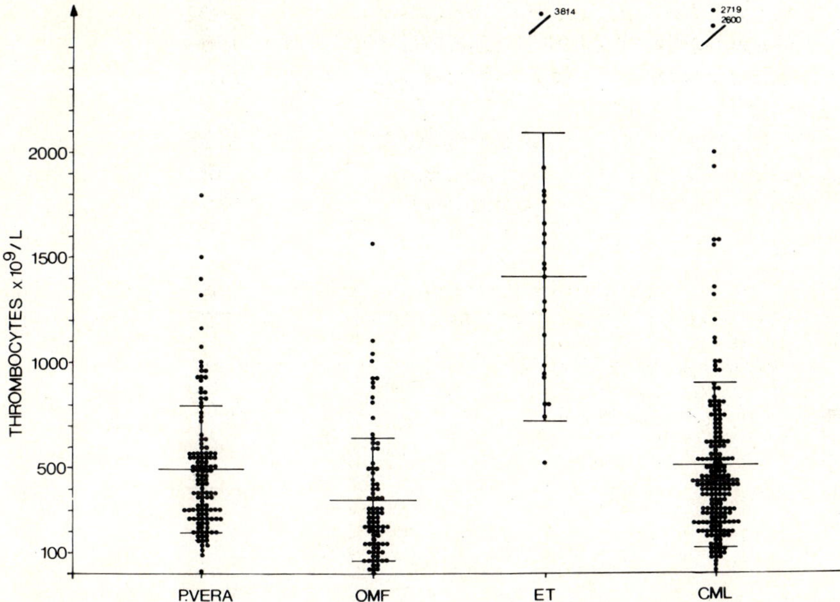

Fig. 3. Platelet count in the four subtypes of chronic myeloproliferative syndrome (c-MPS) at the time of the diagnosis. *P.vera*, polycythemia vera; *OMF*, osteomyelofibrosis; *ET*, essential thrombocythemia; *CML*, chronic myeloid leukemia

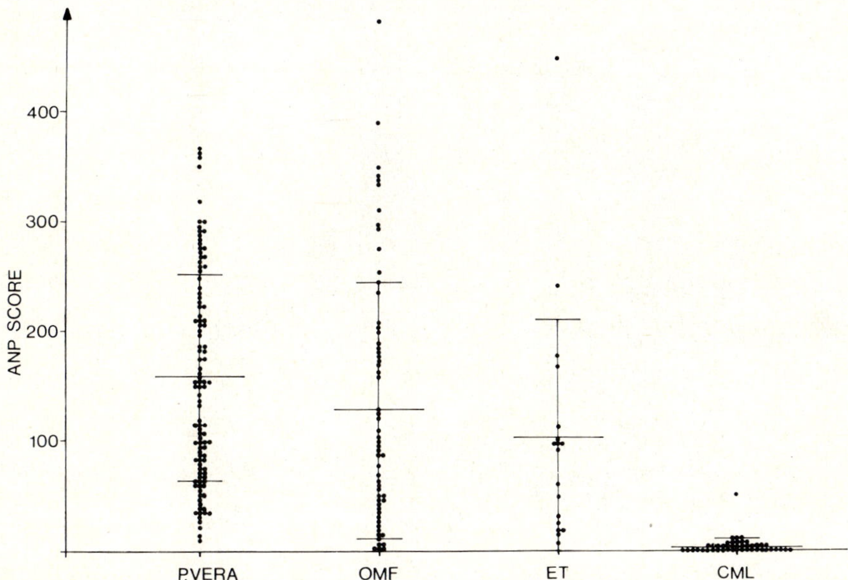

Fig. 4. Neutrophil alkaline phosphatase (ALP) score in the four subtypes of chronic myeloproliferative syndrome (c-MPS) at the time of diagnosis. *P.vera*, polycythemia vera; *OMF*, osteomyelofibrosis; *ET*, essential thrombocythemia; *CML*, chronic myeloid leukemia

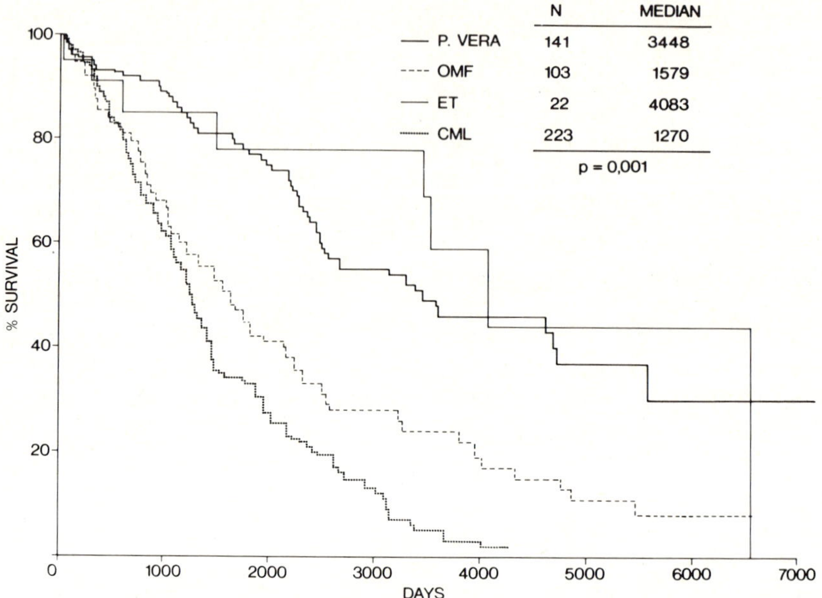

Fig. 5. Survival in the four subtypes of chronic myeloproliferative syndromes

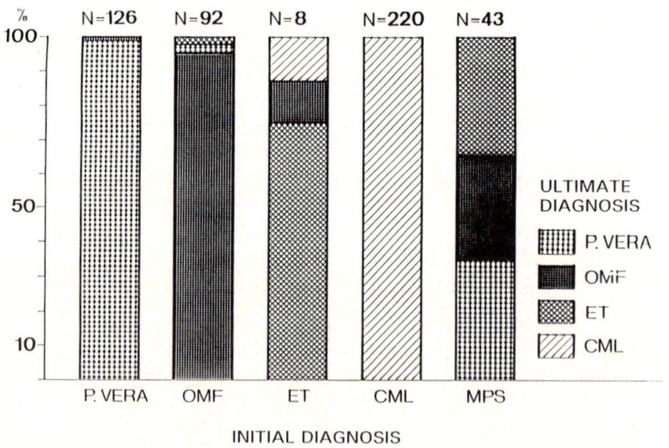

Fig. 6. Initial and ultimate diagnosis in 489 cases of chronic myeloproliferative syndromes. *P.vera*, polycythemia vera; *OMF*, osteomyelofibrosis; *ET*, essential thrombocythemia; *CML*, chronic myeloid leukemia

c-MPS, myelofibrosis was recognized by Gomory stains in most, but not all, patients with the ultimate diagnosis of IMF. It was infrequent in PV patients. By definition the remaining patients with myelofibrosis developed severe myelofibrosis and/or myelosclerosis during the following years, and the same was true for many patients with ET or CML but only for a very few patients with PV. A nonhematological cancer was seen most often in PV patients, as could be expected by the longer survival and observation times in this group.

Initial and ultimate diagnoses are compared in Fig. 6. It is evident that, if the diagnosis of CML was made, switches to other subtypes did not occur. This is due to the fact that the Philadelphia (Ph) chromosome was usually present and served as the unique sifficient and sufficient criterion for CML. In contrast to some earlier reports, we have never observed loss or gain of a Ph chromosome in the course of c-MPS. In patients with a change of diagnosis from ET to CML chromosome analysis had not been performed initially, but was done later in the course of the disease when ALP scores were repeatedly low. Initially unclassified cases showed evolution to PV, ET, or IMF with similar probability.

Discussion

CML has been recognized as a clonal disorder since the Ph chromosome was found to be present in up to 100% of bone marrow cell metaphases. Investigations using X chromosomal coded isoenzymes [1,16] in a small number of patients and molecular markers [3,10,13] in a larger number of patients demonstrated clonality of blood cells also for the majority of patients with the other subtypes. In contrast to CML, cytogenetic or molecular aberrations specific for the other subtypes have not been detected and the factors which govern the phenotypic expression in the different subtypes are not understood.

As shown by the results of this retrospective study, phenotypic characteristics of the chronic myeloproliferative disorders such as neutrophilic leukocytosis, thrombocytosis, erythrocytosis, bone marrow fibrosis, and splenomegaly may be present in all subtypes. If the Ph chromosome and/or the bcr/abl translocation is not present, initial allocation to one of the subtypes may not be possible, and such aptients are referred to as having "unclassified c-MPS." However, if the dieseases are followed, they usually show distinct phenotypic patterns and patients can then be allocated to one of the subtypes. More than one third of initially unclassifiable phenotypes will show evolution towards myelofibrosis. At large, they are identical with what has previously been defined as agnogenic myeloidmetaplasia or the hyperplastic phase of IMF [5,18].

CML, as defined by the presence of the Ph chromosome and/or by the bcr/abl translocation, shows rather definite features which allow one to differentiate CML from the other subtypes. There are few exceptional cases with initial distinct thrombocytosis without leukocytosis but the overwhelming majority show initial neutrophilic leukocytosis and low ALP. ET and PV seem to be closely related, and the phenotypic diagnosis may change with time between these two conditions. Consequently the term "ET/PV syndrome" has been suggested for such cases.

Most relevant for morbidity and mortality are blastic crises with critical organ infiltration and/or consecutive pancytopenia, myelofibrosis with huge spleens and bone marrow failure, and thromboembolic accidents. In CML, a blastic crisis is much more frequent, occurs earlier than in any other c-MPS, and is appearently independent on therapy. This is different from PV, in wich evolution towards acute leukemia is apparently more frequent after cytoreductive treatment with altcylating cytostatics and radiophosphorus. This may also be true in IMF and ET, but statistical evidence is lacking. By definition myelofibrosis with pancytopenia is always present in IMF, but it may be found as an initial marrow abnormality or a later complication in all subtypes, most rarely in PV [9,11,17]. Vascular accidents are the main causes of death in PV and ET but rare in CML and IMF [7,14]. If the subtype diagnoses of ET or PV can be made, the risk of vascular accidents has to be weighted against the risk of therapy-induced secondary leukemia in deciding if and when cytoreductive therapy should be initiated.

Curative therapy is not available for c-MPS, with the exception of allogeneic bone marrow transplantation and possibly of vigorous treatment with interferon in exceptional cases of CML. We have not observed major complications in the initial state of unclassified c-MPS and careful observation is therefore the strategy of choice in such patients. However, chromosomal analysis and/or southern blots for detection of the bcr/abl translocation should always be carried out when phenotypic features suggest the possible diagnosis of CML. This includes patients with very high platelets and only moderately elevated leukocyte counts as well as with other constellations of abnormal blood cell counts if the ALP score is subnormal. Data shown in Fig. 4 confirm earlier reports [8] claiming that low ALP scores are very sensitive but are not specific for CML within the group of c-MPS as a whole.

References

1. Adamson JW, Fialkow PJ, Murphy S, Prchal JF, Steinmann L (1976) Polycythemia vera: stem-cell and probable clonal origin of the disease. N Engl J Med 295:913–916
2. Anger B, Haug U, Seidler R, Heimpel H (1989) Polycythemia vera. A clinical study of 141 patients. Blut 59:493–500
3. Anger B, Janssen JWG, Schrezenmeier H, Hehlmann R, Heimpel H, Bartram CR (1990) Clonal analysis of chronic myeloproliferative disorders using x-linked DNA polymorphism. Leukemia 4:258–61
4. Anger B, Schmeiser T, Heimpel H, Robertson J, Sokal JE, Ganser A, Carbonell F (1990) Evaluation von 196 Patienten mit chronischer myeloischer Leukämie anhand eines Standard-Prognose-Modells. Onkologie 13:109–114
5. Anger B, Seidler R, Haug U, Popp C, Heimpel H (1987) Agnogenic myeloid metaplasia with myelofibrosis (AMM/MF): clinical course and prognosis of 103 patients. Blut 55:283–280

6. Anger B, Seidler R, Haug U, Popp C, Heimpel H (1990) Idiopathic myelofibrosis: a retrospective study of 103 patients. Haematologica 75:228–234
7. Anger B, Seifried E, Scheppach I, Heimpel H (1989) Budd-Chiari syndrome and thrombosis of other abdominal vessels in the chronic myeloproliferative diseases. Klin Wochenschr 67:818–825
8. Bendix-Hansen K, Bergmann OJ (1985) Evaluation of neutrophil alkaline phosphatase (NAP) activity in untreated myeloproliferative syndromes and in leukaemoid reactions. Scand J Haematol 35:219–224
9. Bouroncle BA, Doan CA (1962) Myelofibrosis: clinical, hematological and pathologic study of 110 patients. Am J Med 243:697–715
10. Buschle M, Janssen JWG, Drexler H, Lyons J, Anger B, Bartram CR (1988) Evidence for pluripotent stem cell origin of idiopathic myelofibrosis: clonal analysis of a case characterized by a N-ras gene mutation. Leukemia 2:658–660
11. Ellis JT, Peterson P, Geller SA, Rappaport H (1986) Studies of the bone marrow in polycythemia vera and the evolution of myelofibrosis and second hematologic malignancies. Sem Hematol 23:144–155
12. Hehlmann R, Anger B, Messerer D, Zankovich R, Bergmann L, Kolb HJ, Meyer P, Essers U, Queißer U, Vaupel H, Walther F, Hossfeld DK, Zimmermann R, Heiss F, Mende S, Tigges FJ, Kleeberg UR, Pralle H, Kayser W, Tichelli A, Faulhaber JD, Räth U, Schubert H, Bross K, Schlag R, Schmid L, Weißenfels I, Heinze B, Georgii A, Queißer W, Heimpel H (1988) Randomized study on the treatment of chronic myeloid leukemia (CML) in chronic phase with busulfan versus hydroxyurea versus interferon-alpha. Blut 56:87–91
13. Janssen JWG, Anger BR, Drexler HG, Bartram CR, Heimpel H (1990) Essential thrombocythemia in two sisters originating from different stem cell levels. Blood 75:1633–1636
14. Schafer AJ (1984) Bleeding and thrombosis in the myeloproliferative disorders. Blood 64:1–12
15. Schmeiser T, Arnold R, Wiesneth M, Hertenstein B, Bunjes D, Anger B, Heit W, Heimpel H (1988) Knochenmarktransplantation als Therapie der chronisch-myeloischen Leukämie. Dtsch Med Wochenschr 113:6–10
16. Singal U, Prasad AS, Halton DM, Bishop C (1983) Essential thrombocythemia: a clonal disorder of hematopoietic stem cell. Am J Hematol 14:193–196
17. Thiele J, Simon K-G, Fischer R (1988) Follow-up studies with sequential bone marrow biopsies in chronic myeloid leukaemia and so-called primary (idiopathic) osteo-myelofibrosis – evolution of histopathological lesions and clinical course in 40 patients. Pathol Res Pract 183:434–445
18. Ward HP, Block MH (1971) The natural history of agnogenic myeloid metaplasia (AMM) and a critical evaluation of its relationship with the myeloproliferative syndrome. Medicine 50:357–420

Histomorphological and Cytogenetic Investigations in Chronic Myeloproliferative Diseases

D. Höche,[1] A. Hochhaus, G. Anger, H. Werft, and M. Müller

Essentially, the chronic myeloproliferative diseases comprise the four following diseases: (1) chronic myeloid leukemia, and (2) osteomyelofibrosis (osteomyelosklerosis), (3) primary thrombocythaemia, (4) polycythaemia vera.

A partly retrospective, partly prospective investigation analysed 379 histological biopsies from 301 patients with chronic myeloproliferative diseases. The evaluation was performed mostly semiquantitatively. Important parameters were measured morphometrically. Bone marrow smears were used to supplement the histological study. A comparing histological-cytological consideration was performed for special questions. The clinical data and laboratory findings from all patients were included in the analysis.

The most frequent disease in our group of patients was chronic myeloid leukemia (164 patients), followed by polycythemia vera (59 patients). Osteomyelofibrosis was distinctly rarer in comparison (27 patients). Primary thrombocythemia was found in only 19 patients. The disease of the remaining six patients must be regarded as undifferentiated.

Eighteen patients with primary blast crisis, three with acute myelofibrosis, and five with megakaryoblastic myelosis were included for reasons of differential diagnosis.

A comparatively excellent median survival time of 227 months was found in patients with undifferentiated chronic myeloproliferative disease. In patients with polycythemia vera (184 months) or primary thrombocythemia, the disease showed a favourable course. Patients with a chronic myeloid leukemia clearly died earlier (median survival times 51 months). The survival time for patients with myelofibrosis/osteomyelosklerosis (median 18 months) seemed to be worse, according our examinations.

We differentiate two variants of chronic myeloid leukemia on the basis of bone marrow composition, a predominantly granulocytic variant and a megakaryocytic-granulocytic mixed form. The two subtypes do not differ essentially with regard to survival time, although the megakaryocyte-rich subtype was more inclined to fibrosis. A richness of collagen fibers proved to

[1] Hospital Ohrdruf and Clinic for Internal Medicine, Medical University of Erfurt, O-5807 Ohrdruf, FRG

Fleischer (Ed.) Leukemias

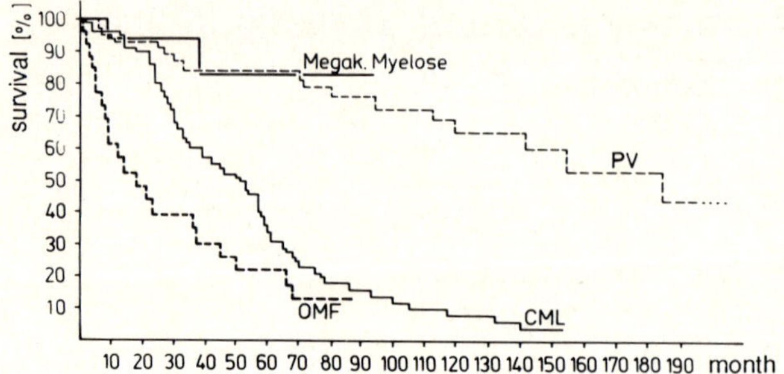

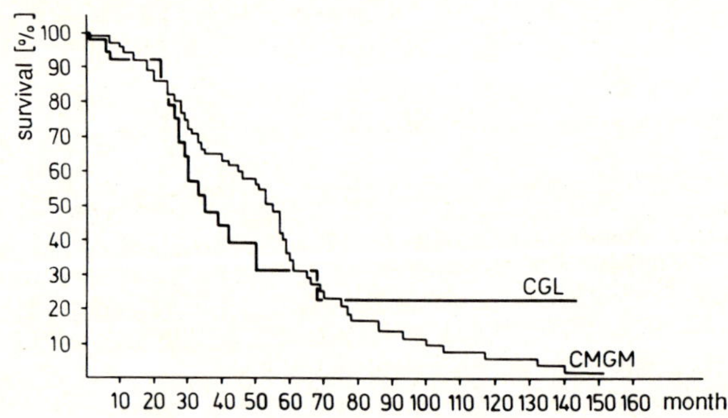

be a negative prognostic sign during the course of chronic myeloid leukemia. A slight reticular fiber formation remains without importance.

The proportion of myeloblasts and promyelocytes in the biopsy is a parameter we have used to estimate of the course of CML. Survival is significantly worse with more than 20% blasts and promyelocytes than below this number.

The blast cell crisis implies the final event in the majority of patients with chronic myeloid leukemia. The prognosis of the primary blast cell crisis is distinctly more favourable (median survival time 28 months) than that of secándary blast cell elevation (median survival time 4 months). A CML-similar type and a AML-similar type of primary blastic transformation can also be characterised which differ in the death date.

Myelofibrosis/osteomyelosclerosis can be differentiated from other myeloproliferative diseases with marrow fibrosis by clinical, haematological,

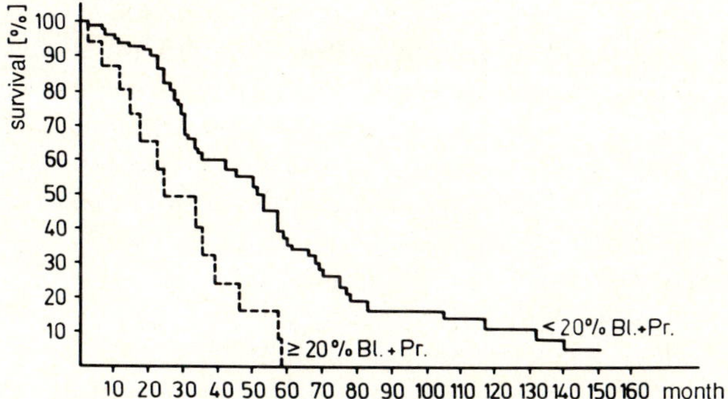

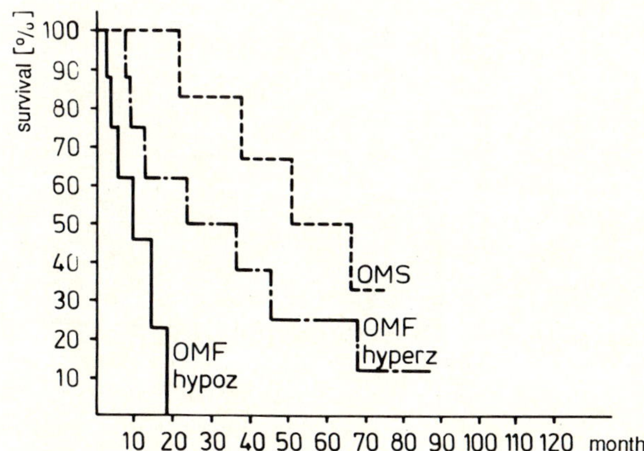

and cytogenetic investigations and biopsies. Osteomyelosclerosis is to a certain extent an independent entity and cannot be seen only as final stage of myelofibrosis. Myelofibrosis shows two patterns, a hypercellular and a hypocellular one.

An idiopathic thrombocythemia develops as a consequence of mature cellular megakaryocytic myelosis. Megakaryoblastic myeloid leukemia corresponds to acute leukemia concerning the appearance and course of the disease.

Bone marrow histology is a valuable resource for the diagnostic of polycythemia vera and gives clues for the prognosis when the proliferating cell rows and the marrow fibrosis are evaluated.

Undifferentiated chronic myeloproliferative disease cannot be classified in any of the four main groups. The disease corresponds quite closely to the so-called agnogenic myeloid metaplasia of the Angloamerican literature.

Cytogenetic analyses constitute a valuable supplement to the histological investigations in chronic myeloproliferative diseases. In particular, the Philadelphia chromosome enables a delimitation between chronic myeloid leukemia and myelofibrosis in many cases. The blast cell crisis is announced by the incidence of additional chromosomal aberrations. Philadelphia chromosome-negative chronic myeloid leukemia proved to be inhomogeneous in detailed examinations.

The delimitation of the individual entities comprising the chronic myeloproliferative diseases demands comprehensive consideration of all aspects of the disease, including past history and clinical and laboratory data, especially bone marrow biopsy and cytogenetic findings. It is thus possible to make a definite diagnosis in nearly all cases. Transformation of one disease into another are not rare during the course of the chronic myeloproliferative diseases, which sometimes causes diagnostic difficulties.

Chronic Megakaryocytic-Granulocytic Myelosis: Accuracy of Clinical Diagnosis of Chronic Myeloproliferative Disorders with Thrombocytosis

H.L. SEEWANN[1] and C. SCHMID

Chronic megakaryocytic granulocytic myelosis (CMGM) is characterized by a bilinear proliferation of granulocyto- and megakaryocytopoiesis originally described by Georgii et al. [1,2]. Histopathological bone marrow examination reveals moderate to high-grade augmentation of megakaryocytes which are polymorphous and extremely atypical. Megakaryocytopoesis shows an abnormal extension towards the osseous trabecula. Neutrophilic granulocytopoiesis is conspicuously increased and hyperplastic. These histopathological features allow one to separate this entity from other chronic myeloproliferative disorders (CMPD) with thrombocytosis such as chronic granulocytic leukemia (CGL) with thrombocytosis, essential thrombocythemia (ETH), polycythemia vera (PV), and agnogenic myeloid metaplasia (AMM). Aim of this study was to compare clinical and histopathological diagnoses of CMPD with thrombocytosis in order to find out how accurately purely clinical diagnosis of CMGM could be carried out.

Material and Methods

Among a total of 81 consecutive patients with CMPD, 43 (53%) were found to have thrombocytosis. In all patients, hematological routine parameters, leukocyte alkaline phosphatase (LAP) score and physical findings were compared with histopathology of methacrylate embedded bone marrow specimens yielded by Jamshidi technique [3]. Thrombocytosis was classified as mild ($450-700 \times 10^3/mm^3$), moderate ($700-1000 \times 10^3/mm^3$) or excessive (more than $1000 \times 10^3/mm^3$). Thrombocytosis was excessive in 16 patients (20%).

According to our prior findings [4,5] CMGM was clinically defined as CMPD with mild to excessive thrombocytosis, leukocytosis lower than $30 \times 10^3/mm^3$, moderate left shift of granulocytes in peripheral blood, high normal to extremely elevated LAP score, the absence of Philadelphia chromosome and red cell mass of low to normal.

---

[1]Medizinische Abteilung III des Landeskrankenhauses und Pathologisch-Anatomisches Institut der Universität, A-8036 Graz, Austria

Fleischer (Ed.) Leukemias
© Springer-Verlag Berlin Heidelberg 1993

Table 1. Comparison of hematological features and spleen size in centimeters below costal margin of ETH, MF, and CMGM

Entity	n	Thrombocytosis			LAP score (range)	Leukocytes (g/l)	Spleen size below costal margin (cm)
		Mild	Moderate	Excessive			
?	21	7	1	13	32–340	8–28	0–15
ETH	−4			4			
MF	−2	2					
?	15	5	1	9	62–340	8–28	0–8
CMGM	10	4	1	5	62–316	8–28	0–8

Results

Purely by hematological criteria all patients with PV and CGL with thrombocytosis could be separated from the whole group. The most important distinctive mark in PV patients was elevated red cell mass. Clinical diagnosis of CGL with thrombocytosis was mainly supported by leukocytosis of more than $30 \times 10^3/mm^3$, pathological left shift and non-existent to low LAP scores. The remaining 21 patients showed overlapping similarities in the criteria of LAP score, leukocytosis, left shift and spleen size. Four patients with excessive thrombocytosis and normal LAP levels could be clinically grouped as ETH, two patients with massive spleen enlargement and/or erythroblastosis as AMM. The remaining 15 patients met the clinical criteria of CMGM (Table 1). Histopathological investigations, however, revealed CMGM in ten of these patients. One patient showed myelofibrosis and four patients, ETH. In summary, in two-thirds of all patients who were clinically expected to have CMGM the histological findings confirmed the clinical diagnosis.

Discussion

CMPD with thrombocytosis are difficult to separate out solely on the basis of clinical methods. Table 1 shows hematological criteria and spleen size below costal margin of patients with ETH, CMGM, and myelofibrosis (MF). Red cell mass was in all cases normal or decreased.

According to our criteria it was possible to make a clinical diagnosis of CMGM in 19% of all cases with CMPD. Histopathology, however, revealed CMGM in only 12% of all cases. This observation means that one-third of "clinical CMGM" was misdiagnosed. We therefore consider histopathology of bone marrow specimens an essential investigation in making the diagnosis of CMPD with thrombocytosis.

References

1. Georgii A, Vykoupil KF, Thiele J (1980) Chronic megakaryocytic granulocytic myelosis – CMGM. A subtype of chronic myeloid leukaemia. Virchows Arch [A] 389:253–268
2. Georgii A (1983) Histopathologie und Klinik der chronischen, myeloproliferativen Erkrankungen. Verh Dtsch Ges Pathol 67:214–234
3. Jamshidi K, Swaim WR (1971) Bone marrow biopsy with unaltered architecture: a new biopsy device. J Lab Clin Med 77:335–342
4. Seewann HL, Lehnert M, Jüttner F (1983) The value of bone marrow biopsy in chronic myeloid leukaemia. Haematologia 16:67–72
5. Seewann HL (1986) Die Jamshidibiopsie in der klinischen Hämatologie. Wien Med Wochenschr 136[Suppl]:100

Morphology of Megakaryocytes in Chronic Myeloproliferative Diseases

J. Dušek,[1] K. Indrák, V. Ščudla, and M. Jarošová

Chronic myeloproliferative diseases are often characterized by proliferation of more than one cell line, which indicates involvement of the pluripotent noncommitted cell in the origin of the disorders. Megakaryocyte proliferation is often remarkable and has been repeatedly described in diseases such as polycythaemia vera, in many cases of chronic myelosis and in myelodysplastic syndromes [1–3]. The proliferating megakaryocytes are often dysplastic especially in cases of so-called granulocytic-megakaryocytic leukaemia [4]. In histological sections, megakaryocytes show increased pleiomorphism with an increase of small, large and senescent megakaryocytes. The usual features of megakaryocyte dysplasia are the presence of large hypolobated nuclei with pale chromatin and prominent nucleoli. The number of megakaryocytic mitoses is increased. Electron microscopy reveals, in addition to the immature appearance of nuclei, abnormalities in the cytoplasm, especially focal absence of the canalicular demarcation system and an uneven distribution of the platelet granules.

A new way of assessing the proliferative activity of bone marrow megakaryocytes could be offered by the visualization of their nuclear organizing regions. These nuclear components containing the ribosomal RNA-related DNA have been studied by several authors [5–7]. The number and size of the nuclear organizer regions (NOR) seem to reflect the degree of cellular immaturity and proliferative activity. In recent years, NOR staining with a colloid silver nitrate solution has been applied in the study of several preneoplastic and neoplastic conditions in various organs. This study compares the morphological appearance and the NORs of megakaryocytes in three types of myeloproliferative diseases.

Material and Methods

Iliac bone trephine biopsies and sternal bone marrow aspirates have been studied in 60 patients with polycythaemia vera, in 58 patients with chronic myelosis and in 50 cases of myelodysplastic syndromes. Paraffin sections

---

[1] Department of Pathology, Department of Clinical Haematology and the Third Medical Clinic, Faculty Hospital, Olomouc, Czechoslovakia

were stained in the modified Ploton's method [6], sometimes in combination with the PAS stain. Megakaryocytes were classified into five groups according to their size and morphological appearance: (a) small (less than 10 µm in diameter), (b) medium-size typical (11–30 µm), (c) medium-size dysplastic, (d) large (more than 30 µm) and (e) senescent megakaryocytes with small remnants of cytoplasm and pyknotic nuclei. Morphologically normal marrow samples from patients with clinically suspected marrow dissemination of various tumours were used as controls. Silver staining was applied in several cases of the three types of myeloproliferative diseases and the number of small and large (composite) NORs was counted.

Results

Compared to control cases, the bone marrow megakaryocytes from cases of chronic myeloproliferative diseases showed pleiomorphism with an increase of cells classified as medium-size dysplastic. There was also an increased

Table 1. Percentage frequency of the megakaryocyte types in myeloproliferative diseases

	Megakaryocytes (%)				
	Small	Medium	Medium dysplasia	Large	Senescent
Controls	0.5	75.1	12.8	5.5	6.1
Polycythaemia vera	2.2	31.3	42.1	9.3	15.8
Chronic myelosis	5.9	41.9	34.7	11.2	6.3
Myelodysplasia	5.3	53.7	16.4	18.7	5.3

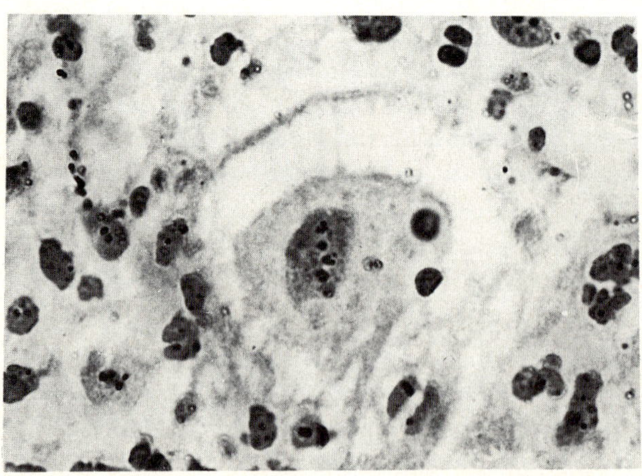

Fig. 1. A medium-size dysplastic megakaryocyte in the case of a myelodysplastic syndrome. Note emperipolesis and several large AgNORs in the nucleus, ×1060

Table 2. AgNOR regions in the bone marrow megakaryocytes

Type	Nuclear area	N/C ratio	NOR	
			Large	Small
Small	43.9	44.2	2.3	1.5
Medium	44.5	21.7	1.7	1.2
Medium dysplasia	119.1	47.3	5.9	6.1
Large	168.9	30.2	1.8	21.1
Senescent	70.5	85.4	0.1	3.1

proportion of small, large and senescent megakaryocytes. The number of medium-size typical megakaryocytes was decreased in all three disorders studied. The percentage values of the megakaryocyte types are summarized in Table 1.

Silver staining of the NOR (Fig. 1) showed numerous positive areas in the nuclei of megakaryocytes. As expected, their number was the lowest in senescent megakaryocytes. Medium-size typical megakaryocytes revealed less NORs than the medium-size dysplastic, small and large forms (Table 2).

Discussion and Conclusions

Morphological analysis of megakaryocytes in the three types of chronic myeloproliferative diseases has shown their abnormality with dysplastic features. The changes in the marrow megakaryocytes may be related to the increased density of reticulin fibers and the evolution of marrow fibrosis. Fibrotic transformation is frequently seen in the terminal phase of polycythaemia vera and in some cases of chronic myelosis, especially in the chronic granulocytic-megakaryocytic type. Recently, fibrosis of the bone marrow has also been reported in myelodysplastic syndromes [8].

Silver staining of the NORs in megakaryocytes has shown an increase in number and in proportion of large clumped NORs in the small and the medium-size dysplastic group. This is likely to be related to the increased proliferative activity of megakaryocytes in chronic myeloproliferative diseases. As expected, senescent megakaryocytes show the lowest number of NORs, mostly of the small type. Silver staining was applied only in a limited number of cases so far. One therefore cannot estimate the value of this method in the study of various aspects of myeloproliferatiove diseases.

References

1. Vykoupil KF, Thiele J (1980) Polycythemia vera. I. Histopathology, ultrastructure and cytogenetics of the bone marrow in comparison with secondary polycythemia. Virchows Arch [A] 389:307

2. Burkhardt R (1981) Bone marrow histology. In: Catovsky D (ed) The leukemic cell. Churchill Livingstone, London, pp 49–86
3. Thiele J, Vykoupil KF, Georgii A (1980) Myeloid dysplasia: a hematological disorder preceding acute and chronic myeloid leukemia. Virchows Arch [A] 389:343
4. Georgii A, Vykoupil KF (1980) Chronic megakaryocytic granulocytic myelosis – CMGM. Virchows Arch [A] 389:253–268
5. Smetana K, Likovský Z (1987) A further study on nucleolar silver stained granules in some mononuclear-lymphoid bone marrow cells. Folia Haematol 114:376
6. Crocker J, Nar P (1987) Nucleolar organizer regions in lymphomas. J Pathol 151:111
7. Crocker J, Boldy DAR, Egan MJ (1989) How should we count AgNORs? Proposals for a standardized approach. J Pathol 158:185
8. Shibata A, Takahashi M, Koike T, Narita M, Moriyama Y (1988) Myelodysplastic syndrome with myelofibrosis: a report of seven cases. Symposium on myelodysplasias. Innsbruck, Austria, June 1988

The Megakaryocytic Myeloid Leukemia: Clinical, Morphological and Functional Aspects

A. Hochhaus,[1] D. Höche, and M. Meyer

Introduction

Megakaryocytic myeloid leukemia is one of the chronic myeloproliferative diseases [3] with nearly isolated hyperplasia of thrombocytopoiesis [2] and concomitant, sometimes massive thrombocythemia in the peripheral blood. Because the terms "essential," "primary" and "idiopathic" thrombocythemia are used only for relatively high thrombocyte numbers [1,7], we prefer to use the more comprehensive notion of megakaryocytic myelosis in order to include less marked thrombocyte increases in the same process.

Megakaryocytic myeloid leukemia is of clinical importance when there are thrombembolic complications and the often simultaneously existing bleeding tendency.

Patients

Twenty-two patients (12 females, 10 males) with megakaryocytic myeloid leukemia, 19–73 years old (mean age 45 years), were included using the following diagnostic criteria:

- Chronic thrombocythemia ($>500 \times 10^9$/l) without a hint of secondary thrombocytosis, with exclusion of a second tumor and of splenectomy
- Megakaryocytosis in the bone marrow with atypical cells; total cell number in bone marrow normal or slightly elevated, fat cell number normal or slightly decreased, erythro- and granulocytopoiesis normal or slightly increased, no or only mild reticulin fibrosis, no collagen fibrosis, no or only slight osteosklerosis in pelvic biospy
- In the course of the disease, haemoglobin $\leqslant$12.0 mmol/l, haematocrit $\leqslant$0.54 (male patients); or haemoglobin $\leqslant$10.5 mmol/l, haematocrit $\leqslant$0.47 (female patients)

[1] Clinic for Internal Medicine of the Medical University of Erfurt, Nordhäuser Str. 74, O-5010 Erfurt, FRG

Fleischer (Ed.) Leukemias
© Springer-Verlag Berlin Heidelberg 1993

- Total leukocyte number during the course of disease $<30 \times 10^9/l$
- Exclusion of Philadelphia chromosome

Methods

Bone Marrow Investigations. The bone casts (Jamshidi technique) were embedded in methacrylate, prepared as normal, and evaluated. Thirteen methacrylate sections were suitable for morphometric investigations. Cell counting was performed at 640-fold microscopic enlargement using an eyepiece grid. Megakaryocytes according were classified to the scheme of Burkhardt et al. [2]. Chromosome studies were carried out with bone marrow cells in four cases using the G-band technique.

Membrane Glycoprotein Diagnosis. Crossed immunoelectrophoresis with polyspecific rabbit antiserum against human thrombocytes [6] and rocket immuno-electrophoresis with monospecific antiglucoprotein-IIb-IIIa antiserum [5,12] were performed in 14 patients with megakaryocyte myelosis. The polyspecific antibodies were prepared according to Herrmann et al. [6] and the monospecific antibodies according to Gogstad et al. [4]. Determinations were carried out three times against a pool of thrombocyte protein extracts from ten healthy blood donors.

Results

Clinical Course

Eleven of 22 patients with megakaryocytic myeloid leukemia developed a bleeding tendency during the course of the disease, including gastrointestinal bleedings (5 cases), inclination to haemorrhages of the skin (5 cases), epistaxis (2 cases), bleeding after injury (1 case), and haemoptysis (1 case). Thrombosis and embolism were observed in 12 patients. Arteries were concerned three times, veins ten times. Two myocardial infarctions, one case of disseminated kidney and spleen infarctions, one arterial leg thrombosis, one thrombosis of the arteria carotis interna, six leg vein, one axillary vein, two splenic vein, one portal vein, and one hepatic vein thrombosis, one case with priapism, and one lung embolism occurred. Three patients claimed disturbances of the acral microcirculation. A bleeding tendency existed parallel to thrombosis and embolism in six cases. In five patients no complications of coagulation could be observed. Hepatomegaly was found in 16 patients clinically, by sonography, or by autopsy, and spleen enlargement in 19 cases.

Three patients died during the observation period. The reasons were related to the tendency towards thrombosis: (1) bleeding of varicose veins of oesophagus; (2) liver failure and coma after portal vein thrombosis (37 months after making the diagnosis); and (3) encephalomalacia with thrombosis of the arteria carotis interna (1 month after making the diagnosis). The follow-up period for the living patients amounted 12–180 months. Calculation of survival probability according the Kaplan–Meier method showed a plateau level of 80.6% between the 37th and 180th month after diagnosis.

Haematological Results

Anaemia developed in 15 patients during the course of the disease and leucocytosis in 16. The highest thrombocyte number ranged from 524 to $2700 \times 19^9/l$. Strongly increased megakaryocytopoiesis with atypical cells was found in the bone marrow in all examined patients. The cellularity and erythro- and granulocytopoiesis were normal or only slightly increased. No or only poorly developed fibrosis was found. Chromosomal investigations performed in four cases produced normal karyograms.

More than one cluster, i.e. the pooling of at least five mature megakaryocytes per square millimeter of bone marrow, was observed in eight of 13 patients who underwent morphometric investigations. Pleomorphic megakaryocytes with irregular cell borders and polyploid, bizarre-shaped nuclei dominated. The distribution density of megakaryocytes in the bone marrow correlated with the number of thrombocytes on the day of biopsy ($r = 0.52$; $p < 0.1$). The frequency of immature cells of megakaryocytopoiesis was inversely correlated with the number of peripheral thrombocytes ($r = -0.51$; $p < 0.1$).

Membrane Glycoproteins

Fourteen patients with megakaryocytic myeloid leukemia showed distinct aberrations on semiquantitative examination of the expression of thrombocytic membrane glycoproteins by crossed-immunoelectrophoresis. A reduction in the glycoprotein IIb–IIIa complex was found in eight patients.

The rocket immunoelectrophoresis of thrombocyte proteins against a monospecific antiglycoprotein IIb–IIIa antiserum showed a glycoprotein content from 96.4% (standard deviation 7.7%) in comparison with pooled thrombocytes from 16 controls. The glycoprotein levels of the patients examined lay between 52% and 121%. They were significantly different from those in the control group ($2p < 0.02$, Wilcoxon test).

There was a inverse correlation between the glycoprotein IIb–IIIa content and thrombocyte number in megakaryocytic myeloid leukemia ($r = -0.66$; $p < 0.01$). Relationships between the glycoprotein IIb–IIIa complex and clinical coagulation complications could not be found.

Discussion

The clinical course of megakaryocytic myeloid leukemia in 22 patients confirmed the incidence of thrombembolic events to be the same or higher than that of haemorrhagic complications [1,8]. The three patients who died as a result of the thrombosis tendency show the prognostic relevance of thrombo-embolic events.

The demonstration of a partial diminution of the glycoprotein complex IIb–IIIa of the platelet membrane is of special interest. The glycoprotein IIb–IIIa content was determined independently from other protein fractions and was compared to that in healthy controls. The inverse correlation between glycoprotein IIb–IIIa content and thrombocyte number supports the assumption that the deficiency is not only the consequence of the defect arising during the stem cell transition but that there is also a reaction to polyploidisation of megakaryocytes with increased release of thrombocytes.

The lack of glycoproteins itself does not explain the bleeding tendency, because comparable levels were found in heterozygote carriers of Glanzmann's thrombasthenia who showed no symptoms of a haemorrhagic diathesis [10].

Because the glycoprotein IIb–IIIa complex acts as a receptor for fibrinogen during aggregation [11], a diminished aggregability would be expected in connection with reduced glycoprotein content. However, this result was not observed in heterozygotes for the Glanzmann's thrombasthenia [9].

References

1. Bellucci S, Janvier M, Tobelem G, Flandrin G, Charpak Y Berger R, Boiron M (1986) Essential thrombocythemias. Clinical, evolutionary and biological data. Cancer 58:2440–2447
2. Burkhardt R, Bartl R, Jäger K, Frisch B, Kettner G, Mahl G, Sund M (1986) Working classification of chronic myeloproli-ferative disorders based on histological, haematological, and clinical findings. J Clin Pathol 39:237–252
3. Dameshek W (1951) Some speculations on the myeloproliferative syndromes. Blood 6:372–375
4. Gogstad GO, Hagen I, Krutnes MB, Solum NO (1982) Dissociation of the glyco-protein IIb–IIIa complex in isolated human platelet membranes. Dependence of pH and divalent cations. Biochem Biophys Acta 689:21–30
5. Herrmann FH, Meyer M, Gogstad GO, Solum NO (1983) Glycoprotein IIb–IIIa complex in platelets of patients and heterozygotes of Glanzmann's thrombasthenia. Thromb Res 32:615–622
6. Herrmann FH, Meyer M, Ihle E (1982) Protein and glycoprotein abnormalities in an unusual subtype of Glanzmann's thrombasthenia. Haemostasis 12:337–344
7. Jabaily J, Iland HJ, Laszlo J, Massly EW, Faguet GB, Brière J, Landaw StA, Pisciotta AV (1983) Neurologic manifestations of essential thrombocathemia. Ann Intern Med 99:513–518
8. Jahn M, Zönnchen B, Köpcke W, Hehlmann R (1988) Klinische Charakterisierung der essentiellen Thrombozythämie im Ver-gleich zu anderen myeloproliferativen Erkrankungen und reaktiven Thrombozytosen. Klin Wochenschr 66:190–198

9. Lusher JM, Barnhart M (1977) Congenital disorders affecting platelets. Semin Thromb Haemost 4:123–186
10. Meyer M, Herrmann FH (1986) Klinik, Diagnostik und Genetik der Thrombasthenie Glanzmann. Z Klin Med 41:520–523
11. Nachman RL, Leung LLK (1982) Complex formation of platelet membrane glycoproteins IIb and IIIa with fibrinogen. J Clin Invest 69:263–269
12. Weeke B (1973) Rocket immunoelectrophoresis. Scand J Immunol 2[Suppl 1]:15–56

Budd-Chiari Syndrome and Other Abdominal Thromboses in the Chronic Myeloproliferative Disorders

B. Anger,[1] E. Seifried, J. Scheppach, and H. Heimpel

Introduction

Bleeding and thrombosis are major causes of morbidity and mortality in a group of clonal diseases of bone marrow stem cells, the chronic myeloproliferative diseases (c-MPD), including polycythemia vera (PV), essential thrombocythemia (ET), and idiopathic myelofibrosis (IMF) [1,5,8–11,13]. The pathogenesis of these thrombotic events is not known. The influence of proposed risk factors like an elevated hematocrit, elevated platelet counts, abnormalities of platelet function, organomegaly due to extramedullary hematopoietic proliferation in liver and spleen, and altered blood flow in the splanchnic circulation has not been clarified [4,6,7,12]. In this report, clinical and laboratory data from 18 patients with thrombosis of major abdominal vessels out of a group of 501 patients with c-MPD will be presented.

Material and Methods

501 patients with documented c-MPD were seen over a 20-year period from May 1967 to March 1987. The records of all patients were examined for evidence of thrombosis of major abdominal vessels including hepatic, portal, splenic, and mesenteric veins, vena cava inferior, and mesenteric veins, vena cava inferior, and mesenteric arter. Eighteen patients (9 females, 9 males) were identified. The diagnosis of the thrombotic event was established by angiography (11 patients), explorative laparotomy (5 patients), or computer tomography (1 patient), or at autopsy (1 patient). The clinical data, blood counts, and results of coagulation tests at the time of diagnosis of the thrombotic event were retrieved from the records. Patients with PV were treated by venesection and/or P32 and/or busulfan. Patients with CML were treated with busulfan or hydroxyurea, followed by bone marrow transplantation if a suitable donor was available. Patients with ET were treated with busulfan if necessary. Patients with IMF received transfusions and/or androgens. Cyclooxygenase inhibitors were not routinely given.

---

[1] Department of Internal Medicine, Division of Hematology, Ulm University Hospital, Robert-Koch-Str. 8, 7900 Ulm, FRG

Fleischer (Ed.) Leukemias
© Springer-Verlag Berlin Heidelberg 1993

Table 1. Thrombosis of major abdominal veins in 501 patients with c-MPS. Distribution of thrombosed vessels (in 10 patients more than one vessel was occluded)

	PV	ET	IMF	CML	Total
No. of patients	141	22	106	232	501
No. with thrombosis	14 (10%)	3 (13%)	1 (1%)	0 (0%)	18
Occluded vessel					
V. portae	7	2	1	0	10 (29%)
V. lienalis	5	3	1	0	8 (24%)
V. mesenterica	4	3	1	0	8 (24%)
Hepatic veins	6	0	0	0	6 (18%)
V. cava	1	1	0	0	2 (6%)

Results

A thrombosis of a major abdominal vessel was documented in 18 of 501 patients with c-MPD (9 males, 9 females, median age 44 years). Thrombosis occurred least often in CML (0%) and IMF (1%). The incidence was much higher in PV (10%) and ET (13%) (see Table 1). In the 18 patients, 34 thrombosed vessels were documented. The portal vein was occluded most often. Occlusion of the vena cava inferior was rare. In three patients the thrombotic event was documented several years before the diagnosis of the c-MPD (-4, -7, and -11 years). In four patients the thrombosis was the first symptom leading to the diagnosis of c-MPD. Common clinical symptoms and signs of the thrombosis were abdominal pain (88%), progressive splenomegaly (88%), ascites (67%), nausea and vomiting (57%), and progressive hepatomegaly (43%). Five of 12 evaluable patients (42%) already had esophageal varices at the time of diagnosis of the thrombosis, indicating that earlier thrombotic events may have gone undetected. Angiography and explorative laparotomy were the diagnostic methods with the highest specificity (83% each). A variety of medical and surgical interventions including fibrinolysis therapy and liver transplantation were tried. A positive response to therapy was obtained in one patient who underwent an early surgical thrombectomy. Seven patients (39%) died within 2 months of diagnosis of the thrombosis, most due to hepatic failure or peritonitis after mesenteric infarction. Those who survived longer than 4 weeks developed a range of complications like liver cirrhosis with portal hypertension, esophageal varices, and gastrointestinal bleeding or the short bowel syndrome after extensive resection of intestine.

Discussion

Thrombosis of major abdominal vessels like occlusion of the hepatic, portal, splenic, and mesenteric veins are rare but highly letal complications of c-

MPD. We detected 18 cases among 501 patients with c-MPD over a 20-year period. Seven of the 18 patients died within 2 months. Most cases were detected in PV (10%) and ET (13%), and no cases in CML. The difference in thrombotic complications between the different subclasses of c-MPD is well known. In our patients, thromboses were fairly evenly distributed among the abdominal vessels, with the portal vein most often affected and the vena cava least often.

The thrombotic event may develop any time during the course of the c-MPD. In four cases the thrombosis was the leading symptom uncovering the c-MPD. The thrombotic event may even precede the clinical diagnosis of a c-MPD by many years: three of our patients had a thrombosis up to 11 years before diagnosis of the c-MPD. Every case of idiopathic thrombosis of major abdominal vessels should be thoroughly evaluated for signs of an occult c-MPD.

A thrombocytosis is often found in patients with c-MPD. However, a clear correlation between the platelet count and the incidence of thrombotic events has not been established. Hematocrit levels and platelet counts in our 18 patients were spread over a range from low to high values. Five of 18 patients had hematocrit and platelet values in the low or normal range, none of them receiving myelosuppressive therapy. Our data do not suggest a significant role of hematocrit or platelet count in the pathogenesis of the thrombosis.

The mortality due to Budd-Chiari syndrome in PV is high. A reasonable prophylaxis should be good medical control of the c-MPD by phlebotomy and/or by myelosuppressive chemotherapy with busulfan or hydroxyurea to keep the hematocrit and the platelet count in or near the normal range. The value of prophylactic therapy with prostaglandin synthetase inhibitors for patients with high platelet counts is controversial. Therapy of established thrombosis should be targeted on clot lysis. Early cases may benefit from thrombolytic therapy with urokinase, streptokinase, or tissue plasminogen activator, followed by anticoagulant therapy.

In our series, only three patients were treated with streptokinase, due to late diagnosis in most cases and associated medical conditions that interfered with thrombolytic therapy in the others. These patients did not respond. A variety of other medical treatment modalities were tried in the 20-year period without detectable benefit. Surgical procedures like splenectomy and resection of necrotic bowel were done in some patients with large splenic infarction or mesenteric infarctions due to mesenteric vein thrombosis. Most of these patients died. One young woman with hepatic failure received a liver transplant but she succumbed to a sepsis. However, liver transplantation and shunt operations may provide the only hope for patients with irreversible liver damage due to hepatic vein occlusion.

References

1. Anger BR, Seifried E, Scheppach J, Heimpel H (1989) Budd-Chiari syndrome and thombosis of other abdominal vessels in the chronic myeloproliferative diseases (c-MPD). Klin Wochenschr 67:818–825
2. Berk PD, Goldberg JD, Silverstein MN, et al. (1981) Increased incidence of acute leukemia in polycythemia vera associated with chlorambucil therapy. N Engl J Med 304:441–447
3. Berk PD, Goldberg JD, Silverstein MN, et al. (1986) Therapeutic recommendations in polycythemia vera based on Polycythemia Vera Study Group protocols. Semin Hematol 23:132–143
4. Buss DH, Stuart JJ, Lipscomb GE (1985) The incidence of thrombotic and hemorrhagic disorders in association with extreme thrombocytosis: an analysis of 129 cases. Am J Hematol 20:365–372
5. Fitzgerald O, Fitzgerald P, Cantwell D, Mehigan IA (1956) Diagnosis and treatment of the Budd-Chiari syndrome in polycythaemia vera. Br Med J 4:1343
6. Kessler CM, Klein HG, Havlik RJ (1982) Uncontrolled thrombocytosis in chronic myeloproliferative disorders. Br J Haematol 50:157
7. Mason JE, DeVita VT, Canellos GP (1974) Thrombocytosis in chronic granulocytic leukemia: incidence and clinical significance. Blood 44:483
8. McCarthy PM, van Heerden JA, Adson MA, Schafer LW, Wiesner RH (1985) The Budd-Chiari syndrome: medical and surgical management of 30 patients. Arch Surg 120:657–662
9. Mitchell MC, Boitnott JK, Kaufman S, Cameron JL, Maddrey WC (1982) Budd-Chiari syndrome: etiology, diagnosis and management. Medicine 61:199–218
10. Murphy FB, Steinberg HV, Shires GT, Martin LG, Bernadino ME (1986) The Budd-Chiari syndrome: a review. AJR 147:9–15
11. Parker RGF (1959) Occlusion of the hepatic veins in man. Medicine 38:369
12. Pearson TC (1987) Rheology of the absolute polycythaemias. In: Lowe GDO (eds) Clinical haematology, vol 1, no 3, Blood rheology and hyperviscosity syndromes. London: Bailliere-Tindall, London, pp 637–664
13. Schafer AI (1984) Bleeding and thrombosis in the myeloproliferative disorders. Blood 1:1–12
14. Tartaglia A, Goldberg JD, Berk PD, Wassermann LR (1986) Adverse effects of antiaggregating platelet therapy in the treatment of polycythemia vera. Semin Hematol 23:172–176

New Therapy of Myelofibrosis with an Antifibrotic Substance and a Macrophage Stimulant

J. Fleischer,[1] H. Wolf, B. Mohr, G. Keck, I. Biester,
J. Irmscher, and C. Kemmer

In an animal experiment liver cirrhosis was induced by thioacetamide (TAA) to assess the influence of drugs on fibrosis. We attached pathological importance to the macrophages, the liver possessing the greatest macrophage population as Kupffer cells in the sinusoids. We had observed an increased proliferation of Kupffer cells after splenectomy in the rabbit in former investigations. Liver cirrhosis induced by TAA developed earlier after splenectomy and more intensively, maybe as a result of hyperplasia of the Kupffer cells [2,3]. The TAA changes were diminished distinctly or inhibited by trypan blue. A Kupffer cell stimulation by trypan blue was evident on electron-microscopic examination (see Fig. 1). Trypan blue is not suitable for the treatment of human beings because of an oncogenic effect. We considered clofazimine, another dye which has an effect on macrophages. Clofazimine is an antiphlogistic substance used in the treatment of leprosy [12]. We examined, by simultaneous administration of clofazimine and TAA, whether changes of the function of Kupffer cells could be correlated with the course of liver damage [4,5,6,13].

A method for Kupffer cell isolation based on collagenase perfusion of the liver and utilization of the adherence capacity of cells was developed. The method yielded Kupffer cells with a purity of 90% and a vitality of more than 95%. The production of oxygen metabolites in respiratory burst with the iodonitrotetrazolium chloride (INT) test and the levels of leukotrienes were taken as functional parameters for Kupffer cells.

The development of TAA damage up to cirrhosis was examined histologically. We determined the amount of hydroxyproline per gram dry tissue as measured for the accumulation of collagen in the liver. Additional parameters of fibrous tissue metabolism were defined for the liver tissue and in serum by A. Müller and D. Jorke (University Clinic for Internal Medicine, Jena, FRG), e.g. N-acetyl-β-D-glucosaminidase. The degree of lipid peroxidation of liver tissue was measured under different conditions.

A distinct inhibition of TAA cirrhosis development (as a consequence of 12 weeks 25 mg TAA/kg body weight daily) by clofazimine could be

[1] Abt. für Hämatologie und Onkologie, Klinik für Innere Medizin, Medizinische Akademie "Carl Gustav Carus", Fetscherstr. 74, O-8019 Dresden, FRG

Fleischer (Ed.) Leukemias
© Springer-Verlag Berlin Heidelberg 1993

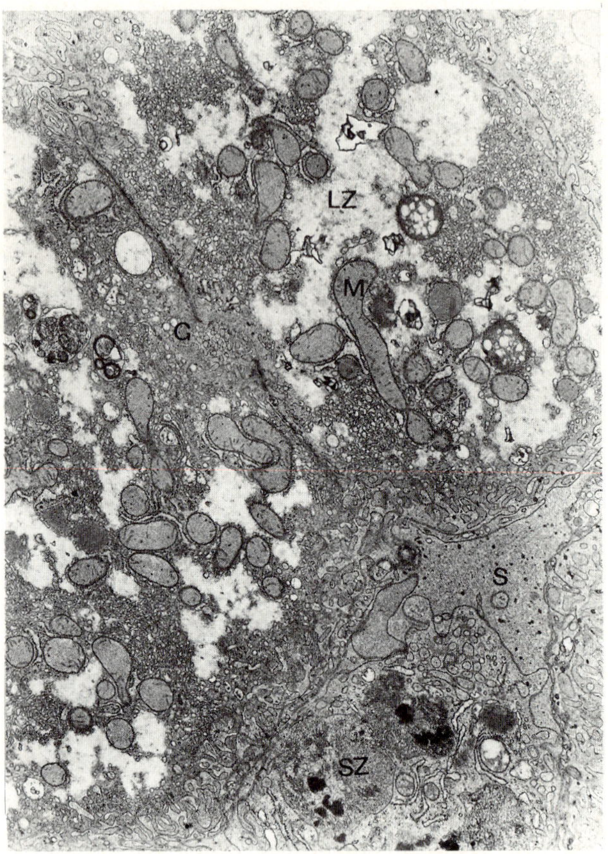

Fig. 1. Liver after intravenous administration of trypan blue. 1:10 000. *LZ*, liver cell; *SZ*, Kupffer cell; *S*, sinuoid. (from [4])

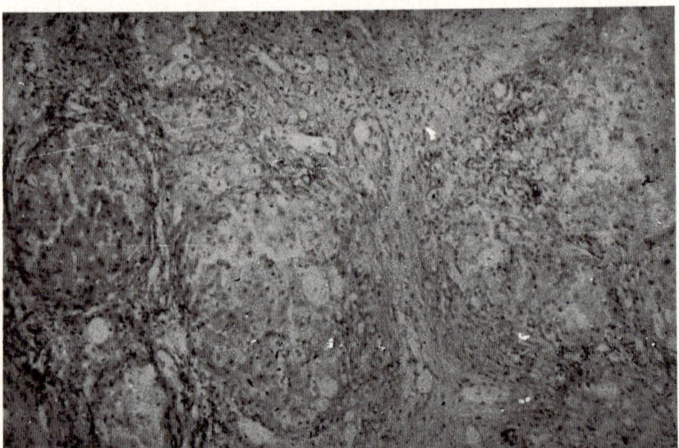

Fig. 2. Thioacetamide induced liver cirrhosis of the rat

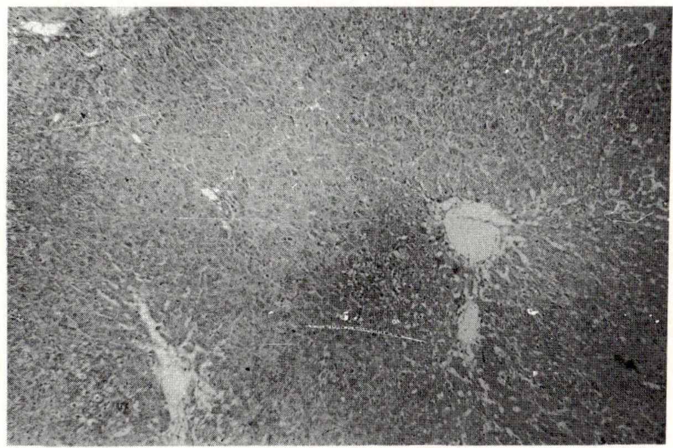

Fig. 3. Rat liver after 12 weeks thioacetamide, clofazimine and zymosan

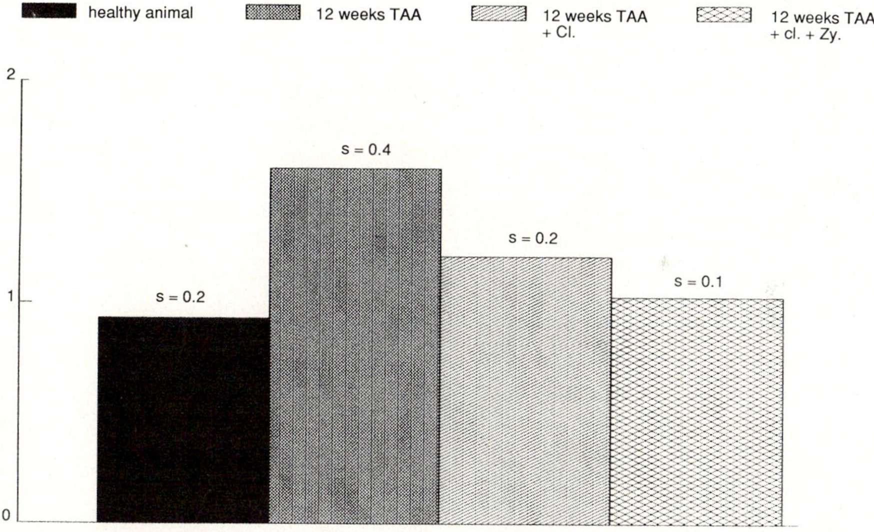

Fig. 4. Hydroxyproline content of liver tissue in mg/g weight of dry liver

observed within a narrow therapeutic range from 0.4 mg clofazimine/kg body weight of animal up to 0.7 mg/kg (best effect with 0.6 mg/kg). According to the histological results (see Figs. 2 and 3), there is a significant decrease of hydroxyproline after 12 weeks TAA and clofazimine (see Fig. 4).

The same was true for *N*-acetyl-β-D-glucosaminidase. The levels after 12 weeks TAA rose to 72.2 (U/g protein) in comparison to 58.7 in normal animals. After the additional administration of clofazimine and zymosan only an increase of 0.5 could be observed (see Table 1). The lipid peroxidation reflects the extent of liver damage by reactive oxygen radicals: after 12 weeks TAA, 215 mU (absorbance) in comparison with 164 mU of the normal animals; after 12 weeks TAA, clofazimine and zymosan 176 mU (see Table 2).

The INT test with Kupffer cells shows the superoxide anion (O^-_2) production capacity. The stimulation factor F is the quotient of stimulated and spontaneous extinction. After 12 weeks TAA the Kupffer cells demon-

Table 1. N-acetyl-β-D-glucosaminidase levels in liver tissue in U/g protein

Normal animals	58.7 + 10.0 ($n = 6$)
Experimental animals	
After 12 weeks TAA	72.2 + 12.6 ($n = 12$)
After 12 weeks TAA and 8 weeks without therapy	63.6 + 7.1 ($n = 4$)
After 12 weeks TAA and simultaneously 8 weeks clofazimine and zymosan	61.2 + 11.4 ($n = 12$)
After 12 weeks TAA, clofazimine and zymosan	59.2 + 13.4 ($n = 6$)

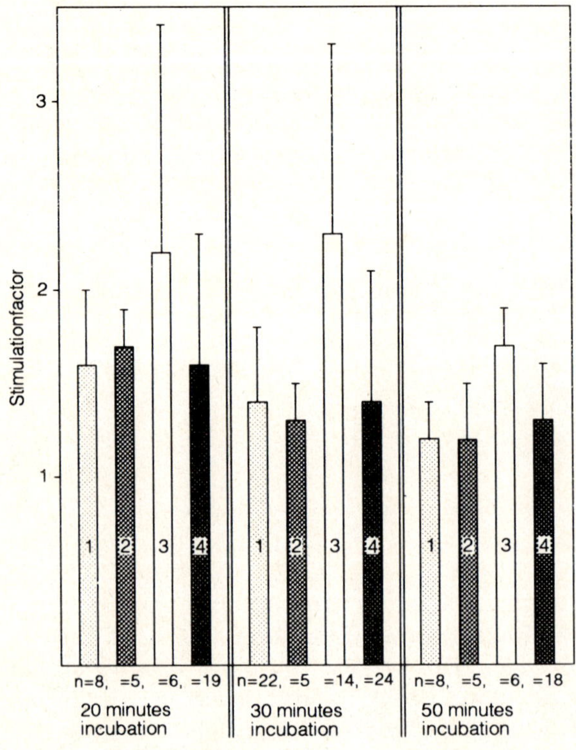

Fig. 5. Factor of stimulation for O_2 generation (reduction of INT) by macrophages of the liver (Kupffer cells). Group *1*, untreated animals; group *2*, 12 weeks zymosan, clofazimine, drinking water; group *3*, 12 weeks TAA; group *4*, 12 weeks zymosan, clofazimine, TAA

Table 2. Lipid peroxidation of liver tissue

	Absorbance (mU/g protein)	SD	n
Normal animals	165	25.7	9
Experimental animals			
After 12 weeks TAA	215	61	14
After 12 weeks TAA and 8 weeks without therapy	221	90	4
After 12 weeks TAA, simultaneously 8 weeks clofazimine and zymosan	172	29	12
After 12 weeks TAA, clofazimine, and zymosan	176	24	8

strate the highest 0^-_2 production, with a significant difference to all other 12-week groups. The results of the animal group treated with all three drugs (TAA, clofazimine, zymosan) concerning Kupffer cells corresponded to those of the untreated animals in activation ability of respiratory burst after stimulation (see Fig. 5).

We had pointed out already that prostaglandin (PG) E_2 is a favorable indicator of the inhibition of liver changes, because levels increase and decrease suddenly at a certain point. Knook and Brouwer [9] were able to prove the rise and gradient of PG E_2 with increasing doses of lipopolysaccharide in Kupffer cell culture. Now we believe that a leukotriene supports the process of development of fibrosis until macrophage function by an antileukotriene after massive Kupffer cell stimulation is inhibited. The antileukotriene produced by macrophages could be a different substance. The final result is a stop in the process of fibrosis development. Mackenzie demonstrated an increase of leukotriene B_4 by stimulation of macrophages with *S. epidermidis* [10]. Instead of the assumed antileukotriene, an anti-transforming growth factor could be responsible for stopping the development of fibrosis.

Because of the assumed importance of macrophages in the development of fibrosis it is reasonable to add a second macrophage-stimulatory substance to clofazimine to inhibit TAA-induced changes. We decided to use zymosan, which is able to increase phagocytosis and cytokine production in macrophages and to augment Kupffer cells. The intraperitoneal (i.p.) administration of zymosan was chosen because of quick resorption into the portal vein. After 12 weeks TAA (orally daily 25 mg/kg), clofazimine (orally daily 0.6 mg/kg), and zymosan (i.p. weekly 20 mg/kg), we found definite inhibition of TAA cirrhosis. We measured hydroxyproline levels in liver tissue, which are lower than those after TAA and clofazimine administration (see Fig. 4). This result is important because only few substances are known as antifibrotic drugs. Manabe et al. (Osaka) described in detail an effective antifibrotic substance with malotilate [11]. Traditional drugs like *Rheum palmatum* from China and *Tinospora cordifolia* from India posses a certain antifibrotic effect.

Kivirikko found that prolylhydroxylase metabolizes proline into hydroxyproline and the blocking of the enzyme by pyridine dicarboxylate suppresses the collagen synthesis in an animal model. Wildhirt treated patients with chronic aggressive hepatitis, some with cirrhosis in the early stage, with glycyrrhizioacid infusions which have an antiphlogistic effect and induce production of interferon; only 10% of 150 patients did not respond to treatment. Feher [1] uses an antioxidant which interrupts radicals in the stimulation process. The antioxidant silybin (Silibinin) is the act substance

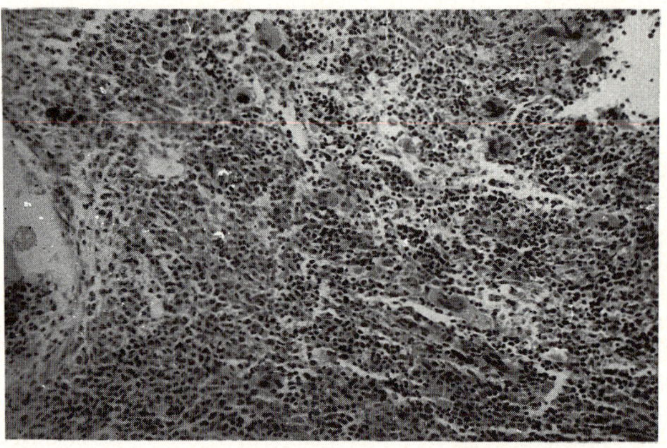

Fig. 6. Primary myelofibrosis before treatment (high cellularity, atypical megakaryoblasts)

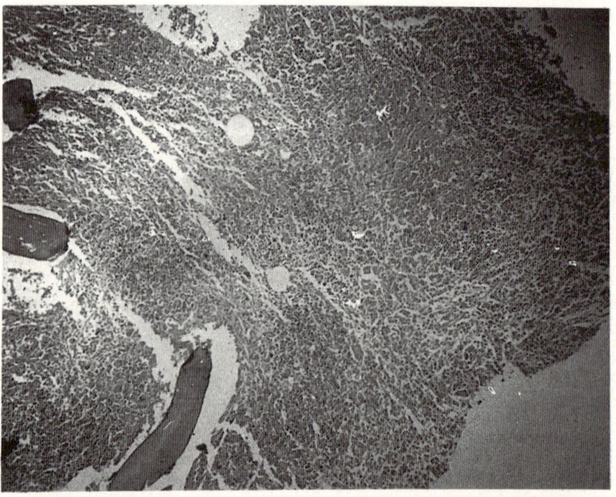

Fig. 7. Primary myelofibrosis after 12 weeks clofazimine (diminished cellularity, no atypical megakaryoblasts)

of milk thistle (*Silybum marianum*) and the main isomer of a group of flavonoid compounds, the silymarin-group. Thirty-six liver cirrhosis patients were treated with silymarin (Legalon) for 6 months; procollagen III peptide decreased and the histological picture improved distinctly [1].

We transferred these procedures to myelofibrosis [7,8] in spite of the fact that fat-storing cells do not exist in bone marrow, but there is a close connection between thrombocytopoiesis and fibrosis development (platelet-derived growth factor). We studied early primary disease, convinced that in advanced-stage disease with extremely enlarged spleen there would be only an insignificant response or none at all. It was necessary, before combining the administration of clofazimine with an additional macrophage stimulant, to examine clofazimine alone.

Before administering clofazimine to patients with primary myelofibrosis we registered its side effects. They arise nearly always with the administra-

Table 3. Results in six patients with primary myelofibrosis before and after 3 months clofazimine (Lampren)

Bone marrow histology
   No change of degree of fibrosis
   Cellularity decreased ($n = 2$)
   Megakaryocytosis decreased ($n = 2$)
Bone marrow cytology
   Cellularity decreased ($n = 2$)
   Erythrocytopoiesis
      No change ($n = 3$)
      16%–31% ($n = 1$)
      4%–41% ($n = 1$)
      12%–22% ($n = 1$)
   Megakaryocytosis decreased ($n = 2$)
Peripheral blood picture
   Hemoglobin
      No change ($n = 4$)
      From 5.7 to 6.5 mmol/l ($n = 1$)
      From 5.8 to 6.7 mmol/l ($n = 1$)
   Reticulocytes
      No change ($n = 3$)
      From 21‰ to 46‰ ($n = 1$)
      From 15‰ to 34‰ ($n = 1$)
      From 17‰ to 27‰ ($n = 1$)
   Leukocytes
      No change ($n = 4$)
      From 35.1 to 27.3 GPT/l ($n = 1$)
      From 9.3 to 19.3 GPT/l ($n = 1$)
   Thrombocytes
      No change ($n = 2$)
      From 207 to 371 GPT/l ($n = 1$)
      From 354 to 613 GPT/l ($n = 1$)
      From 560 to 395 GPT/l ($n = 1$)
      From 29 to 112 GPT/l ($n = 1$)

GPT, gigaparticle.

tion of 300 mg and more daily, especially in the gastrointestinal tract, and are dose related. Reversible pink discoloration of the skin, skin dryness, or skin rash may arise. A cornea pigmentation was observed in 0.5% of the leprosy patients treated, which also was reversible, and which did not necessitate interrupting the therapy. Macula pigmentations have only developed very rarely up to now.

Ciba-Geigy's (Basel) has reasonably recommended a restricted dosage of 100 mg daily for 12 weeks for reasons of safety. We treated six patients with the mentioned clofazimine dosage for 12 weeks in a pilot study. The hyperplastic bone marrow showed reduced cell numbers histologically twice (see Figs. 6, 7; Table 3). The cellularity was diminished cytologically in these two cases too. Megakaryocytosis and eosinophilia was found to have disappeared twice. Cytologically the erythrocytopoiesis increased in three of the six patients. The increase from 4% up to 41% in one case correlated with the disappearance of the necessity for blood transfusions clinically. The thrombocyte count normalized in two patients. The size of the spleen did not decrease with respect to the size measured by sonography.

The patients had no complaints with clofazimine. Ophthalmologically a mild one-sided disturbance was found at examination with the Nagel anomaloscope and the pseudoisochromatic tables (color vision test) according to Ichikawa in two of the six patients which were age related and not drug acquired (M. Marré, unpublished observations).

In summary one advantage of the clofazimine therapy has been recognized. A second pilot study using higher daily doses and a longer administration time has been initiated. The combination with the macrophage stimulant muramyl tripeptide seems to be possible; a second arm using alpha-interferon is planned for a national study.

References

1. Feher J (1990) Therapie der alkoholinduzierten Leberzirrhose mit Silymarin. 25 ster EASL-Kongreß, 3–6 Okt 1990, Budapest
2. Fleischer J (1978) Das "Mononuclear Phagocyte System" (früher "RES") aus experimenteller und klinischer Sicht. Dtsch Gesundheitswes 33:1171–1175
3. Fleischer J, Irmscher J (1969) Der Einfluß der RHS-Blockierung auf die tierexperimentelle Leberzirrhoseentwicklung. Allerg Asthma 15:44–48
4. Fleischer J, Irmscher J, Kemmer C (1981) Folgen der teilweisen Blockierung des Makrophagensystems. Folia Haematol 108:289–293
5. Fleischer J, Keck G, Wolf H, Reinhardt U (1984) Die Beeinflussung der Enzymproduktion in Makrophagen. Folia Haematol 111:146–148
6. Fleischer J, Keck G, Wolf H, Mundra J (1989) Beeinflussung der Enzymaktivitäten von peritonealen Makrophagen und von Kupfferzellen im Tierversuch. Folia Haematol 116:9–15
7. Fleischer J, Wolf H, Mohr B, Keck G (1989) A new therapy of myelofibrosis with an antifibrotic substance and a macrophage irritant. Blut 59:269
8. Fleischer J, Wolf H, Mohr B, Biester I, Müller A, Jorke D, Ehrenlechner U, Löwel U (1990) Additional experimental investigations to the new therapy of myelofibrosis and liver fibrosis. Blut 61:132

9. Knook DL, Brouwer A, et al. (1986) Functional characteristics of isolated and cultured human Kupffer cells, 7th international congress of liver diseases, 16–18 Okt 1986, Poster Abstracts Nr 14, Cirrhosis, Basel
10. Mackenzie RK, Coles GA, Williams JD (1990) Eicosanoid synthesis in human peritoneal macrophages stimulated with *S. epidermidis*. Kidney Int 37:1316–1324
11. Manabe N, Katoh M, et al. (1986) Effects of malotilate on cellular immunological responses in rats with liver fibrosis induced by egg yolk sensitization. 7th international congress of liver diseases, 16–18 Okt 1986, Poster Abstracts Nr 6, Cirrhosis, Basel
12. Thangaraj RH, Yawalkar SJ (1989) Leprosy for medical practitioners and paramedical workers, 4th edn. Ciba-Geigy Limited, Basel, Switzerland
13. Wolf H (1988) Die Rolle der lysosomalen Enzyme der Kupfferzellen bei der thioazetamidinduzierten Leberzirrhose der Ratte. Habilitationsschrift. Medizinische Akademie Dresden

Preliminary Results of a Multicenter Study of Chronic Myelogenous Leukemia Comparing Busulfan/6-Mercaptopurine with Dibromomannitol/6-Mercaptopurine

W. Helbig,[1] R. Krahl, M. Kubel, F. Fiedler, U. Schattmann, and R. Rohrberg

In 1985 a randomized study was introduced to compare busulfan (Bu; $2.5\,mg/m^2$) with dibromomannitol (DBM; $150\,mg/m^2$), each being combined with 6-mercaptopurine (6-MP; $30\,mg/m^2$) in the initial therapy of chronic myelogenous leukemia (CML). These dosages were used at the beginning of the therapy daily and reduced gradually until the stable chronic phase (CP) was reached. This means the fixed combination of an alkylating agent with 6-MP was stable and only the number of days of administration was reduced, to just a few per week.

The aim of the study was:

- First, to give indirectly more patients the option of an allogeneic bone marrow transplantation (BMT), if a human leukocyte antigen (HLA)-matched donor is available, since this is the only way to cure this disease
- Second, to prove the effectiveness of the seldom combination of two commonly used alkylating agents with the same antimetabolite in CML

Cytostatic treatment was initiated immediately after diagnosis. So far 282 patients have been included in this study. In 83% of the patients the Philadelphia (Ph^1) chromosome was investigated and 93% of them proved to be Ph positive.

To establish the phases of the disease the criteria of the International Bone Marrow Transplant Registry (IBMTR) were used. It is remarkable that 35% of the patients were initially in an accelerated phase (AP).

When using the prognostic criteria of Sokal [3] for classification we found a significant difference between the East German and the US population for CML (Table 1). East German patients were diagnosed evidently later. There is no explanation for this, because CML was diagnosed in many patients by chance while being treated for other ailments.

The duration of the initial therapy with respect to the initial phase and both regimens is illustrated in Table 2. A stable CP was reached in 76% of

[1] Division of Hematology and Oncology, Department of Internal Medicine, University of Leipzig, Johannisallee 32, O-7010 Leipzig, FRG

Fleischer (Ed.) Leukemias
© Springer-Verlag Berlin Heidelberg 1993

Table 1. Staging and prognosis in CML according to Sokal et al. [3]

	East Germany	Sokal et al.
Relative risk		
<0.8	67	114
0.8 –1.2	84	145 ($p < 0.025$)
>1.2	104	102
Mean values		
Age (years)	48	43
Spleen size (cm below costal arch)	6.52	7.51
Platelet count ($\times 10^9$/l)	332	(525)
Circulating blasts (%)	3.74	2.1

Table 2. Duration of initial therapy regarding the initial phase and therapy

Initial phase	Treatment regimen	Response (n)				Median time to stable CP (days)
		Total patients	R	PR	NR	
CP	CP/Bu + 6-MP	86	71	15	0	64 (13–248)
CP	CP/DBM + 6-MP	82	63	18	1	54 (12–225)
AP	CP/Bu + 6-MP	53	36	17	0	84 (7–259)
AP	CP/DBM + 6-MP	37	27	9	1	83 (13–308)

CP, chronic phase; AP, accelerated phase; R, remission; PR, partial remission, i.e., no complete hematological or clinical remission; Bu, busulfan; DBM, dibromomannitol; MP, mercaptopurine.

the patients although 35% of them were initially in an AP. The median duration of initial therapy was about 2 months for both schemes; patients in AP needed 3–4 weeks longer to reach the stable CP.

So far for scheme 1 (Bu + 6-MP) there are no differences in patients with initial CP or AP (Fig. 1) regarding the duration of stable CP or the probability of survival. Median survival has not yet been reached for patients with initial CP. In patients treated with scheme 2 we generally found the same, i.e., no differences between patients with initial CP or AP. If we compare all patients treated with scheme 1 or 2 there are no differences between the duration of stable CP and survival as yet either but the median follow-up is only 15 months for all groups. Concerning the Sokal criteria it is striking that the survival curves of the two groups with the intermediate and high stage at diagnosis do not differ as yet.

So far there is no difference in survival regarding the sex of the patients, but survival rates in patients between 30 and 60 years of age tend to be better than those in younger or older patients. The diagnosis of AP by the participating physician is an obstacle in evaluating the efficacy of the treatment in this phase because the doctors were obviously not willing to accept that the patient's disease had accelerated. As a rule they were not willing to

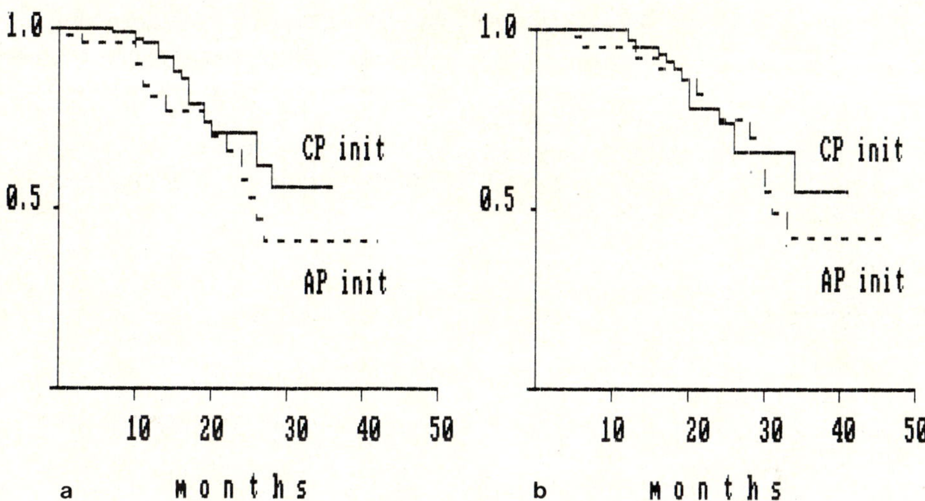

Fig. 1a,b. Scheme 1: Development of initial chronic phase (*CP init*) to CP (*n* = 82) vs. initial accelerate phase (*AP init*) to CP (*n* = 43). **a** Duration of CP, *p* = 0.332. **b** Survival, *p* = 0.662

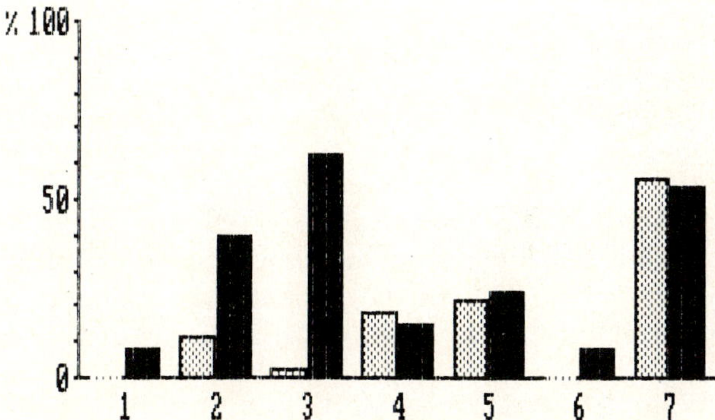

Fig. 2. Relative frequencies of the International Bone Narrow Transplant Registry (IBMTR) criteria for AP (IBMTR; *stippled bars, n* = 55) and AP marked (*solid bars, n* = 31). *1*, WBC difficult to control; *2*, ≥ 10% blasts in blood or marrow; *3*, ≥ 20% blasts plus promyelocytes in blood or marrow; *4*, ≥ 20% basophils plus eosinophils in blood; *5*, anemia or thrombocytopenia unresponsive to therapy; *6*, persistent thrombocytosis; *7*, increasing splenomegaly

accept AP until the hard criteria of AP were evident (Fig. 2), i.e., when the counts of blast and promyelocytes increase in the blood and marrow into the range of the defined count for CP. Thus, it is not astonishing that we could observe a delay of AP diagnosis in a median of 8.5 months. Some 58% of the patients suffered from an AP before reaching the blast phase (BP); in the others, CP led immediately to BP.

Patients below the age of 40 years tend to survive longer if transplanted in CP ($n = 13$) than patients treated by chemotherapy. The probability of leukemia-free survival (LFS) in transplated patients is 56%, but so far no significant difference could be reached because of the limited number of allografted patients. Only six patients could be grafted in AP and only one patients is still alive. Thus, 23% of CML patients in this age-limited group were transplanted, two thirds of them in CP.

Conclusions

1. Probably neither CT regimen is superior or inferior to the monotherapy in the literature [1,2].
2. More than one third of the patients fulfilled the IBMTR criteria of an AP at diagnosis, but had similar success with the initial therapy including survival as patients in initial CP.
3. BMT shows a trend towards an increased probability of survival.
4. The short median follow-up of 15 months allows only preliminary conclusions. Thus, the study has to be continued.

Summary

A multicenter study comparing the fixed combinations of busulfan/6-MP and dibromomannitol/6-MP was conducted. There was no difference in the results of the two regimens in reaching a stable chronic phase or in the duration of this phase or the probibility of survival. Neither was there a difference compared to the results in the literature. In the group up to 40 years of age, 23% of the patients were allografted. These patients tend to survive longer. Because of the short median observation time of only 15 months these results are preliminary.

References

1. Champlin RE, Golde DW (1985) Chronic myelogenous leukemia: recent advances. Blood 65:1039–1047
2. Kardinal CG, Bateman JR, Weiner J (1976) Chronic granulocytic leukemia, review of 536 cases. Arch Intern Med 136:305–313
3. Sokal JE, Baccarami M, Russo D, Tura S (1988) Staging and prognosis in chronic myelogenous leukemia. Sem Hematol 25:49–61

Ag-NOR in B-Cell Chronic Lymphocytic Leukemia: Pathomorphological Subtypes of the Disease

G. KELÉNYI[1]

In the diagnosis of B-cell chronic lymphocytic leukemia (B-CLL) lymph node biopsy is not of primary importance. Although views widely differ in this respect, lymph node biopsy seems to be indicated in patients under 50 years of age, if lymph nodes increase in size rapidly, or if on the basis of clinical findings other non-Hodgkin's malignant lymphomas (ML) may be suspected [18].

The prognostic value of the lymph node biopsy in B-CLL is not clear. From the three types of lymph node histology (diffuse, pseudofollicular, tumour-forming) described by Lennert et al. [13], the prognosis of the tumour-forming type is poor. The histological features of the lymph nodes in prolymphocytic transformation of B-CLL, as well as of those in B-cell prolymphocytic leukemia are not well characterized [1,11,13]. In spite of these circumstances the diagnosis of B-CLL in our lymph node biopsy material is quite frequent; it represents 27% of all non-Hodgkin's ML cases registered in the Lymphoma Reference Center (1987–88: 167 cases). Consequently, the study of this material for the prognosis of possible subtypes seemed to be warranted. For the evaluation of the cases, to establish possible relationship between morphological pattern and prognosis besides routine procedures the silver nucleolar organizer region (Ag-NOR) method was also used.

The NOR consists of deoxyribonucleic acid (DNA) loops, corresponding to ribosomal ribonucleic acid (RNA) genes (rDNA) [10]. The Ag-NOR reaction demonstrates some NOR-associated proteins, nucleolin being the most important nucleolar non-histone protein [12]. In the course of the reaction black granules appear over the nuclei; the size, number and shape of these granules is indicative of the transcription activity and potential of rDNA, or in a more general sense, of cellular activities [7]. According to recent publications [4,8] there is a correlation between the number of the Ag-NOR granules and proliferative activity of cells (cells in the S phase of the cycle, Ki-67 positive cells). In benign and malignant lesions of identical

[1] Department of Pathology, University Medical School of Pécs, Szigeticut 12, H-7643 Pécs, Hungary

Fleischer (Ed.) Leukemias
© Springer-Verlag Berlin Heidelberg 1993

histogenesis (nevi and melanoma [14], low and high grade ML-S [3,5]) the malignant cells contain more granules than the more benign ones.

In our study of lymph node biopsies of B-CLL patients both the diffuse and the pseudofollicular type showed a more mature and an immature subtype with significantly different Ag-NOR granule numbers. Besides, a very immature and a nodular variant of the pseudofollicular type was distinguished with characteristic Ag-NOR granule numbers.

Material and Methods

We analysed 64 lymph node biopsies of B-CLL patients. *Pseudofollicular CLL* (CLL-PF, 37 cases): In fields of small lymphocytes with round nuclei smaller or larger groups of prolymphocytes and paraimmunoblasts (pseudofollicles or proliferation centres) are present. On the basis of their size, cellular composition, number of mitoses, a mature and an immature subtype may be distinguished (PF_{mat} and PF_{imm}, 20 and 17 cases, respectively). In eight further cases the PFs were very large, nearly confluent with a very low number of small lymphocytes between them ("inter-pseudofollicular area"; PF → D). In seven cases the distribution of the reticulin fibres showed a more or less nodular pattern (PF-N).

Diffuse CLL (CLL-D, 12 cases): In fields of small lymphocytes there were either no prolymphocytes or paraimmunoblasts or they were seen as single cells scattered among the small cells. Accordingly, a mature and an immature subtype ($CLL-D_{mat}$ and D_{imm}) were distinguished.

The Ag-NOR granules were visualized in 6- to 7-μm thick formaldehyde-paraffin sections by the one-step method of Howell and Black [9] and of Ploton et al. [16]. In each section the Ag-NOR granules of between 100 and 300 nuclei were counted. In CLL-PF the number of granules of the PFs and of the inter-pseudofollicular areas (IPF) were evaluated separately.

Clinical data: In 24 cases the initial clinical stages were noted and in 22 patients who died, the survival times were registered.

Results

1. *Mature and immature pseudofollicular CLL* ($CLL-PF_{mat}$, $-PF_{imm}$): Of the 37 cases 20 belonged to the mature and 17 to the immature subtype. The number of Ag-NOR granules was significantly different ($p < 0.01$; Table 1).
2. *Very immature pseudofollicular CLL* (CLL-PF → D, eight cases): The PFs of these biopsies were very large and confluent and the IPF small lymphocytic areas inconspicuous (the number of Ag-NOR granules of these cells was difficult to assess). The average number of Ag-NOR granules in these eight cases was higher than in the PF_{mat} cases (3.36 vs.

Table 1. Number of Ag-Nor granules and histological subtypes in 37 patients[a]

PF_{mature}	IPF_{mature}	$PF_{immature}$	$IPF_{immature}$
	$(n = 20)$		$(n = 17)$
3.14 ± 0.35 SD*	1.59 ± 0.20 SD	3.61 ± 0.38 SD*	1.65 ± 0.18 SD
(2.51–3.99)	(1.24–1.88)	(3.02–4.49)	(1.28–2.04)

PF, pseudofollicles; IPF, fields of small lymphocytes between PF
*$p < 0.01$
[a] Average age of patients was 64.9 years and included 25 men and 12 women.

3.14); the difference, however, was not significant. The relatively low number of Ag-NOR granules in this subtype might be due to the intermingling of prolymphocytes and paraimmunoblasts with remnants of the IPF areas. i.e. with the small lymphocytes (with low granule numbers). The average patient age in this group was 4 years younger than that of all patients. Five of the eight patients died; the average survival of these patients was 39 (7–66) months.

3. *Nodular pseudofollicular CLL* (CLL-PF-N, seven cases, four women, three men): In the lymph node biopsies of typical CLL-PF cases the reticulin fibre distribution is homogeneous [13]. In seven out of the 64 cases the reticulin fibre distribution was more or less nodular. The number of remnants of follicles was very low, similar to the other CLL-PF cases with diffuse fibre distribution. All these cases showed PFs of the mature subtype. However, the number of Ag-NOR granules was higher than in the PF_{mat} (3.47 vs. 3.14; $p < 0.05$). The average age of these patients was 69.5 years, 4 years older than that of all the patients.

4. *Mature and immature diffuse CLL* (CLL-D_{mat} and CLL-D_{imm}): In the 12 cases of this group the number of Ag-NOR granules in the mature (1.57 ± 0.17 SD) and immature (2.42 ± 0.15 SD) subtypes were quite different.

Discussion

The lymph nodes analysed in the present study were removed at the time of clinical diagnosis. That means a certain degree of patient selection since the disease was detected at clinical stages A II, B I-II or C III-IV [2]. That might partly explain the male predominance in the present patient material (43 males, 21 females).

In repeated biopsies (interval 1 month to 5 years, six cases), the number of Ag-NOR granules did not change significantly. In two further cases the number increased with a more immature cytological pattern of the pseudofollicles.

The number of Ag-NOR granules of PF_{mat} and PF_{imm} differed significantly ($p < 0.01$); the values were near to those observed in high grade ML-S [5].

In the near diffuse pseudofolliclular type (PF → D), the relatively short survival in five out of eight cases speaks for an unfavourable prognosis.

In the CLL-D, the number of Ag-NOR granules and the morphological picture were indicative of two clearly separated subtypes.

The PF-N group represents a special subtype. In CLL-D we did not see such a nodular reticulin fibre pattern. The high number of Ag-NOR granules in the PF-N subtype may be explained by assuming that in these cases cells are closer in their differentiation to cells of follicles than in the others ("borderline cases"). The higher number of Ag-NOR granules in centrocytes than in the small round lymphocytes supports this assumption. It should also be mentioned that prolymphocytic leukemic lymph node biopsies may show a nodular pattern, and the presence of cleaved cells (centrocytes?) was also described [1,11]. The higher average age of the patients in the PF-N group is also peculiar (patients with prolymphocytic leukaemia are usually older than those with B-CLL).

Our studies seem to indicate that the lymph node biopsies in B-CLL may show, in addition to the well-known types, further subtypes. In a disease with very different survival rates the possible prognostic relevance of these sub-types may be interesting. In the present series most of the patients are still under clinical observation and only the follow-up might clear up the possible correlation of lymph node morphology and survival. The very immature pseudofollicular subtype (PF → D) seems to be of poor prognosis and similar to the tumour-forming type of Lennert et al. [13] or to the recently described "paraimmunoblastic variant" of B-CLL described by Pugh et al. [17].

References

1. Bearman RM, Pangalis GA, Rappaport H (1978) Prolymphocytic leukemia. Clinical, histopathological and cytochemical observations. Cancer 42:2360
2. Binet JL, Catovsky F, Chandra P. et al. (1981) Chronic lymphocytic leukemia: proposals for a revised prognostic staging system. Br J Haematol 48:365
3. Crocker J, Egan MJ (1988) Correlation between NOR sizes and numbers in non-Hodgkin's lymphomas. J Pathol 156:233
4. Crocker J, Macartney JC, Smith PJ (1988) Correlation between DNA flow cytometric and nucleolar organizer region data in non-Hodgkin's lymphomas. J Pathol 154:151
5. Crocker J, Nar P (1987) Nucleolar organizer regions in lymphomas. J Pathol 151:111
6. Endrédi, J (1991) Lymphoma Reference Centre 1987–88. Oru Hetil 132:739
7. Falkan S, Hernandez-Verdun D (1986) The nucleolus and nucleolar organizer regions. Biol Cell 56:189
8. Hall PA, Crocker J, Watts A, Stansfeld, AG (1988) A comparison of nucleolar organizer regions staining and Ki-67 immunostaining in non-Hodgkin's lymphoma. Histopathol 12:373

9. Howell WM, Black DA (1980) Controlled silver staining of nucleolar organizer regions with protective colloidal developer: a 1-step method. Experientia 36:1014
10. Jordan G (1987) Transcription: at the heart of the nucleolus. Nature 329:489
11. Lampert I, Catovsky D, Marsh GW, et al. (1980) The histopathology of prolymphocytic leukemia with particular reference to the spleen: a comparison with chronic lymphocytic leukemia. Histopathol 4:3
12. Lapeyre B, Bourbon H, Amalric F (1987) Nucleolin, the major nucleolar protein of growing eukaryotic cells: an unusual protein structure revealed by the nucleotide sequence. Proc Natl Acad Sci USA 84:1472
13. Lennert K, Mohri N, Stein H, et al. (1987) Malignant lymphomas other than Hodgkin's disease Springer, Berlin Heidelberg New York
14. Leong ASY, Gilham P (1989) Silver staining of nucleolar organizer regions in malignant melanoma and melanocytic nevi. Human Pathol. 20:257
15. O'Connor SJ, Delay DT, Weisenburger DD (1989) Pseudofollicular proliferation centers in small lymphocytic lymphoma lack dendritic reticulum cells. Lab Invest 60:67A
16. Ploton D, Menager M, Adnet JJ (1984) Simultaneous high-resolution of Ag-NOR proteins and nucleoproteins in interphase and mitotic nuclei. Histochem. J. 16:897
17. Pugh WC, Manning JT, Butler JJ (1987) Paraimmunoblastic variant of small lymphocytic lymphoma. Lab. Invest. 56, 61A
18. Rossi GD, Mandelli F, Covelli A, et al. (1989) Chronic lymphocytic leukemia (CLL) in younger adults: a retrospective study of 133 cases. Hemat. Oncol. 7:127

Flow Cytochemical Analysis of Lymphoid Cells in B-Chronic Lymphocytic Leukemia (B-CLL)

F. Lanza[1] and G.L.Castoldi

Introduction

In chronic lymphocytic leukemia (CLL) a great number of prognostic factors have been isolated. Some of them were grouped together by Rai et al. [8] in a clinical staging system that has been extensively accepted and verified. However, there may still be considerable variation in the course of the disease, even in patients presenting in the same clinical stage. In view of this fact, several attempts to improve this classification have been carried out by various authors. The prognostic role of the size and morphology of peripheral blood lymphocytes has been the object of debate for a long time. The presence of large lymphocytes resembling prolymphocytes or lymphoblasts was correlated by some authors with a poor prognosis [1,2, 5,6], while others have suggested the opposite [7]. Yet others did not find any significant relationship between cell morphology and clinical course [4].

In order to morphometrically evaluate the lymphocytic population, an analysis of peripheral blood samples from 118 consecutive patients with B-cell CLL was performed using a new generation automated hematology analyzer (Technicon H∗1). Data obtained were therefore compared with clinical staging and other well-defined prognostic factors. The use of this instrument in monitoring the response to the administration of cytostatic drugs will be further discussed in the present paper.

Material and Methods

Patients. One hundred and eighteen patients with CLL of B-cell type were included in the study (66 males and 46 females). The median age of the patients was 65 years (range: 48 to 88 years). The patients were staged according to Rai et al. [8] and the IWCLL (International Workshop on Chronic Lymphocytic Leukemia) [3] staging system, concomitantly with Techicon H∗1 analysis. Patients entered in the study did not receive any

[1] Hematology Section, University of Ferrara, S. Anna Hospital, Cso Giovecca 203, I-44100 Ferrara, Italy

Fleischer (Ed.) Leukemias
© Springer-Verlag Berlin Heidelberg 1993

previous treatment for the disease. For each patient H∗1 analysis was subsequently performed at monthly intervals, over a follow-up period of 22 months. During the follow-up analysis, 48 patients underwent chemotherapy [32 were treated with a single agent (chlorambucil associated or not with prednisone); 16 received polichemotherapy (COP, CHOP courses – cyclophophamide, hadriblastin, vincristine, prednisone)].

Automated Flow Cytochemistry Analysis. Technicon H1 (Technicon Inst. Corp. Tarritown, N.Y.) is an automated hematology analyzer that performs a full blood count and WBC five-part differential (percentage and absolute cell numbers) by counting 10000 cells per sample of whole blood. WBC are classified and measured using white light [(at two wavelengths) and laser technology on two separate channels: the peroxidase channel identifies, through tungsten based optics and cytochemistry, the different types of leukocytes (neutrophils, monocytes, eosinophils, lymphocytes and "large unstained cells," LUCs)]; and the basophil manifold, totally revised with respect to its predecessor H6000, distinguishes basophils from mononuclear and polymorphonuclear cells by stripping the cytoplasm from all WBC except basophils which are resistant to the reagent treatment. The basophil/lobularity channel, indeed, provides information about the degree of maturity of each WBC nucleus by a laser beam measurement of nuclear lobularity and density. The range of expected values of the different types of WBC were determined in a control group composed of 200 healthy adults. The values of the principal hematology parameters are as follows: lymphocyte count, 900–5200/cmm; LUCs count, 10–400/cmm; % LUCs to WBC, 0.1%–4.0%; basophil count, 0–200/cmm; % blasts, 0%–1.2%.

Results

Table 1 shows the distribution of hematological parameters as determined by the H∗1 system in the different Rai clinical stages. A progressive increase in the mean percentage of LUC, LUC count, lymphocyte count and proportion of blasts with advancing stage can be observed. A statistical analysis clearly demonstrated that patients in Rai III and IV clinical stages and

Table 1. Technicon H∗1 data of 118 B-CLL patients

Rai clinical stage	Patients (n)	Lymphocytes (n)	LUC (n)	% LUC to WBC	% LUC to lymphocytes	% Blasts
O	46	14 447	678	2.65	4.2	1.5
I	33	24 319	1470	4.52	6.2	2.0
II	23	28 349	2269	6.79	10.6	4.9
III + IV	16	38 612	9273	18.69	36.8	9.9

Values are means in the different Rai clinical stages.
LUC, large unstained cells.

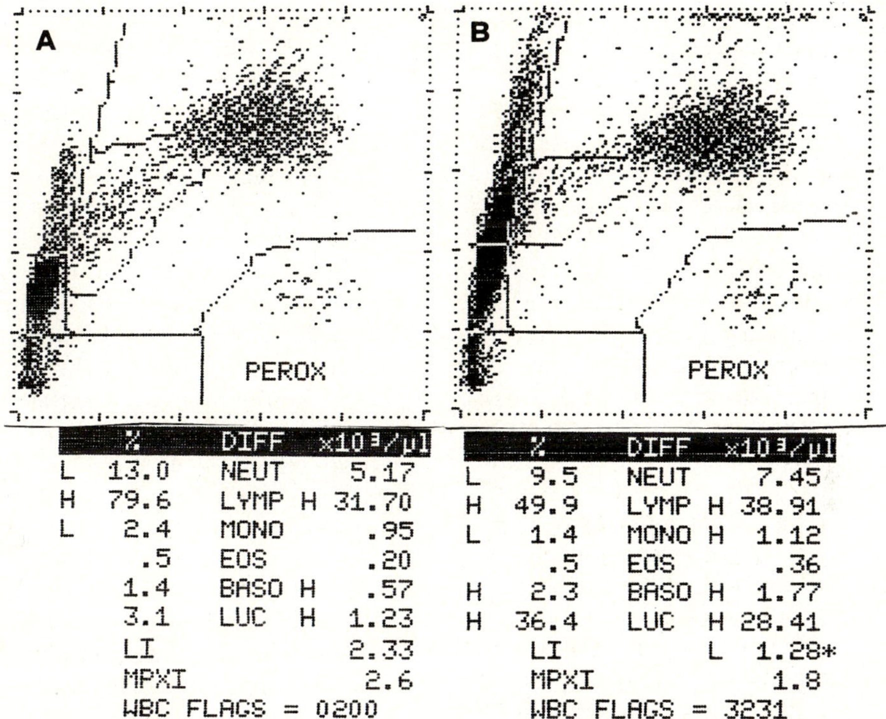

Fig. 1. Peroxidase channel display of H*1 system showing the distribution of the different types of leukocytes from (A) a patient in an initial Rai clinical stage (I), and (B) a patient in advanced (IV) Rai stage

IWCLL stage C had the highest percentage and count of both LUC and blast. In contrast, patients in Rai stages O and I and IWCLL stage A exhibited, statistically, LUC and blast percentages and counts very similar to those observed in the control group. Furthermore, LUC and blast proportions positively correlated with the following prognostic factors: peripheral lymphocytosis (>60 000/cmm), marked splenomegaly (>10 cm under costal margin), higher percentages of peripheral prolymphocytes. Our data analysis further revealed that chemotherapy produced a greater reduction of the LUC count than of that of small lymphocytes. Finally, an increase in LUC and blast counts were observed in conjunction with deterioration of the clinical status (i.e., progressive changes in clinical stages, occurrence of prolymphocitoid transformation and/or of Richter's syndrome).

Discussion

Automated flow cytochemistry represents a new approach to the study of blood cells and their related pathological conditions. Besides its usefulness in detecting abnormalities in routine blood blood samples, some applications in hematological research may also be obtained by the use of such instruments. This study represents a detailed analysis of the possibilities of an automated differential leukocyte counter (Technicon H*1 system) to assess the size and nuclear characteristics of the lymphocytic population from a series of 118 consecutive patients with B-CLL. Our data confirmed previous studies about a close relationship between the presence of higher percentage and count of large lymphoid cells (LUC, as measured by the analyzer) and advanced Rai and IWCLL clinical stages of the disease. Indeed, an increase was observed in cells classified as blasts by the H*1 system with advancing clinical stages. These data, together with the demonstration that the LUC population was more sensitive to cytostatic drugs with respect to the small lymphocytes, lead us to suggest that the presence of a higher proportion of large lymphoid cells with peculiar nuclear characteristics may play a negative prognostic role in B-CLL due to the different biological properties of the cells.

References

1. Binet JL, Vaugier G, Dighiero G, et al. (1977) Investigation of a new parameter in chronic lymphocytic leukemia: the percentage of large peripheral lymphocytes determined by the Hemalog D. Am J Med 63:683–688
2. Drewinko B, Bollinger P, Brailas C, et al. (1987) Flow cytochemical patterns of white blood cells in human hematopoietic malignancies: II. Chronic leukemias. Br J Haematol 67:157–165
3. International Workshop on CLL (1981) Chronic lymphocytic leukemia: proposals for a revised prognostic staging system. Br J Haematol 48:365–367
4. Kuse R, Schuster S, Shubbe H, et al. (1985) Blood lymphocyte volumes and diameters in patients with chronic lymphocytic leukemia and normal controls. Blut 50:243–248
5. Lanza F, Castoldi GL (1988) Basophil count in samples from chronic leukaemia patients analyzed by the automated flow cytochemistry technology. Br J Hematol 68:495–499
6. Lanza, F, Scapoli GL, Spanedda R, et al. (1985) Automated assessment of lymphoid cells in chronic lymphocytic leukemia: correlation with prognostic features. Hematol 70:212–220
7. Peterson L, Bloomfield C, Brunning R (1980) Relationship of clinical staging and lymphocyte morphology to survival in chronic lymphocytic leukemia. Br J Haematol 45:563–567
8. Rai K, Sawitsky A, Cronkite E, et al. (1975) Clinical staging of chronic lymphocytic leukemia. Blood 46:219–234

Immunodiagnosis of Leukemic Blood Cells of Patients with Chronic Lymphocytic Leukemia and Other Non-Hodgkin's Lymphomas by Monoclonal Antibodies of the *Biowissenschaften Leipzig* Series

K. MALBERG,[1] L. SCHÄFER, M. LÖBNITZ, M. HEROLD, and K. WUTKE

Problems

Lymphoproliferative diseases are to be identified by cell membrane antigens. These surface markers can be used to differentiate between leukemic T- and B-cell non-Hodgkin's lymphomas (NHLs) and to subclassify various entities [1]. Our aim was to determine the marker profile of different leukemic NHLs with monoclonal antibodies (mabs) of the *Biowissenschaften Leipzig* (BL) series.

Material and Methods

The diagnosis of the 56 NHLs was confirmed by clinical, cytological, and cytochemical means. All patients had leukaemic cells in their peripheral blood. Mononuclear cells were isolated from heparinized blood using Ficoll/Visotrast density gradient centrifugation [2]. The slide technique was applied to subtype lymphocytes by using anti-human leucocyte mabs from the BL series (Table 1) in an indirect immunofluorescent technique [4]. Fluorescein isothiocyanate (FITC) conjugated goat anti-mouse serum was taken as a secondary antibody. The cells were examined with a microscope equipped with fluorescent illumination and phase contrast. A minimum of 200 cells was evaluated.

Discussion and Results

All leukemic cells were of the B-cell type, because T-cell antigens, for instance CD2, and the natural killer (NK) cell antigen CD16 were not to be found on their surface. The antigen Ia4 was expressed constantly except in the cells of three of nine immunocytoma patients (Table 2). B-cell chronic lymphocytic leukemia (B-CLL) patients had heterogeneous cell marker combinations of the antigens CD5, CD6, CD10, CD22, sIg and cIg (Table

[1] Department of Medical Immunology, Medical High School, Nordhaüser Str. 74, O-5010 Erfurt, FRG

Fleischer (Ed.) Leukemias
© Springer-Verlag Berlin Heidelberg 1993

Table 1. Reaction spectrum of the murine monoclonal BL antibodies used

BL antibody	CD	Lymphocytic specificity
B22	22	Mature B cells
Ia4	–	MHC class II antigen on B cells and activated T cells
CALLA	10	Early B cells
TP5	5	Most T cells and some B cells
TP6	6	Like TP5
TP2	2	Sheep erythrocyte rosette receptor (T cells)
TP3	3	Mature T cells
TH4	4	Helper/inducer T cells
TS8	8	Suppressor/cytotoxic T cells, some NK cells
LGL	16	Most NK cells
M11c	11c	Some B cells
Tac	25	Activated T and B cells
Ac 38	38	Activated T and B cells, plasma cells
IgM	–	Mµ chains
IgL	–	Ig light chains
kappa	–	Ig kappa chains
lambda	–	Ig lambda chains

MHC, major histocompatibility complex; CALLA, common acute lymphocytic leukemia antigen; NK, natural killer; Ig, immunoglobulin; LGL, large granular lymphocytes.

Table 2. Monoclonal BL antibody reaction patterns with leukemic blood cells from different lymphocytic leukemia and other NHL patients

BL antibody	CLL	Pro-LL	Hairy cell leukemia	Unicentric blastoma or cytoma	Unicentric cytoma	Immunocytoma
B22	11/32	0/3	1/1	1/6	4/5	4/9
Ia4	31/31	3/3	1/1	6/6	5/5	6/9
CALLA	7/35	0/3	1/1	0/6	1/5	2/9
TP5	16/33	1/3	0/1	2/6	2/5	2/9
TP6	13/24	1/2	0/1	4/5	3/4	2/5
TP2	0/18	0/1	0/1	0/1	0/1	0/2
Ac38	0/23	0/2	ND	1/5	0/3	2/4
LGL	0/22	0/3	0/1	0/4	0/4	0/5
sIgM	9/26	2/3	ND	3/6	3/5	1/8
sIgL	6/26	1/3	ND	2/5	3/4	0/6
s-kappa	6/26	1/3	1/1	0/1	0/1	0/3
c-kappa	5/11	0/1	ND	ND	ND	1/1
c-lambda	0/7	0/1	ND	ND	ND	0/1

Numbers indicate positive reactions per number of examined patients.
S, surface; C, cytoplasmic.

3). Prolymphocytic leukaemia (Pro-LL) should de sIg-positive typically, but only two of three patients showed sIg in high density (Table 2).

The BL antibodies used make it possible to distinguish between B- and T-cell type leukemic NHL cells. But the actual panel of BL mabs is not

Table 3. Distribution of the BL antibody-determined markers on the leukemic cells of individual CLL patients

Patient number	BL markers				
	B22	CALLA	TP5/6	sIg	cIg
1	+				
2			+		
3			+		
4			+		
5		+	+		+
6				+	+
7	+		+	+	+
8					
9			+	+	
10		+	+		
11					
12				+	
13	+				
14					+
15			+		
16			+		
17	+	+	+	+	
18					
19			+	+	
20	+		+		+
21				+	
22		+	+	+	+
23					
24					
25			+		
26	+	+	+	+	
27	+	+	+		
28				+	
29	+		+		
30					
31	+	+		+	
32				+	
33				+	
34				+	
35	+				
36	+				

suitable for the further differentiation of leukemic B-NHLs into various immunologic entities. Presently it is not clear whether any particular combination of leukemic cell markers in B-CLL patients offers better prognosis. The leukemia immunophenotyping has to be continued with more and different mabs–especially for B-cells–and with a greates number of patients.

References

1. Bernard B, Boumsell L, Dausset J, Milstein C, Schlossmann SF (eds) (1984) Leucocyte typing. Springer, Berlin Heidelberg New York
2. Boyum A (1968) Isolation of mononuclear cells and granulocytes from human blood. Scand J Clin Lab Invest 21:77–89
3. Gale R, Rai KR (eds) (1987) Chronic lymphocytic leukaemia: recent progress and future direction. Liss New York
4. Kupper H, Typlt H, Grimmecke P, Fiebig H (1983) Objektträgertest zur immunfluoreszenzmikroskopischen und enzymologischen Erfassung von Zellmembran-antigenen. Allerg Immunol 29:223–228

Advanced and Terminal Phase of B-Cell Chronic Lymphocytic Leukemia

K. Rak,[1] A. Kiss, and B. Telek

Chronic lymphocytic leukemia (CLL) is a heterogeneous group of diseases among the low-grade malignant lymphomas [8]. B-cell CLL (B-CLL) is the most common form of CLL in Hungary. There is still a considerable range of variability within this category itself. The course of disease is chronic and monotonous, at least morphologically, in most cases, but may be very different and varying in a minority of cases. The factors that determine the rate of advance are unknown and features associated with a poor prognosis are those reflecting advancing stage. Progress from a static phase to a more advanced and finally terminal stage may be of very different duration. While taking care of more than 200 B-CLL in- and out-patients during the last 14 years (1975–1988) in our haematologic department, several cases of different forms of advanced and terminal B-CLL were observed. It is important to distinguish two types of development of a new malignant event in B-CLL: (a) the *transformation of the leukemic B-cell* to a cytologically less differentiated, and clinically more agressive, cell type, representing the malignant evolution of the B-CLL clone [1–5,7,9–11,14]; and (b) the appearance of a *new malignancy* whose cell type is different and unrelated to that of CLL [12,13,15]. Only the first type represents a true transformation of the disease and is analogous to the well-known transformation of chronic granulocytic leukemia (CGL; the accelerated and blastic phase). This change could take different forms and we should like to summarize these forms of malignant events. The development of secondary neoplasia, usually carcinoma or acute myeloid leukemia, may relate indirectly to the immunodeficiency of CLL or reflect a genetic predisposition and is an additional but separate problem.

Which are the known prognostic features in CLL syndrome?

1. *Size of leukemic cell mass* (clinical stage – *Rai* or *Binet* –, and number of circulating leukemic cells).
2. *Biology of disease*, static (indolent) or progressive? (Lymphocyte doubling time, lymphoid cell morphology, number of prolymphocytes, bone marrow histology, prognostic score – immunological or enzymological –, cytogenetics, age, sex, lymph node histology).

---

[1] Second Department of Medicine, University Merdical School, H-4012 Debrecen, Hungary

Table 1. A brief characterization of the three variants of the B-CLL syndrome

Variant	Reference	Characteristics
B-CLL	[10]	A disease with relatively homogeneous features Patients on average 65 years old Predominant lymph node involvement WBC highly variable with a mean of 100 g/l Small lymphocytes (median volume 212 ± 23 fl) Low-density SmIg, high mouse (M)-rosette formation High expression of T1 (CD5) antigen Low reactivity with the McAb FMC7 Less than 10% PROL in peripheral blood, progressive increase at least beyond this limit Median survival is 8 years (worse prognosis for those older than 74, beyond stage II or with WBC >200 g/l)
B-PLL	[6]	Distinct disease entity Patients on average are 8–10 years older than those with CLL A minimum of 55% PROL in peripheral blood among the lymphoid cells Median volume of PROL is variable (280–354 fl) Mean WBC 176 ± 143 g/l Massive splenomegaly, lymph node involvement negligible High-density SmIg, PROL usually do not form M-rosette formations Strong reactivity with the McAb FMC7 Median survival significantly shorter (3 years)
B-CLL/PL	[10]	"Intermediate" between CLL and PLL Closer to the typical CLL groups in that age incidence is the same, and lymph node involvement and surface markers are similar, but splenomegaly and high-density SmIg in one-third of patients Mean WBC 120 g/l Double population of small and large cells, the small-cell component is predominant (258 fl) 10–55% PROL in PB, proportion is stable in most cases Progressive PROL transformation in some cases with a change to PLL phenotype Median survival significantly longer with PROL <15 g/l Approximately 3 years, like in PLL, with PROL >15 g/l Heterogeneous group, with may be variously interpreted: 1. Prolymphocytoid transformation (progressive disease) 2. Cases of genuine CLL and PLL (end of the "tail") 3. Third disease entity (?)

3. *Response to treatment* (individual observations, former clinical experiences).

Table 1 reviews briefly the main clinical and laboratory features of the three variants of B-CLL syndrome, i.e. B-CLL, B-cell prolymphocytic leukemia (B-CLL) and B-CLL/PL (intermediate between CLL and PLL).

The several transformations are described in Table 2. Development of a diffuse large cell lymphoma (Richter syndrome), prolymphocytoid trans-

Table 2. Transformations of B-CLL

Transformations	Characteristics
Richter syndrome	Richter 1928 – lymphoma of large pleomorphic cells 3–15% of the total cases of CLL. Reticulum cell sarcoma, diffuse histiocytic lymphoma. Immunoblastic (large cell) lymphoma arising from a single transformed clone of B lymphocytes. But: in some cases cells display different heavy and light chains, as well as different rearrangements of heavy chain genes, suggesting distinct B cell malignancies (independent large cell lymphomas in B-CLL, similar to that observed in other immune deficiency states). Histology could be confused with that of Hodgkin's disease!
CLL/PL as a progressive disease	Transformation to prolymphocytoid leukemia occurs gradually over several years and in associated with increasing anaemia, thrombocytopenia, adenomegaly, splenomegaly and resistance to treatment. PROL express the same Ig isotype as the CLL cells. Incidence about 10%. Represents malingnant evolution of the B-CLL clone.
Development of ALL (L2)	Incidence less than 1%. Clinical and laboratory features of acute lymphocytic leukemia (ALL; blast crisis). Treatment is usually ineffective. Transformation of the leukemic cell clone to a cytologically less differentiated, and clinically more aggressive, cell type.
Multiple myeloma	Rarest form of transformation involves differentiation into MM. In most cases, the heavy and light chains of the myeloma cells have been reported to be identical to the CLL cells. Two separate clones were identified with anti-idiotypic antibodies in a limited number of cases, suggesting the occurrence of two unrelated diseases.

Table 3. Distribution of patients with CLL and related disorders in the 2nd Department of Medicine, University Medical School, Debrecen (1975–1988)

Disorder	Patients (n)	Transformations	
		Type	n
B-CLL	202	Diffuse large cell lymphoma	1
		Prolymphocytoid transformation	4
		Blast crisis (ALL)	1
B-CLL/PL	1		
B-PLL	2		
B-HCL	9		
T-CLL	2		

formation, acute or blast crisis, and progression into multiple myeloma are specified in short.

Finally, the distribution of patients with CLL and related disorders observed and cared for in our department is shown in Table 3.

The *treatment* of patients suffering from any form of transformation is almost always difficult. It is associated with resistance to the conventional therapy used in CLL (e.g. chlorambucil with or without prednisone) and has therefore a bad prognosis. Some responses have been reported for the combination chemotherapy used for large cell lymphoma in Richter syndrome, and for the usual combination treatment for acute lymphocytic leukemia (ALL) in blastic transformation.

References

1. Brouet JC, Preud'homme JL, Seligmann M, et al. (1973) Blast cells with monoclonal surface immunoglobulin in two cases of acute blast crisis supervening on chronic lymphocytic leukaemia. Br Med J 4:23
2. Enno A, Catovsky D, O'Brien M, et al.(1979) Prolymphocytoid transformation in chronic lymphocytic leukemia. Br J Haematol 41:9
3. Flandrin G. (1988) Richter's syndrome. In: Polliac A, Catovsky D (eds) Chronic lymphocytic leukemia. Harwood, Chur, p 209
4. Foucar K, Rydell RE (1980) Richter's syndrome in chronic lymphocytic leukemia. Cancer 46:188
5. Ghani AM, Krause JR, Brody JP (1986) Prolymphocytic transformation of chronic lymphocytic leukemia. Cancer 57:75
6. Galton DAG, Goldman JM, Wiltshaw E, et al. (1974) Prolymphocytic leukemia. Br J Haematol 27:7
7. Hamblin TJ, Oscier DG, Gregg EO, et al. (1985) Cell markers in a large single centre series of chronic lymphocytic leukemia the relationship between CLL and PLL. Br J Haematol 61:556
8. Hamblin TJ (1987) Chronic lymphocytic leukemia. Baillieres Clin Haematol 1:499
9. Jacobs AD, Schroff RW, Gale RP (1984) Acute transformation of chronic lymphocytic leukemia. Med Pediat Oncol 12:318
10. Melo JV, Catovsky D, Galton DAG (1986) The relationship between chronic lymphocytic leukemia and prolymphocytic leukemia. I. Clinical and laboratory features of 300 patients and characterisation of an intermediate group. Br J Haematol 63:377
11. Ostrowski M, Minden M, Wang C, et al. (1989) Immunophenotypic and gene probe analysis of a case of Richter's syndrome. Am J Clin Pathol 91:215
12. Pines A, Ben-Bassat I, Selzer G, et al. (1984) Transformation of chronic lymphocytic leukemia to plasmocytoma. Cancer 54:1904
13. Richter MN (1928) Generalised reticular cell sarcoma of lymph nodes associated with lymphatic leukemia. Am J Pathol 3:285
14. Trump DL, Mann RB, Phelps R, et al. (1980) Richter's syndrome: diffuse histiocytic lymphoma in patients with chronic lymphocytic leukemia. A report of five cases and review the literature. Am J Med 68:539
15. Videbaek A (1988) Chronic lymphocytic leukemia associated with other malignancies. In: Polliack A, Catovsky D (eds) Chronic lymphocytic leukemia. Harwood, Chur, p 219

Subject Index

Printing: Druckerei Zechner, Speyer
Binding: Buchbinderei Schäffer, Grünstadt